ESSENTIALS OF

# Research Methods in Health, Physical Education, Exercise Science, and Recreation

## Third Edition

# ESSENTIALS OF
# Research Methods in Health, Physical Education, Exercise Science, and Recreation

## Third Edition

**KRIS E. BERG, EdD**

*Professor*
*School of Health, Physical Education, and Recreation*
*University of Nebraska at Omaha*
*Omaha, Nebraska*

**RICHARD W. LATIN, PhD**

*Professor*
*School of Health, Physical Education, and Recreation*
*University of Nebraska at Omaha*
*Omaha, Nebraska*

 Wolters Kluwer | Lippincott Williams & Wilkins
Health

Philadelphia · Baltimore · New York · London
Buenos Aires · Hong Kong · Sydney · Tokyo

Acquisitions Editor: Emily J. Lupash
Managing Editor: Karen M. Ruppert
Marketing Manager: Christen D. Murphy
Production Editor: Sally Anne Glover
Designer: Stephen Druding
Compositor: Aptara, Inc.

Third Edition

**Library of Congress Cataloging-in-Publication Data**

Berg, Kris E., 1943-
   Essentials of research methods in health, physical education, exercise science, and recreation / Kris E. Berg,
Richard W. Latin.—3rd ed.
     p. ; cm.
   Includes bibliographical references (p. 279–280) and index.
   ISBN-13: 978-0-7817-7036-1
   ISBN-10: 0-7817-7036-X
   1. Research—Methodology.    2. Technical writing.    3. Medical sciences—Research—Methodology.    4. Physical
education and training—Research—Methodology.    5. Recreation—Research—Methodology.    I. Latin, Richard Wayne,
1953-    II. Title.
   [DNLM: 1. Physical Education and Training.    2. Research—methods.    3. Exercise.    4. Recreation. QT 255 B493e 2008]
Q180.55.M4B417 2008
001.4'2—dc22
                                2007025367

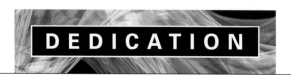

# DEDICATION

Writing a dedication for my friend, colleague, and coauthor, Rick Latin, I knew would be the most difficult writing in this third edition. This book meant a great deal to him. We had many a conversation prior to writing the first edition because of our strong mutual belief that a class in research methods was valued dimly by many students. To counter this, we wrote the initial book hoping to make it as practical and user friendly as possible so that our students could master the fundamentals and perhaps even enjoy some of the content. While I tend to be detailed and descriptive in my writing, Rick was more succinct and to the point. The first edition turned out to be shorter and user friendly largely because of his influence. I think that helped the overall effectiveness of the book. This philosophy was carried out in the second edition, and I have attempted to do so in the third edition as well but without his presence to remind me.

Rick passed away on February 14, 2006. The memorial service held in the HPER Building was a testimony to the strong influence he had on so many of his students. The many e-mails and conversations I have had with these students confirm the strong influence that good teachers can have on people's lives. I have been moved many times by thoughts of these expressions from his colleagues and students.

Rick and I coauthored a good number of papers over the years. I think we were a good team, as we could be entirely open and frank with each other; his strengths supplanted my weaknesses and together we did so much more than either of us could have done alone. Although Rick was not here to work directly with me on the third edition of our book, his thoughts and philosophy are still represented very strongly. Many a time I sat pondering over a point while writing, and simply asking myself what Rick's response would likely have been usually led to a quick decision.

Thanks, Rick, for the great friendship we enjoyed.

—K.B.

# PREFACE

The third edition of *Essentials of Research Methods in Health, Physical Education, Exercise Science, and Recreation* has been written specifically for students and professionals in these disciplines. The overall aim of the book is to enhance the reader's abilities to conduct research and for practitioners to be able to use research in their professional work. Numerous examples of research are cited across the various academic areas to demonstrate how various research techniques have been used to address specific problems and concerns in the disciplines. The approach in writing this book has been to be user friendly with an emphasis on being practical and application-oriented rather than encyclopedic and theoretical.

The authors are experienced teachers and researchers who have taught a required research methods class for many years. The attempt was made to pare content to a level that allows covering fundamentals within the traditional semester in such a class. A basic competency of the content should allow students to write sound research proposals and theses, to read and better understand research published in the discipline, and to conduct research. In addition to these essentials, we have included several topics not commonly presented in other texts, such as the role of research in higher education; quality control; historical background and need for informed consent; ethics; and tips in interpretation of research. It is hoped that presentation of these additional topics will enhance understanding the entirety of the research process and make readers better able to interpret and critique research. As a result, the reader will hopefully feel more comfortable and competent in reading research.

## FEATURES

Certain pedagogical features to facilitate learning have been used throughout the text. Each chapter begins with a brief list of **key concepts** that will be covered and a statement of **learning objectives.** We suggest that students read these before and after reading each chapter. Additional **learning activities** appear at the end of each chapter. These activities suggest supplementary means of learning about research such as attendance at thesis meetings and examining articles for certain characteristics covered in a chapter. Within each chapter, selected main points are restated or rephrased in the margin for emphasis. Lastly, cartoons are used to bring humor to a subject that typically is viewed as dry.

Section III, Statistics, emphasizes interpretation rather than mathematics. Numerous examples are integrated with various types of experimental and nonexperimental designs so that students can more easily understand the application of statistics to specific research questions. The chapters in this section provide problems and their solutions reflecting research questions from the various subdisciplines. At the end of each chapter, **statistics exercises** offer the opportunity to practice solving problems via hand or computer. The answers appear in an appendix. Instructors are provided PowerPoint slides for each chapter on the connection companion website **(http://connection.lww.com)**.

## SUMMARY

We hope the third edition will meaningfully enhance the reader's knowledge and appreciation of research. The growth and development of our professions as well as the effectiveness of each professional seemingly require a greater utilization and understanding of research than in the past. To these ends we hope the journey through this book will be pleasant, informative, and useful.

# ACKNOWLEDGMENTS

I wish to express appreciation to my wonderful wife, Carolyn, and my sons, Eric and Steve, for their support during the revising of this book. The strong support base they have provided throughout my academic career and numerous writing projects, including writing and, more recently, revising this book, has been constant and of immeasurable help. I am also fortunate for the love of my parents, Richard and Frederica, who always made me feel like a winner. Other key players in my life are my sister, Diana, my brothers Chuck, Steve, Bob, and Brian, and my parents-in-law, Nancy and Bill Heard. They contributed more than they realize.

I would also like to thank the many fine students in my classes at the University of Nebraska at Omaha. Their questions, concerns, helpful feedback, enthusiasm, and patience with my many attempts at different teaching techniques have always been a source of inspiration. That inspiration has provided me with a continual source of energy to "do it better." Good teaching requires a lot of time, energy, and caring about people. My students have always made it seem very worthwhile.

I thank my colleague, Rick Latin. His linear thinking and high level of efficiency have helped me "cut to the chase" in many joint writing endeavors. For some 20 years, we worked together in numerous research and writing projects, and I am the better for it. It has always been a joy working with him.

I would also like to acknowledge the contributions of Dr. Manoj Sharma, University of Cincinnati, for authoring the chapter on Qualitative Research Methods. His expertise filled a void in our knowledge and experience. This chapter is a welcome addition to the book.

Lastly, I would like to express my gratitude to the staff at Lippincott Williams & Wilkins. Karen Ruppert, Managing Editor, Emily Lupash, Acquisitions Editor, and Pete Darcy, Editor, have been wonderful to work with. They have provided much guidance, generated numerous ideas to consider in the revision, and were forever patient in answering my many questions. Their facilitation made the writing a good deal easier and more enjoyable.

—K.B.

# CONTENTS

Dedication *v*
Preface *vii*
Acknowledgments *ix*

## PART I: INTRODUCTORY CONCEPTS   1

**1** Introduction to Research.................................................................*3*

**2** Ethics in Human Subject Research......................................*17*

## PART II: RESEARCH WRITING   25

**3** Getting Started: Information Retrieval................................*27*

**4** The Research Paper and Proposal........................................*35*

**5** Completing the Research Paper: Results, Discussion, Conclusion, and References........................................*48*

**6** Research Writing........................................................................*57*

## PART III: STATISTICS   71

**7** Basic Statistical Concepts.....................................................*73*

**8** Central Tendency, Variability, and the Normal Curve.......*85*

**9** Probability and Hypothesis Testing...................................*102*

**10** Relationships and Predictions...........................................*121*

**11** Comparing Mean Scores.......................................................*145*

**12** Selected Nonparametric Statistics.....................................*170*

## PART IV: MEASUREMENT AND RESEARCH DESIGN    185

**13**  **Measurement and Data Collection Concepts**.........................................................*187*

**14**  **Experimental Validity and Control**.....................................................................*201*

**15**  **Experimental Research and Designs**...................................................................*216*

**16**  **Nonexperimental or Descriptive Research**.........................................................*229*

**17**  **Qualitative Research Methods**...........................................................................*245*

## PART V: QUALITY CONTROL AND APPLICATION OF RESEARCH    257

**18**  **Quality Control in Research**.............................................................................*259*

**19**  **Assessment and Application of Research**...........................................................*268*

Appendix A:   Statistics Tables                                *291*
Appendix B:   Answers to Statistics Exercises                 *301*
Appendix C:   Sample Consent Form and Sample Letters   *305*
Glossary                                                      *311*
References and Selected Readings                              *317*

Index                                                         *319*

# EXPANDED CONTENTS

Dedication  *v*
Preface  *vii*
Acknowledgments  *ix*

## PART I: INTRODUCTORY CONCEPTS  1

### 1  Introduction to Research ........................................................................3

Primary Purposes of Research  *4*
A Common Misconception About Research  *4*
Research in Our Daily Lives  *6*
The Scientific Method  *7*
Inductive and Deductive Reasoning  *9*
Fact, Theory, and Principle  *9*
Less Scientific Methods  *11*
Basic and Applied Research  *11*
Location of Research  *12*
Internal Validity  *12*
External Validity  *13*
Independent and Dependent Variables  *13*
Characteristics of the Researcher  *13*

### 2  Ethics in Human Subject Research ........................................... 17

Codes and Guidelines  *17*
The Institutional Review Board  *18*
Informed Consent  *18*
Confidentiality and Anonymity  *21*
Invasion of Privacy  *21*
Safe and Competent Treatment  *22*
Knowledge of Results  *22*
The Researcher's Role in Ethical Treatment  *22*

## PART II: RESEARCH WRITING  25

### 3  Getting Started: Information Retrieval ................................... 27

Sources of Information  *27*

Bibliographies    *28*
Abstracts    *28*
Indexes    *29*
Research Reviews    *30*
Journals    *30*
Computerized Information Retrieval    *30*

**4  The Research Paper and Proposal**..................................................................*35*
Components of the Thesis    *36*
Chapter 1: Introduction    *38*
Chapter 2: The Problem    *39*
Chapter 3: Review of Literature    *43*
Chapter 4: Procedures or Methods    *44*

**5  Completing the Research Paper: Results, Discussion, Conclusion,
and References**..................................................................*48*
Chapter 5: Results    *48*
Chapter 6: Discussion    *49*
Chapter 7: Summary and Conclusions    *52*
References    *53*
Appendix    *55*

**6  Research Writing**..................................................................*57*
Getting Started    *57*
Collating Reference Material and Writing    *59*
Tips for Good Writing    *60*
Common Faults in Writing    *63*

## PART III: STATISTICS    71

**7  Basic Statistical Concepts**..................................................................*73*
Measurement Scales    *74*
Parametric and Nonparametric Statistics    *76*
Descriptive and Inferential Use of Statistics    *77*
Selected Sampling Procedures    *78*
Some Computational Notations and Tips    *81*

**8  Central Tendency, Variability, and the Normal Curve**..................................................................*85*
Central Tendency    *86*
Measures of Variability    *87*
The Normal Curve    *90*

The *Z* Score   *97*
Nonnormal Distributions and Curves   *98*

**9** **Probability and Hypothesis Testing** ..................................................................... *102*

Probability   *102*
Hypothesis Testing   *106*
Interpretations After the Hypothesis Test   *117*
Practical Hypothesis Testing   *118*

**10** **Relationships and Predictions** ..................................................................... *121*

Concepts in Correlation   *122*
Pearson Correlation   *124*
Prediction: Simple Linear Regression   *131*
Prediction: Multiple Regression   *136*
Partial Correlation   *139*
Factor Analysis   *140*

**11** **Comparing Mean Scores** ..................................................................... *145*

Statistical Assumptions   *146*
Correlated or Dependent *t* Tests   *146*
Independent *t* Test   *149*
Analysis of Variance   *152*
Analysis of Covariance   *165*

**12** **Selected Nonparametric Statistics** ..................................................................... *170*

Chi Square   *171*
Restrictions and Assumptions for Chi Square   *178*
Spearman *r*   *179*
Some Other Nonparametric Tests   *181*

**PART IV: MEASUREMENT AND RESEARCH DESIGN   185**

**13** **Measurement and Data Collection Concepts** ..................................................................... *187*

Validity   *188*
Reliability   *191*
The Relationship Between Validity and Reliability   *194*
Interpreting Validity and Reliability Coefficients   *195*
Validity: Is There Really Such a Thing?   *197*
Measurement Error   *197*

**14** **Experimental Validity and Control** ................................................................. *201*

Internal Validity   *201*
External Validity   *208*
Controlling for Threats to Internal Validity   *210*
Controlling for Threats to External Validity   *212*
Internal versus External Validity: Which Should Be the Focus
and Which Is More Important?   *213*

**15** **Experimental Research and Designs** ............................................................... *216*

Experimentation and Cause-and-Effect Relationships   *216*
Experimental Control Revisited   *217*
Experimental Research Designs   *218*
True Experimental Designs   *220*
Quasi-Experimental Designs   *222*
Pre-experimental Designs   *225*

**16** **Nonexperimental or Descriptive Research** ................................................. *229*

Nonexperimental Research and Cause-and-Effect Relationships   *230*
Survey Research   *232*
Other Survey Methods   *238*
Informed Consent and Surveys   *239*
Other Nonexperimental Methods   *239*

**17** **Qualitative Research Methods** ........................................................................ *245*

Quantitative vs. Qualitative Research   *246*
Case Studies   *247*
Focus Groups   *248*
Nominal Groups   *250*
Content Analysis   *251*
Qualitative Design, Sampling, Data Collection, Analysis, and Interpretation   *251*

**PART V: QUALITY CONTROL AND APPLICATION OF RESEARCH   257**

**18** **Quality Control in Research** .............................................................................. *259*

Internal Quality Control   *259*
External Quality Control   *263*
Publish-or-Perish and Research Quality   *265*
Research Dishonesty   *266*

**19** **Assessment and Application of Research** ................................................... *268*

Assessing the Quality of Research   *269*
Interpreting and Summarizing the Results of Research   *276*

Tips for Interpretation of Research    *279*
Application of Research    *284*


Appendix A:    Statistics Tables                                      *291*
Appendix B:    Answers to Statistics Exercises                        *301*
Appendix C:    Sample Consent Form and Sample Letters    *305*
Glossary                                                              *311*
References and Selected Readings                                      *317*

Index                                                                 *319*

# PART I

# Introductory Concepts

1. Introduction to Research

2. Ethics in Human Subject Research

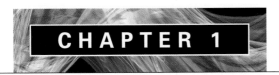

# CHAPTER 1

# Introduction to Research

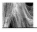

## KEY CONCEPTS

- The scientific method
- Inductive and deductive reasoning
- Fact, theory, and principle
- Basic and applied research
- Field research
- Laboratory research
- Internal validity
- External validity
- Independent and dependent variables
- Characteristics of the researcher

## AFTER READING THIS CHAPTER YOU SHOULD BE ABLE TO:

- Explain the role of research training in graduate education.
- State the primary purpose of research.
- Describe common misconceptions about research.
- Explain the importance of staying current with new knowledge in one's field.
- Define the scientific method and explain each step.
- Describe inductive and deductive reasoning.
- Explain how fact, theory, and principle are interrelated.
- Understand the limitations of making decisions based on tradition, trial and error, bias, and superstition.
- Differentiate between basic and applied research.
- State the pros and cons of field versus laboratory research.
- Define internal and external validity.
- Define and give an example of an independent and a dependent variable.
- Describe desirable characteristics of the researcher.

Nearly all graduate degrees offered by universities and colleges in the United States require a course in research design or methods. There must be a good reason why such a requirement is so common. Tradition may be one reason, but a more persuasive rationale may be because research is so much a part of modern life that students need to understand the process—for general knowledge as well as for professional training. Newspapers, television, radio, magazines, and the Internet regularly report research in some form. Research data are quoted to describe and justify expenditures. The local school board quotes figures about increasing enrollment and teachers' salaries as a means to justify a bond levy. The city council cites traffic density data to justify widening the streets or to construct new entrance and exit ramps from an interstate. Advertisements proclaim that "9 out of 10 doctors recommend..." and so on.

We are bombarded during election years with surveys indicating the support and rank order of candidates. The media quote the latest study on cholesterol, fiber, and so on. While watching a ball game on television, we are inundated with sports trivia such as batting averages, win–loss records against certain opponents, passing and running yardage, percent of third downs converted, and more. Nearly everything we do is quantified by someone to facilitate making a decision. The decision may involve the products we purchase, how we eat and exercise, whether or not we smoke, and many other facets of our lives.

So, whether or not we like it or even realize it, we live in a world of statistics and research. Consequently, it is logical that an educated person today, particularly with an advanced degree, should possess a basic knowledge of the research process.

## PRIMARY PURPOSES OF RESEARCH

Research, simply put, is a way to gather information and make a sound decision or judgment or develop new knowledge. A recreation therapist wishes to find a better way to encourage participation in recreational activity in patients with physical limitations. A coach wants to know how to safely and effectively build strength in her athletes. A health teacher isn't sure how much time to spend lecturing and transmitting information versus letting students discuss, watch films, or listen to guest speakers. An athletic trainer wonders how much flexibility is needed to reduce hamstring pulls. To find an answer and make a decision in each of these examples, an understanding of research could be very helpful.

## A COMMON MISCONCEPTION ABOUT RESEARCH

Many people, including graduate students early in their programs, view research as dull, theoretical, and impractical. Researchers are viewed as overly cerebral intellectuals with IQs surpassing 180, wearing white lab coats and working in highly sophisticated laboratories using extremely complex and expensive equipment. They are thought to deal only with such esoteric topics as subatomic particles, the distance of the farthest galaxies, and other matters that the average person barely understands or can relate to. What people may not realize is that many professional people use research techniques in their daily work. They may do their research work in far less technical environments, including schools, hospitals, parks, and businesses. They typically are not concerned with

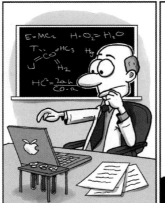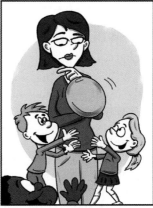

Rocket scientist versus researcher in the "real world."

splitting atoms but are interested in and deal with everyday problems and questions. For example, health educators may use research to study the causes, prevention, and treatment of drug abuse, marital stress, and eating disorders. Physical educators investigate when it is safe and effective for children and adolescents to train with weights, how to develop the abdominal musculature without injuring the back, how to create student interest in personal physical fitness, and what fitness tests to use. Recreation professionals investigate what activities to offer in a summer recreation program, the effects of recreational services on people's use of leisure time, and the leisure time practices and needs of people. All of these are real problems that professionals in health, physical education, recreation, and associated specialties in exercise science and athletic training can address, and sound research methods typically provide the best way to find a sound answer.

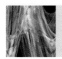 In the fields of health, physical education, and recreation (HPER), where is most research performed?

Most of the research done by professionals in HPER is application-oriented simply because our disciplines evolved from a host of other traditional, longstanding academic fields. Sport psychology is derived from psychology; exercise physiology from biology, chemistry, and physiology; and kinesiology from anatomy and physics. Health and recreation/leisure studies are even broader than the various subdisciplines in physical education. They incorporate knowledge across a wide array of academic disciplines. These fields draw their base of knowledge from many disciplines related to health, lifestyle, and use of leisure time. Consequently, the disciplines and their related problems and questions are highly applied.

## RESEARCH IN OUR DAILY LIVES

### Staying Current and Being Professional

Staying reasonably up to date with the rapidly developing knowledge of today is a demanding task even for the most dedicated professional. Toffler's book *Future Shock* describes the rapidity of change in every facet of modern society and suggests that the rate of change is forever accelerating. To carry out our daily work as effective professionals, we must all be consumers of a certain amount of research. Doing something well in this day and age implies doing it based on the best and most recent knowledge available. Therefore, we need to stay current, which requires a certain amount of professional reading, some of which should be research reports.

Few of us would go to a dentist who uses outdated techniques. Similarly, people with whom we work should expect to receive accurate, current information. An expectation of reasonable quality should be held for any professional, and part of that quality can be attained and maintained only by reading research journals in your field. However, a bit of understanding is needed to distinguish legitimate research from pseudo-scientific research. Advertisements cleverly overstate the benefits of a product and tout it as being better than the product of a competitor. Professionals with research training should be able to detect the limitations of such statements. Much of the public may not have the background to do so effectively.

As an example, some of the lay literature exaggerates the benefits of the healthy lifestyle. Well before research data were available to document the cost-effectiveness of corporate fitness and health promotion programs, numerous articles claimed fantastic savings for corporations. Few if any data actually existed to support the claims. So it is with vitamin and mineral supplements. Articles abound with claims of reduced illness, cures of disease, improved energy, and even reversal of aging. Research data simply don't support such dramatic effects. However, note how frequently pseudo-health authorities appear on television espousing their fantastic claims to the American public.

False and misleading advertising is rampant. Perhaps people would rather watch and listen to a glamorous celebrity than be informed by a knowledgeable professional in the allied health sciences. This makes our work a little more challenging, since we may have to correct some of the notions people have picked up from such sources. We need to be able to differentiate sound from unsound sources of information and facts from fantasy and misconceptions.

Although sound nutritional habits and health promotion programs certainly are important, well-informed professionals need to be able to distinguish fact from fiction. We need to know what characterizes sound research and the limitations of a study (and every study has limitations). We then can provide people with facts rather than let them search for information from the wrong sources. The Internet is widely used, and incredible amounts of information are easily available to the lay person. Yet, not all of the information is factual and sound. Misinformation is consequently a problem in this technological age.

## Being a Consumer of Research

With a good understanding of the fundamentals of research, you are not only more likely to read research on your own but also far more likely to comprehend it. Becoming a consumer of research should be a goal of any graduate student. Making frequent use of research may well be a factor that separates the more successful professional from the average one. Reading research and thinking about ways to use some of the findings allow one to grow and to be stimulated. This enhances job performance and may even contribute to job satisfaction.

Research skills can be useful even in your daily life. It can affect the way you plan your finances, organize for a summer vacation, plan for a career move, or even choose a graduate school. An educated person is often said not merely to know facts but also to know how to obtain and use facts and information. Knowing how to efficiently access sources of information is a critical skill for the modern HPER professional. A well-trained student or professional can perform this function quickly and easily.

The research process isn't perfect, but for most of us it is superior in terms of maximizing the soundness of our decisions. The process, with regular use, becomes an invaluable skill that carries over into much of your professional life. In short, you should become more productive professionally by using a well-organized scientific approach.

## THE SCIENTIFIC METHOD

The time-honored procedure used by scientists and most researchers to solve problems or discover new knowledge is the **scientific method**. It is a logical basis for answering questions and interpreting data. Because of its application to all academic disciplines and potentially any real world problem, it is considered the foundation of the research process.

The scientific method involves several steps described next. An example study dealing with two strategies to lower blood cholesterol levels is used for illustrative purposes.

## State the Problem

Does diet or exercise have a greater impact on reducing blood cholesterol level?

## State a Testable or Measurable Hypothesis

Diet has a greater effect on blood cholesterol than does exercise.

## Plan the Methods to Be Used in Carrying Out the Study

1. Who will be the subjects? What will be their characteristics regarding age, sex, diet, physical activity, initial blood cholesterol levels, medical history, and so on?
2. What measurements will be made? How and when will they be made?

3. Define exactly what the two groups will actually do. What will each group eat? How will adherence to the diet be assessed? Exactly what will the exercise group do in regard to intensity, duration, frequency, and type of exercise? How will their adherence be determined?
4. How will the data be treated statistically?
5. Carry out the study. The two groups follow the guidelines for exercise and diet.
6. Analyze the data using appropriate statistics.
7. State the conclusion or conclusions. Diet and exercise are equally effective in reducing serum cholesterol.

What the subjects actually did with their diet and exercise was carefully identified. The change in blood cholesterol levels was then judged to be noteworthy, or statistically significant, based on a predetermined criterion, that is, a significance level of .05, which means that there is a 5% probability that the finding was in error but a 95% probability that the finding was correct. This is different from eyeballing the results and drawing a conclusion.

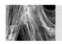 Are researchers ever 100 percent sure of their findings?

Most people looking for answers to a problem or trying to make a decision probably have some bias favoring one answer or outcome. For example, a dietitian may have expected that the influence of diet exerted a greater effect on blood cholesterol levels, whereas a physical educator may have hoped for the reverse. Without using an objective statistical approach, it is all too easy for the dietitian or physical educator to pronounce small differences noteworthy. For example, if the blood cholesterol levels in the exercise group dropped from 190 mg/dL to 180 and that of the diet group dropped from 195 to 183, is the difference in change between the two groups really meaningful? Is it valid for the physical educator to proclaim that exercise has a greater effect than diet?

Given the potential bias that many of us may have when making comparisons, statistics are needed to reduce the subjectivity in analyzing data. If the difference between the two groups is too small to be statistically significant, one can be reasonably confident that the difference is not real and is most likely the result of other factors, such as chance and measurement error. Consequently, the scientific method allows one to make a bias-free judgment. This does not mean it is always the best decision, but it certainly tends to be better.

Research should not be viewed as a mere compilation of results from many independent studies. Rather, it should be thought of as an ever-changing mass of information that may yield different interpretations over time. New results engender new hypotheses, which are tested in accordance with the scientific method. Former "facts" may no longer be supported but rather replaced by new results. Consequently, the state of knowledge of a topic at any time must be thought of as a temporary state, with future modifications "baking away in the research oven."

## INDUCTIVE AND DEDUCTIVE REASONING

Inductive reasoning is one method of reasoning that researchers use. It is based on making a conclusion or generalization based on a limited number of observations. Thus, it proceeds from the specific to the general. All research that makes inferences or generalizations about the results of a study uses inductive reasoning. For example, if 40 vegetarians were studied and all were found to be introverts, one might conclude that all vegetarians are introverts. Obviously, the conclusion, though logical, may not characterize all vegetarians. One can readily understand why researchers prefer to have a reasonable number of subjects in a study; the conclusion reached is more likely to be true. The formation of theory from fact is also based on inductive reasoning because a generalization is made on a limited number of observations.

Deductive reasoning is the reverse of inductive reasoning: It proceeds from the general to the specific. A foreigner who visited the United States and was taken to tryouts for a professional basketball team could easily conclude that most men in this country can dunk a basketball. The logic would go something like this: All American men can dunk a basketball. Joe is an American man. Therefore, Joe can dunk a basketball.

The application of research is also based on deductive reasoning. We assume or deduce that what occurred in a sample of subjects in a study may also occur in other people similar to the subjects. If estrogen replacement therapy was found in a study to increase bone density of postmenopausal women, you might deduce that a similar change might occur in your 60-year-old aunt and encourage her to see her physician about it.

Inductive reasoning and deductive reasoning obviously do not always produce sound conclusions. The soundness of either method of reasoning is only as good as the premise used. For example, most American men cannot dunk a basketball, as a movie title once suggested; generalizing from a limited number of cases or to dissimilar people places severe limitations on deductive reasoning.

 Is reasoning necessarily sound because it is inductive or deductive?

## FACT, THEORY, AND PRINCIPLE

### Fact

The scientific method is used to obtain facts. Facts can be thought of as consistently observed events. For example, changes in blood cholesterol levels associated with dietary changes or alteration in mood before and after recreational activity can be measured to see how consistently they are changed by selected variables. The consistency is determined with statistics that indicate whether the change is more likely to be due to the

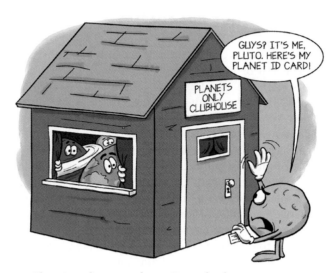

Pluto is no longer a planet. Facts do change.

effect of the variable or to chance. If the balance of studies detect similar change in a variable, at some point a fact has been engendered.

## Theory

Theory is the integration of many facts into the explanation of a phenomenon. This complex process attempts to address most facts associated with the phenomenon. For example, a theory of obesity must include knowledge about food intake (type, amount, fiber content), physical activity (occupational and leisure), resting metabolic rate, and family history of obesity. As new information becomes available, theory must be modified accordingly. As stated previously, because new information is continually produced, fact and theory may be revised periodically. Consequently, it is important to understand that knowledge perpetually changes. Once again the rationale for training all graduate students to become consumers of research is supported.

## Principle

One of the most vital reasons for conducting research besides simply understanding ourselves and the world we live in is to guide behavior. Guides to behavior that are based on fact and theory are called principles. Many things we do professionally as well as personally are based on fact and theory. Examples include weight-training principles, dietary guidelines, and learning principles. Professions obviously strive to develop guidelines for practitioners as a means of improving the lives of people served. Consequently, research and the weaving together of fact, theory, and principle will always be a vital component in the work of allied health professionals.

## LESS SCIENTIFIC METHODS

Compare decision making with the use of the scientific method, including statistics, with that of making decisions based on **tradition, trial and error,** and **bias.** Many of the purchasing decisions we make are done on an emotional basis. Madison Avenue spends billions of dollars creating designs, colors, shapes, and sizes that they hope we will find attractive enough to buy. Think of the number and variety of cereal boxes in the supermarket. Consider the great number of shoes for runners, walkers, aerobic dancers, tennis players, and so on. They are aimed largely at the visual and emotional regions of our brains. Incidentally, how do you think they actually select the various colors, shapes, words, and pictures? Through research, naturally!

Although the scientific method is not perfect, it probably will yield the best information in most situations. It is common for people to base many decisions on tradition, emotions, and overall limited logic. How many coaches switch to the offense or defense of the top-rated team after completion of the bowl games? How much vitamin C does the average American think is needed for good health? Why is a book about a new means of weight loss likely to sell so many copies? Is a Hollywood star qualified to write a book on physical fitness? Is a former professional athlete an authority on physical fitness for children?

Although most of us realize how common these examples may be, we are less likely to imagine how often we base decisions at our jobs on similar criteria. Think about the last time you made a fairly important change in something you do at the workplace or in your personal life. Have you altered your eating habits or exercise program? Have you added, deleted, or changed certain exercises in an exercise class you teach? Have you altered some procedure in your professional work? Have you used any facets of the scientific method in helping to make a decision about any of these changes? If not, you are a particularly good candidate for improving the effectiveness of your decisions through application of the scientific process.

## BASIC AND APPLIED RESEARCH

**Basic research** typically deals with theoretical concepts and has no immediate concern with application. This research is conducted primarily for the sake of knowledge alone. In contrast, **applied research** is done with a specific question or application in mind. Consider a health educator who wishes to know whether a 6-week unit on drug education will change drug usage and attitudes in high school students. The researcher wishes to address a specific question. In comparison, imagine a researcher in particle physics who designs an experiment to accelerate subatomic particles to a velocity previously never reached. The purpose? Perhaps it is simply to see what happens. This somewhat vague approach demonstrates basic research.

Although it is typically viewed that basic research is done with no specific purpose in mind, one might question whether this is actually so. The physicist in the example cited may have some fairly specific hunches as to what may happen and why. Observing what does actually happen may develop more links among observations, theories, and hunches. So, is it really research without a purpose? Perhaps it is not so important to answer the question as it is to realize that both types of research may exist on two ends of a continuum with neither one necessarily at the absolute end.

## LOCATION OF RESEARCH

**Field research** is done outside the tightly controlled environment of the laboratory. The location may be a school, classroom, gymnasium, park, hospital, or any location in the real world. **Laboratory research** is conducted under more "sterile" conditions, which allows researchers to exert tighter control over an experiment. This facilitates sound research but somewhat limits the application of the results. In real life, many factors affect learning other than the experimental variable, and field research allows these other factors to operate. Some mistakenly feel that field research is inferior to laboratory research. This is not the case. Some settings make experimental research difficult or impossible. This is the case in many environments in which allied health professionals work. It would be more accurate to state that both experimental and field research have their strengths and limitations. These are explained later.

## INTERNAL VALIDITY

Internal validity is the soundness or overall quality of research. Were measures accurately and reliably made? Were appropriate statistical techniques used to analyze the data? Was the study conducted in a way that allows the possible effect of an independent variable to be demonstrated adequately? Were the effects of factors other than the independent variable minimized? Good research deals with all factors that allow a research question to be soundly tested.

Laboratory research generally is characterized by higher internal validity than field research because of the relatively tight controls that may be placed on a study. For example, the lifestyle of mice can be regulated strictly with regard to diet, physical activity, temperature, and so on. The lifestyle of people living and working in a variety of environments makes regulation of their lifestyle rather difficult. Demonstrating that a low-fat diet reduces blood cholesterol levels would thus be easier in mice than in a group of people who may not fully adhere to the dietary regimen.

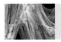 What are the characteristics of an internally valid study?

## EXTERNAL VALIDITY

External validity deals with the potential application of the results of a study, or its generalizability. No statistic provides a simple answer as to when and what can be applied. Rather, application is justified to the degree that the people and conditions involved in the potential application are similar to the subjects and conditions of the original experiment. For example, results of a study comparing two methods of teaching the tennis serve to 12-year-old novices may not be applicable to older, more experienced players. Similarly, the effects of a drug on subjects with high cholesterol levels may not be applicable to people with normal cholesterol levels.

Field research often allows greater potential for application than laboratory research because it is conducted in an environment more likely to be similar to conditions outside the experiment.

## INDEPENDENT AND DEPENDENT VARIABLES

An **independent variable** is one that is manipulated or controlled by the researcher, whereas the **dependent variable** is the behavior that is measured to determine whether it is affected by the independent variable. For example, in a study examining the effect of consuming caffeine on anxiety level, caffeine is the independent variable, and anxiety level is the dependent variable. It thus will be determined whether the behavior (anxiety level) is dependent on caffeine (manipulated variable).

## CHARACTERISTICS OF THE RESEARCHER

Certain traits appear to be common to competent researchers, which suggests that development of these traits is important in people training to become researchers. Awareness of such characteristics may help you to enhance your educational goals and to understand some of the requisites for success in research.

### Open-Mindedness

Researchers should keep their minds open to all possible options in deciding what questions to ask, strategies to use in studying a problem, and possible explanations for results. One shouldn't pigeonhole his or her thinking, as it tends to narrow one's options. Limiting the breadth of one's thinking reduces the likelihood of examining all possibilities. Many great scientific theories probably emerged largely because someone could view a concept in an open, unobstructed manner.

## Knowledge of a Specific Subject

The researcher must know a given field fairly well to ask appropriate questions. What problems or controversies exist? What problems have limited the study of a given topic? Such limitations may affect methodology, such as inability to assess something accurately. Measurement of body fat even today is limited by the fact that calculation of body fat from underwater weighing is based on the dissection of a small number of cadavers decades ago. Equations were developed to predict body density based on the findings from these few cadavers, so use of the same equations to other people with widely varying ages and physical activity levels is not strongly justified.

## Intellectual Curiosity

Few people muster the time and energy to do research without a reasonably good amount of intellectual curiosity. One cannot develop much knowledge of a topic without considerable reading. Strong curiosity leads to reading and desire to learn. As they accumulate knowledge, intellectually curious people tend to want to know even more. Details become more important as the mind strives to connect and relate concepts and bits of information.

This curiosity probably explains why many researchers do much of their work in one specific topic. As a few research questions are answered, more questions are raised, and curiosity leads to more research on the topic.

## Perseverance

As previously stated, developing the knowledge and insights needed to do research takes time and effort. The research process itself involves numerous detailed steps often requiring several years for completion. Perseverance is obviously needed. Formulating the exact research question may take many hours of reading and discussion with other researchers. Writing the documents that are required by most universities to obtain approval to perform a study takes time. The study must be planned and explained in detail. The actual collection of data may take months, depending on the nature of the study. Then the data are analyzed statistically and the final portions of the research paper are written.

Typically, researchers submit the study in an abstract form to be presented at a professional meeting. The manuscript is prepared and submitted to a research publication, then reviewed by several expert researchers on the topic, who suggest revisions to the author or authors (peer review). The manuscript is revised accordingly and resubmitted in hopes of it being accepted for publication. It may or may not be accepted, however. Some HPER research journals reject more than 80% of submitted manuscripts. If the paper is rejected, the author will most likely submit the manuscript to a different publication. It is no wonder that the time from developing the research question to the date of publication in a journal typically is several years. This does require perseverance.

## Honesty

In writing the manuscript of a study for publication or presentation, a researcher has ample opportunity to be dishonest. A person may plagiarize or, even more likely, alter data to support a given hypothesis or line of reasoning. Considerable pressure to publish and obtain funding for grants exists in many universities. Also, to gain a professional reputation, a person could decide to cut corners and do something unethical.

Another example of academic dishonesty is the placement of a faculty member's name before that of a graduate student under the faculty member's supervision. Graduate students who write theses or dissertations should always be the first author of a study. This breach of ethics occurred often in the past, and many professional groups and universities have a written policy declaring that the student's name must be placed first.

Developing the state of knowledge in a discipline is seriously hindered by those who may falsify data. If the work is published, it has the potential to mislead many other scholars and students, who may base their work in part on the false findings, throwing them off the track and causing considerable waste of time. Also, much of the information presented in textbooks is based on research findings. Falsification of findings can ultimately lead to students learning erroneous information. Consequently, a bit of misinformation may lead to considerable compounding of the act.

## Summary

Training in research has been a hallmark of graduate education for many years. It is considered a key trait of a professional with advanced training because it encourages work that is logical, analytical, and competent and produces a person who is likely to read and understand professional literature. Consequently, it can improve the overall quality of one's professional work. Although not all HPER professionals actually conduct research, all of us should view ourselves as consumers of research.

The scientific method is an orderly and logical means of addressing problems and answering questions. Consequently, it is a practical tool. Unscientific methods, such as tradition, superstition, trial and error, and mimicking the champions, are illogical and less useful.

Research, though sound and useful, isn't easy to do. It requires a high degree of open-mindedness, specific knowledge in a field, intellectual curiosity, perseverance, and honesty.

## Learning Activities

1. Have you accomplished the objectives stated at the beginning of the chapter? If not, reread the concepts you're uncertain about.
2. Examine a textbook in a discipline that tends to change fairly rapidly, such as athletic training, motor learning, health problems and issues, recreation therapy, or exercise physiology. Identify several facts or theories that have been altered

over the years because of new research findings. Topics might include some of the following:

- Fluid replacement guidelines in warm weather
- Theories or models that explain health behavior
- Guidelines for aerobic or strength training
- Dietary guidelines

3. Cite several studies in your field and identify the independent and dependent variable or variables.

4. Identify several theories or principles in your academic field. Locate an article that was published at the time the theory or principle was initially presented. Carefully read the article, noting the number of references made to justify the theory or principle. Is a strong rationale made in defense of the theory or principle?

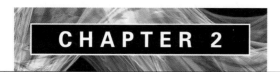

# CHAPTER 2

# Ethics in Human Subject Research

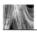

## KEY CONCEPTS

- Codes and guidelines
- The Institutional Review Board
- Informed consent
- Confidentiality and anonymity
- Invasion of privacy
- Safe and competent treatment
- Knowledge of results
- The researcher's role in ethical treatment

## AFTER READING THIS CHAPTER YOU SHOULD BE ABLE TO:

- Explain the major concerns for ethical treatment of research subjects.
- Describe the process of informed consent and the components of an informed consent document.
- Discuss the issues of confidentiality, invasion of privacy, safe and competent treatment, and knowledge of results regarding research subjects.
- Explain the role of the researcher concerning the ethical treatment of subjects.

Research subjects have intrinsic rights that allow them to make informed decisions about participating in a study, and during and after participation to be treated in a safe, humane, and professional manner. The design of a study, the characteristics of the subjects, the methods used in an investigation, and the disposition of the researcher all may influence the ethical treatment of the participant. Furthermore, the public (i.e., potential research subjects) has become much more sensitive to and opinionated about controversial human subject research, such as organ transplantation and stem cell and embryo investigations. Therefore, before we delve into more detailed discussions of these and other research topics, it is important to examine some of the basic considerations and rights of human research subjects.

## CODES AND GUIDELINES

In 1974, the U.S. Congress formed the National Commission for the Protection of Human Subjects of Biomedical and Behavioral Research to address guidelines for ethical treatment of human subjects. The Belmont Report (1979) was published as a result of the commission's deliberations and is one of the keystone documents for research ethics in the United States. Federal agencies involved in human subject research, such as the Food and Drug Administration and the Department of Health and Human Services, have regulations that reflect the recommendations of the Belmont Report. Many international codes, such as the Code of Nuremberg (1949) and the Declaration of Helsinki (1974), also address the protection of research subjects. Today, almost every journal that publishes human subject and animal research has a policy statement regarding obtaining informed consent and ethical treatment of subjects, and investigators must declare that they have complied with that policy.

 *The Belmont Report is one of the keystone documents for research ethics in the United States.*

Many of these codes and guidelines have evolved from noted abuses of human subjects' rights in the not-so-distant past. One of the most prominent of these is the Nazi experimentation on World War II prisoners, who were subjected to "studies" involving exposure to war chemicals, environmental extremes, medicines, and food and sleep deprivation. Another example is studies conducted by the U.S. Air Force in the 1950s in which Alaskan Eskimos were allegedly fed radioactive iodine pellets to determine their effect on thyroid gland function and cold survival. A final example is the long-running Tuskegee, Alabama, study that was exposed in the 1970s in which men with syphilis were "treated" with a placebo instead of a standard drug.

In the preceding examples, subjects participated either involuntarily or without informed consent, both violations of their principled rights. It should be obvious: Ethics in research on human subjects is a serious matter that requires our attention.

## THE INSTITUTIONAL REVIEW BOARD

An institutional review board (IRB) is a panel of research experts that pass judgment on the quality and safety of studies before they can be conducted. Most institutions that conduct studies on human subjects have an IRB. The IRB serves primarily as a means of protecting the rights of subjects and is an important research quality control measure. The IRB also protects researchers and the institution. Among the many functions of the IRB are the evaluation and approval of proposed studies and obtaining informed consent documents that will be used in an investigation. We will discuss the IRB in much more detail in Chapter 18, but for now simply note that the IRB serves as a vital means of ensuring that sound and ethical research practices are used at an institution.

## INFORMED CONSENT

An investigator has an ethical commitment to ensure that a potential subject has sufficient information and comprehension to make a sound decision about participating in a study. The right to give informed consent is one of the subject's most important rights. Typically, the informed consent process involves the prospective subject reading a simple but thorough written document that provides the essential details of the study. After reading the document and discussing any questions with the investigator, the subjects are usually well enough informed to determine whether it is in their best interest to consent to participate.

*Informed consent is one of the subject's most important rights.*

Informed consent statements vary in terms of language, length, and detail. Studies that pose little or no risk may use very simple and brief consents, whereas investigations involving greater risk (even life-threatening in some cases of medical research) need to use much more elaborate consent forms and practices. The consent form must be written at the comprehension level of the subject without using unnecessarily big words or technical jargon. This means that a consent form geared for medical students would be considerably different from one aimed at fourth graders. This is probably the most significant problem and challenge for researchers preparing these documents. What seems like everyday language to the professional may be foreign to the subject. The document must be written in a noncoercive and straightforward manner that is respectful of the prospective subject. Finally, for subjects under the legal age of consent, parental consents and youth and child assents serve as consent documents. Examples of some consent forms may be seen in Appendix C.

## Components of Informed Consent

Consent forms vary considerably in terms of content, language, and length. What follows are descriptions of some of the basic elements of an informed consent document. Check with your university for specific information regarding its consent form requirements. A summary of the elements of an informed consent document appears in Table 2-1.

**Background and Invitation to Participate** This brief statement provides some background about the study, the need to conduct it, and why the subject is being asked to participate. This is an important section, since the researcher is trying to stimulate interest in and inform the subject about why it is important to become involved.

| TABLE 2-1. Elements of an Informed Consent Document |
| --- |
| ***Background and Invitation to Participate*** |
| Explanation of procedures |
| Potential risks and discomforts |
| Potential benefits |
| Rights of inquiry and withdrawal |
| Signatures of subject and witness |

**Explanation of Procedures**  The investigator must describe all of the procedures that the subject will be asked to perform or submit to and where the procedures will be conducted. Sufficient details must be provided for each aspect of the study, including all pre- and post-assessments, intervention of a treatment, time commitment, and so on. Failure to provide critical components and characteristics such as risks, unpleasantness, and costs could be regarded as an act of unethical deception. Imagine a researcher approaching a subject during a study and saying, "We forgot to tell you that we'll need to perform a muscle biopsy. Sorry!"

**Potential Risks and Discomforts**  In this section, the investigator must describe any apparent risk or discomfort that may occur during the study that may affect the subject's decision to participate. Risks may be classified as physical (e.g., heart attack, pain, bruised skin, nausea), psychological (e.g., distress, anxiety, fear), legal (possible criminal action), economic (loss of job), or social (invasion of privacy). In addition to these descriptions, many universities and agencies require a statement of the type of medical treatment the subject may receive if injured or if he/she becomes ill during the research. The federal and international codes previously mentioned also mandate the disclosure of foreseeable risks. It is best to be detailed and inclusive in their description.

**Potential Benefits**  Two types of benefits may result from the research. One is the possible benefits to the **subject** and the other is to **society.** Therefore, in this section any benefits that are likely to be expected are described. These descriptions must be written in a way that does not guarantee or exaggerate the benefits, so the subject is not misled. The possible benefits of the proposed research may or may not have direct value to the subject. So if there are no direct benefits to the subject, it must be clearly stated. There always must be some benefit to society, such as advancement of knowledge, for a study to be ethically conducted. The societal benefit should be stated in this section as well.

**Rights of Inquiry and Withdrawal**  Subjects must be informed that they have the right to ask questions and have them answered by the investigator at any time. This is true particularly during the consent process, when clarification of uncertainties clearly affects the subject's ability to make an informed decision. The subject also has the right to withdraw from the study at any time. Therefore, subjects must be informed that they are free to withdraw at any time without fear of reprisal or future prejudice on the part of the researcher or the sponsoring institution. This may raise debate relative to requiring students to participate in a research study as a class requirement or other such academic situations.

  Also, when subjects provide their consent, it is unethical to ask them to waive any legal rights or privileges. Therefore, there cannot be any language in the consent form that requires the subject to relinquish any of these rights. This is also true for any language that absolves the researcher or the institution from any liability for negligent actions.

## Valid Informed Consent

We all have probably read and signed documents that we didn't understand, such as a bank loan contract or an insurance policy. We sign on the good faith that the loan officer or agent is not trying to take advantage of us. All too often a subject hastily reads a consent document and agrees to participate with that same good faith. The point is that a signature from a subject doesn't necessarily mean that valid informed consent was obtained. Actually, the consent form serves only to assist the investigator in negotiating valid consent from the subject. To help verify that prospective subjects comprehended what they just read and are prepared to provide a valid consent, it is suggested that the investigator ask them several questions about the document before signatures are obtained. Normally signatures of the **subject** and a **witness** appear at the end of the document.

 *To assist in securing valid consent, the investigator should ask subjects questions prior to signing the document.*

## CONFIDENTIALITY AND ANONYMITY

All observations of research subjects should be treated in as confidential a manner as possible. This typically implies that only the investigators or possibly those involved in gathering the research information have access to or knowledge of the identity of the subjects and their related information.

When possible, codes or identification numbers should be assigned to subjects and their research records to protect their anonymity. Reporting of research results is usually done with group rather than individual data, which further masks the identity of singular observations. Individual results may be disclosed or reported only with the subject's permission.

## INVASION OF PRIVACY

It is acceptable to make research observations of many public acts that would normally be viewed by others. However, it is unethical and an invasion of privacy to make clandestine observations of acts that are considered personal or sensitive. That is not to say that research of this type can't be ethically conducted. For instance, many such studies in human sexual activities have been done. Before doing any research on highly personal behaviors or use of covert observational techniques, it is essential to explain the rationale to the subjects and obtain their permission and consent before any data collection.

## SAFE AND COMPETENT TREATMENT

A subject should expect the investigator or participating personnel to have a high degree of skill in making research assessments. The measurements should be made in a competent manner that respects the dignity of the subject and minimizes any risk or discomfort. Practicing new or unfamiliar skills during a study may expose a subject to unnecessary risk, diminish the validity of the data collected, and reduce the credibility of the investigator in the eyes of the subject or others involved in the project.

## KNOWLEDGE OF RESULTS

A researcher's responsibility to the subject doesn't end after the last measurement is made. An investigator has a professional obligation to provide the subjects with feedback about their own outcome and the general results of the study and to fulfill any other promises that were made for consideration for participating in the study. Failure to provide knowledge of outcome conveys a negative, impersonal message about the researcher and is a breach of common courtesy. Be assured that subjects prefer to work with polite researchers, so providing feedback in a gracious and timely manner not only enhances the investigator's reputation but also may help in recruiting subjects for future studies.

## THE RESEARCHER'S ROLE IN ETHICAL TREATMENT

It should be apparent that the investigator is the person who is primarily responsible for the ethical treatment of research subjects. No IRB, federal agency, or international code can directly oversee the research process; therefore, it is incumbent on the researcher to use safe, honest, and fair practices. Unfortunately, a few researchers feel that some guidelines and review boards are so restrictive that they limit their academic freedom. Those adopting this viewpoint sometimes attempt to justify some unethical research practices to promote their own research agenda. Usually, there is little merit to these claims. We discussed the characteristics of a researcher in Chapter 1, and it

 *The investigator is the entity that is primarily responsible for the ethical treatment of research subjects.*

should be evident that these traits play an important role in relation to ethical protection of subjects and research conduct.

 **Summary**

Many boards, agencies, and codes exist to protect human research subjects. Among the ethical research rights are informed consent, confidentiality, anonymity, privacy, safe and competent treatment, and knowledge of results. Even though there are many external sources for the protection of subjects, the investigator is the individual directly

| **TABLE 2-2. Summary of Human Subject Research Rights** |
| --- |
| *Informed Consent* |
| Confidentiality |
| Anonymity |
| No invasion of privacy |
| Safe and competent treatment |
| Knowledge of results |

responsible for providing professional and ethical treatment of research participants. A summary of the research subject's rights is presented in Table 2-2.

 **Learning Activities**

1.  Have you accomplished the objectives stated at the beginning of the chapter? If not, go back and reread the concepts you're uncertain about. Also, ask your professor questions about these topics.
2.  Suggest a class discussion about some timely and/or controversial issues regarding human subject research.
3.  Read some selected research articles (perhaps focus on the methods section) to determine any possible breaches in research ethics.

# PART II

# Research Writing

3.  Getting Started: Information Retrieval

4.  The Research Paper and Proposal

5.  Completing the Research Paper: Results, Discussion, Conclusion, and References

6.  Research Writing

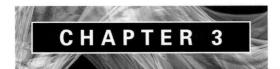

# CHAPTER 3

# Getting Started: Information Retrieval

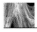

## KEY CONCEPTS

- Sources of information
- Bibliographies
- Abstracts
- Indexes
- Research reviews
- Journals
- Computerized information retrieval

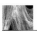

## AFTER READING THIS CHAPTER YOU SHOULD BE ABLE TO:

- Identify several reasons for reviewing the literature before writing a proposal.
- Describe why researchers should read primary rather than secondary references.
- List and define several sources of reference information and give examples of each.
- Describe how computer information retrieval systems operate and several advantages of them.
- Name several data-based computer systems and the indexes they search.

Before beginning to write a research proposal, you should do some general and specific reading to develop a general state of knowledge of the topic. This knowledge should include areas of controversy, designs, methods, characteristics of topics studied and not yet studied, and recommendations made by others. Viewing the literature with some of these aspects in mind will enhance the results of your reading.

## SOURCES OF INFORMATION

### Primary and Secondary References

References or sources of information can be classified as either **primary** or **secondary.** Primary references are the original article, report, or book, whereas secondary references are those in which the original work is described or mentioned by someone other than the author of the original work. In the latter case, one is informed secondhand. Much of the information in textbooks is based on original work that is described, cited in the text, and referenced. The text is thus a secondary reference for that particular information. The difference should be understood because it is assumed that references cited in a research paper or proposal were read firsthand to provide the best possible understanding of the original work. Restriction to secondary references increases the probability that opinion and bias from author to a reader is transferred. The effect is analogous to whispering a secret in someone's ear and having him or her whisper the secret to another person. With each person involved in the chain of communication, accuracy potentially decreases. To ensure the highest level of accuracy in reporting information, read the original or primary reference so that the references cited in the paper indicate that you did read the

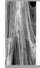 *Primary references are the original article, report, or book; secondary references are those in which the original work is described or mentioned by someone other than the author of the original work.*

primary reference rather than an interpretation or summary by another author. Secondary references should be used only when the original work is not available. It is tempting but less sound to do otherwise. Some sources of reference information are briefly discussed.

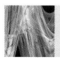 Why is it important to read an original work or primary reference rather than a secondary reference?

## BIBLIOGRAPHIES

Bibliographies offer information from books, articles, and documents. However, no summary or abstract is included, so the use to the reader is limited to the title. Examples of bibliographies related to HPER appear in Table 3-1.

## ABSTRACTS

An abstract is a compilation of information on a given topic; it provides a bibliographic entry and a summary for each source. Typically, publications from dozens and even hundreds of journals are included in an abstract. The sole purpose of reading an abstract is to decide whether to read the original work. Abstracts are a source of information for previously published information and work yet to be published and so provide the most recent work being done on a topic. The process of writing, submitting a manuscript, revising it, and having it published typically takes a year or two. Therefore, the most recent work usually appears in abstracts. Examples of abstracts pertinent to HPER are provided in Table 3-1.

**TABLE 3-1. Examples of References in Health, Physical Education, and Recreation (HPER)**

| Type | Example |
|---|---|
| Abstracts | Current Index to Journals in Education |
| | Abstracts in hygiene |
| | Dissertation abstracts |
| | Medical abstracts |
| | Physiologic abstracts |
| | Completed research in HPER |
| | Sociological abstracts |
| | Annual meeting abstracts of the American College of Sports Medicine (published annually as a supplement to *Medicine and Science in Sports and Exercise*) |
| | Annual meeting abstracts of the Research Consortium of the American Alliance of Health, Physical Education, Recreation, and Dance (published annually as a supplement to the *Research Quarterly for Exercise and Sport*) |
| Bibliographies | Sociological information retrieval for leisure studies |
| | Bibliography of biomechanics |
| | *Physical Fitness/Sports Medicine Quarterly* |
| | Bibliography of research using female subjects |
| Indexes | *Education Index* |
| | *Index Medicus* |
| | Index to literature in leisure, recreation, parks, and recreational services |
| Research reviews | Review of educational research |
| | Physiologic reviews |
| | Psychological reviews |
| | College health reviews |
| | Annual review of public health |
| | Exercise and sport sciences reviews |

The term *abstract* as used here refers to a compilation of sources of information. It should not be confused with the brief summary of a research article, which commonly appears on the first page of a journal article below the title.

## INDEXES

An index is identical to a bibliography except that it is limited to periodicals, that is, journals and magazines. Usually, no summary or abstract is provided. See Table 3-1 for examples.

## RESEARCH REVIEWS

Research reviews are thorough summaries and interpretations of a topic written by an expert in the field. Reviews typically include the historical development of a specific area of research, limitations in the existing research, suggestions for future research, and topics that should be addressed. Numerous references are cited, which provides a good list of initial references to consult. Consequently, reviews are helpful to the student searching for a possible research topic. Examples appear in Table 3-1.

## JOURNALS

The disciplines of health, physical education, and recreation are fairly specific today, and consequently a wide variety of journals are available. Selected research journals in HPER appear in Table 3-2. Most professional organizations publish one or more journals, with one of them focused on research in the discipline. Examples are the *Research Quarterly for Exercise and Sport,* published by the American Alliance of Health, Physical Education, Recreation, and Dance; *Medicine and Science in Sports and Exercise,* published by the American College of Sports Medicine; and the *Journal of Strength and Conditioning Research,* published by the National Strength and Conditioning Association.

## COMPUTERIZED INFORMATION RETRIEVAL

Use of the computer to speed information retrieval began in the 1970s. A massive number of references are instantly available on the Internet, which saves a great deal of time. Locating references manually in indexes, bibliographies, and other sources used to involve many hours in the library. Today, key words or descriptors are typed on a computer terminal, and the system searches for these terms in a database. The references containing these terms can then be printed. The entire process is fast and can be done in the convenience of one's office or home. In many cases, on-line abstracts and full-text documents can be obtained. A fee is typically charged for each full-text document or article. A list of electronic resources related to HPER is provided in Table 3-3.

The origin of World Wide Web sites is designated by various terms at the end of the site address. The .com indicates a primarily commercial site; .org indicates nonprofit sites; .edu is an educational site; and .gov is a site developed by a government agency. Be cautious in selecting websites, because many commercial sites may be more interested in selling products than providing sound information. The Internet is a fast and easy way to access information, but researchers and students need to be cautious about whether the sites are valid sources of information. If the website is commercial, the accuracy of information may be biased, and the user should beware. Sound, reputable sources tend to be those sponsored by a professional organization or national health agency, such as the American Heart Association or American Cancer Society.

## TABLE 3-2. Selected HPER Journals

| | |
|---|---|
| Health | *American Journal of Clinical Nutrition* |
| | *Annual Review of Health Education* |
| | *College Health Review* |
| | *Death Education* |
| | *Educational Gerontology* |
| | *Health Education* |
| | *Journal of the American School Health Association* |
| | *Journal of Environmental Health* |
| | *Journal of Health Promotion* |
| | *Wellness Perspectives* |
| Physical education | *Adapted Physical Activity Quarterly* |
| | *Dance Annual* |
| | *Dance Perspectives* |
| | *Dance Research Journal* |
| | *International Journal of Sport Sociology* |
| | *International Journal of Sports Biomechanics* |
| | *Journal of Biomechanics* |
| | *Journal of Educational Psychology* |
| | *Journal of Motor Behavior* |
| | *Journal of Physical Education, Recreation, and Dance* |
| | *Journal of Sport Psychology* |
| | *Journal of Sports Medicine and Physical Fitness* |
| | *Journal of Strength and Conditioning Research* |
| | *Journal of Teaching Physical Education* |
| | *Journal of Philosophy of Sport* |
| | *Medicine and Science in Sports and Exercise* |
| | *Perceptual and Motor Skills* |
| | *Physical Educator* |
| | *Quest* |
| | *Research Quarterly for Exercise and Sport* |
| Recreation | *Adapted Physical Activity Quarterly* |
| | *American Corrective Therapy Journal* |
| | *Journal of Leisure Research* |
| | *Journal of Health, Physical Education, Recreation, and Dance* |
| | *Park Maintenance* |
| | *Recreation Management* |
| | *Parks and Recreation* |
| | *Therapeutic Recreation Journal* |

Another virtue of Internet databases and websites is that they are likely to be more current than printed documents because they can be updated with new references more easily. Table 3-4 lists selected websites pertinent to disciplines in HPER.

Selecting appropriate terms to use in a search for a topic is important. Terms may be found in published journal articles. The words are typically listed after the abstract

| TABLE 3-3. Electronic Resources | |
|---|---|
| *Resource* | *Areas Covered* |
| Basic Biosis | Life sciences, including nutrition, physiology, and public health (1994–present) |
| CINAHL | Nursing and allied health 1982–present; includes biomedical and consumer health |
| Dissertation Abstracts | Theses and dissertations with abstracts from 1980–present |
| Electronic Library | Broad coverage of academic areas |
| ERIC | All areas of education, 1966–present |
| Health Service Plus | Consumer health, 1990–present |
| Medline | All areas of medicine, including sports medicine, fitness, and athletic training |
| PsycINFO | Psychology and related disciplines, such as medicine, nursing, education, and physiology |
| Sport Discus | Sports, fitness, training, sports injury, physical education, 1975–present |
| Women's Resources International | Women's studies, 1972–present |
| World Almanac | Biographies, encyclopedia entries, facts, and statistics |

of the article on the first page under the side heading key words. Care must be taken in selecting descriptors to obtain usable references. One of the unique benefits of the computer approach is that several options, such as combining two or more terms, for example *and, or,* and *not,* can help to limit the references. Quotation marks can also be used to limit the search, for example, "calcium and bone metabolism." This eliminates

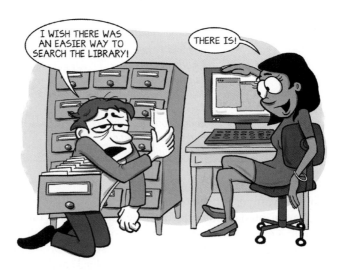

## TABLE 3-4. Websites in HPER

| | |
|---|---|
| American Cancer Society | www.cancer.org |
| American College of Sports Medicine | www.acsm.org/sportsmed |
| American Dietetic Association | www.eatright.org |
| American Diabetes Association | www.diabetes.org |
| American Heart Association | www.amhrt.org |
| American Medical Association | www.AMA-assn.org |
| American Psychological Association Sport & Exercise Psychology Division (APA Div. 47) | www.psyc.unt.edu/apadiv47/ |
| American Public Health Association | www.apha.org |
| American College of Sports Medicine | www.acsm.org/sportsmed |
| American Society of Exercise Physiologists | www.css.edu/users/tboone2asep/toc.htm |
| American Society of Biomechanics | www.asb-biomech.org/ |
| American Alliance for Health, Physical Education, Recreation, and Dance | www.aahperd.org |
| Association for the Advancement of Applied Sport Psychology | www.aaasponline.org |
| Association for Worksite Health Promotion | www.awhp.org |
| Centers for Disease Control and Prevention | www.cdc.gov/ |
| Centre for Activity and Aging | www.uwo.ca/actage |
| Council on Physical Education for Children | www.aahperd.org/naspe/ specialinterest-copec.html |
| Go Ask Alice (health info) | www.columbia.edu/cu/healthwise/alice.html |
| Merck Manual of Medical Information | www.MerckHomeEdition.com |
| National Association for Sport and Physical Education | www.aahperd.org |
| National Strength and Conditioning Association | www.nsca-lift.org |
| National Wellness Association | www.nationalwellness.org |
| National Dance Association | www.aahperd.org |
| National Athletic Trainers Association | www.nata.org |
| National Education Association | www.nea.org |
| North American Society of the Psychology of Sport and Physical Activity | www.naspspa.org |
| Nutrition Navigator (Tufts University) | www.navigator.tufts.edu |
| President's Council on Physical Fitness and Sports | www.fitness.gov |
| Sport Quest | http://sportquest.com |

sources dealing with all aspects of calcium or bone metabolism and limits the search to calcium and bone metabolism together. These options are important because they greatly influence the number of references listed. For example, a recreation therapist who is seeking information on recreational fitness activities in paraplegic children would want to narrow the topic so that references only minimally related would not be listed. Key words might include *fitness, paraplegic children,* and *recreation.* However, *fitness* may be too broad; so instead more specific terms, such as *strength* and *flexibility,* may be used if appropriate. Articles not having *strength* or *flexibility* in the title would be omitted. Thus, one could limit the articles to only those having all of the key words, three of the four key words, etc.

*A good source of terms to use in a search for a topic may be found in published journal articles. The words are typically listed after the abstract of the article on the first page under the side heading key words.*

Typically, it is more difficult to limit the search than it is to achieve a good number of references. Reference librarians are most helpful in getting started on a computer search and explaining special features that may enhance your search. You may even work with a reference librarian who is a subject matter specialist in your discipline. A reference librarian will be able to assist you in selecting key words.

## Summary

Begin reading with at least a general direction as to what type of information you are seeking. A wide variety of resources, including abstracts, bibliographies, indexes, research reviews, and computer searching are available. Secondary references may be used to identify publications you want to read, but primary references should be read to enhance understanding and accuracy.

## Learning Activities

1. Have you accomplished the objectives stated at the beginning of the chapter? If not, reread the concepts you are uncertain about.
2. Conduct a computer search for a topic. Compare the listings obtained using different combinations of key words.
3. Read a paragraph in a textbook that cites several references. Read several of these references and compare the information in them with the paragraph in the text. What information did the author of the text choose not to use from the original work?

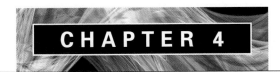

# CHAPTER 4

# The Research Paper and Proposal

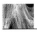

## KEY CONCEPTS

- Title
- Abstract
- Chapter 1: Introduction
- Chapter 2: Problem
- Chapter 3: Review of literature
- Chapter 4: Procedures or methods

## AFTER READING THIS CHAPTER YOU SHOULD BE ABLE TO:

- List and summarize the components of each chapter.
- State the components of the proposal that are not seen in a published article.
- Explain why such detail is required in the methods chapter.
- Explain why all studies have limitations.
- Explain how the body of the chapter on review of literature should be written.
- Define and state examples of speculation.

The typical research proposal written for a class and graduate degree thesis or dissertation is explained in detail here and in Chapter 5. Examples are given throughout to facilitate understanding not only the content that is to be included but the manner in which it is to be written.

There is no single universal protocol regarding the numbering of chapters or even the exact components of each chapter. There is, however, a definite trend as to what is recommended or required at most institutions. One finds considerable variation within and between departments on a single campus, which indicates that the faculty members on a thesis committee determine the specific content of each chapter. Furthermore, the components explained here hold true for most types of research in health, physical education, exercise science, recreation, and leisure studies.

With these institutional, departmental, and academic idiosyncrasies in mind, we proceed to cover here the comprehensive thesis. The research paper or journal manuscript is brief and does not include all aspects of the thesis. The thesis format is explained

| TABLE 4-1. Timetable for a Thesis | |
|---|---|
| **Step** | **Estimated Time** |
| 1. Obtain committee chair and committee | 1 week |
| 2. Write proposal and revise after advisor feedback | 2–3 months |
| 3. Distribute copies to committee | 1 week ahead of meeting |
| 4. Prepare for and present proposal to committee | 1 week |
| 5. Revise proposal | 1–2 weeks |
| 6. Write IRB document | 1 week |
| 7. IRB review and approval | 1–4 weeks |
| 8. Conduct study | Several months |
| 9. Analyze data and write final chapters | Several weeks |
| 10. Prepare for and defend thesis (see steps 3 and 4 above) | 2 weeks |
| 11. Revise thesis | 1 week |
| 12. Submit for final approval | 5 minutes! |

IRB, institutional review board.

chapter by chapter, and, where appropriate, omissions or variations in the journal article are noted. The research proposal ends with the methods chapter. Very often students enrolled in a research methods class write a proposal but never carry out the study. This is not all bad, because it ensures that all graduate students have participated in the planning of a study, which provides considerable insight into the research that is inherent in much graduate work. The chapters that follow the Methods section (Results, Discussion, Summary, and Conclusion) are explained in Chapter 5 in the same detail as the chapters in the proposal, because students writing a thesis need this information explained in detail and because it adds to every student's general understanding of the purposes and features of the results, discussion, and so on. This knowledge should be helpful in reading these sections in a journal article.

For students considering writing a thesis, we urge you to plan ahead. It takes about a year to accomplish the numerous steps, including discussing a topic with a professor who might chair the committee, writing and presenting the proposal to your committee, obtaining the approval of the institutional review board, and so on. Table 4-1 elaborates the steps and estimated time to complete each. Note how many steps depend on the motivation of the student. One's self-discipline, motivation, and need to graduate at some predetermined date all appear to vary considerably in our experience. We advise developing a timeline early in the process. It seems to help.

## COMPONENTS OF THE THESIS

The chapters of a thesis are similar to the plans and specifications for building a house. Numerous details must be considered and written to ensure that all facets of the project are considered. The sequence and content of the chapters are reminiscent of the steps

| **TABLE 4-2. Components of the Thesis and Research Paper** |
| --- |
| Title |
| Abstract |
| Chapter 1: Introduction |
| Chapter 2: The Problem |
| Chapter 3: Review of Literature |
| Chapter 4: Procedures or Methods |
| Chapter 5: Results |
| Chapter 6: Discussion |
| Chapter 7: Summary and Conclusions |
| References |
| Appendix |

in the scientific method. As a matter of fact, the thesis is an elaboration of the scientific method. If the recommendations here are followed, the writing of a thesis or proposal should be a logical, step-by-step cookbook affair. Division of the various chapters into components allows working on various sections of each chapter in limited blocks of time rather than having to work for long, tiresome periods. This permits a good level of flexibility while working on a proposal and may even enhance work efficiency.

The components of the thesis and research paper are listed in Table 4-2. Note that the introduction and problem chapters are often combined into a single chapter, as are the results and discussion chapters.

Research writing is usually done in the second or third person, that is, he, she, or they. Much of the proposal is written in the future tense because the research has yet to be done. In the thesis, the review of literature, results, and discussion chapters are written in the past tense because they deal with work already done.

## Title

A title should describe what a paper is about so that readers may decide whether or not to read it. Computer searches to identify related published information are based on identification of key words in titles. Consequently, it is important to use meaningful words to describe a work. Typically titles are about 10 to 15 words, with nouns as key words. Jargon is avoided to ensure clarity. If the title of a published article is vague or too broad, it may not be read by many people. An overly brief title makes it difficult for readers to decide whether the study is related closely enough to their needs and interests. Although students preparing a research proposal should not be overly concerned with these aspects, they should understand why the title is important for works that eventually are published. It also provides insight into the highly specific titles seen in journal articles. Below are some titles with comments regarding their suitability.

*Health Risks in Children.* This title is too general and too short. It does not describe any specific traits of the children, such as age, sex, or socioeconomic level. It also fails to indicate any specific aim of the study: Was it comparative? Were risks measured before and after some experimental variable was administered? Compare the former title with the second one to determine whether it meets the criteria of being precise as well as concise: *Substance Abuse in 12- to 15-Year-Old Latchkey vs Non–Latchkey Students.*

Another example of a title of a study is *Hematologic Changes Occurring as a Result of Exposure to Various High-Altitude Environments.* This is adequately descriptive, but some of the words are unnecessary. A revised title is *Hematologic Changes Occurring at High Altitude.* This conveys as much information as the first one in far fewer words. A good rule of thumb for effective research writing is to strive for brevity. If something can be communicated clearly in 100 words, then doing so in 150 words is less efficient. Most readers prefer getting the facts as quickly as possible. Newspaper articles are written with this in mind, as are journal articles, to minimize the length and cost of printing each issue.

## Abstract

An abstract is a summary of the proposal or article that very briefly describes the purpose of the study, subjects, methods, results, and conclusions. It is not part of the proposal because no data have yet been collected and analyzed. In journal articles, the abstract is usually printed in italics or boldface immediately below the title and is limited to about 100 to 300 words.

## CHAPTER 1: INTRODUCTION

The introduction is treated as a brief chapter in this text, although it is often combined with Chapter 2 as described here, the statement of the problem. The main purpose of the introduction is to justify the need for the study. To do this, cite key studies from the literature that document the need for the study. For example, if there is disagreement about the results of several studies on a topic, which is typical in research, studies supporting each side of a point should be referenced. Conflicts or varying findings in the results of research abound, since researchers gravitate to topics of disagreement and controversy. Existence of conflict by itself nearly justifies research that attempts to resolve the problem. Textbooks and articles often point out areas of unsettled knowledge, as do professors teaching their classes. Articles in research journals review the state of knowledge on a specific topic. Specific recommendations for future research are typically provided, and they highlight the direction of future research and offer suggestions for improving the methods used to study a topic. Also, a wealth of references is immediately available in review articles.

 What is the primary purpose of the introduction?

Years ago, many studies published in the allied health professions were performed using only college-age male subjects. Although these studies described the response or characteristics of young men, the responses of older and younger males and females were relatively unknown. Since then, these other populations have been more commonly used as subjects. Consequently, 10 and 20 years ago the study of these other groups often was the main rationale or purpose of a number of investigations.

Improved research techniques open the door to replicate old methods to verify the results. Use of modern strength assessment equipment has caused researchers to re-evaluate techniques to improve muscular fitness. Computer software is now widely available to perform complex statistical analyses that previously were infrequently used because without computers they were too labor intensive. These limitations can now be overcome and consequently allow researchers to re-examine problems and questions that even today may not be resolved.

In summation, the introduction is critical to understanding the overall meaning and value of a study. This chapter should emphasize the importance of asking good research questions and documenting the need to answer the question. It is analogous perhaps to a lawyer presenting a client's case in a trial. If your professor does not buy the reason for doing the study, the remainder of a proposal is obviously of lesser meaning. When researchers submit their work to a journal in hopes of having it published, they too must clearly substantiate the reason for it. Failure to accomplish this task may result in the paper being rejected for publication.

It may be helpful at this point to refer to a fairly recent copy of a research publication in your field. Read the first several paragraphs of the article. The term *Introduction* may not appear as a central or side heading, but it is assumed that these initial paragraphs of a paper are in fact the introduction. References are cited to make the reader aware of the state of knowledge on a particular topic. The section is often quite short, typically several paragraphs. But do not confuse brevity with lack of importance. The last paragraph is commonly phrased something like "The purpose of this study is to...." Scan several articles and see how similar they are as to length, content, and even the wording of the last sentence. A definite pattern emerges.

In some research papers or theses, the introduction is a separate chapter because it may place greater attention to substantiating the need for the study. It is helpful to read the introductions of several papers or theses to better understand how the need for a study is justified.

Most of the introduction is written in the past tense because it cites and describes the results of previous studies. Only the last sentence, "The purpose of this study..." is written in the future tense. After a study is actually conducted and completed, the sentence is changed to the past or present tense.

## CHAPTER 2: THE PROBLEM

The chapter on the problem provides an overview of the study and usually includes subsections such as statement of the purpose or problem to be addressed, hypothesis, delimitations (scope), limitations (variables that could not be controlled), and significance of the study. In writing a proposal, the future tense is typically used in most sections because at that time the study is merely a plan that is to be critiqued by a professor or committee. If the proposal is written with the intention of using it for a thesis rather than a project for a class, a thesis committee consisting of several faculty will examine the plan and most likely suggest revisions that will be used for the actual study. At the completion of the study, the verbs must be changed to past tense, reflecting the fact that the work was completed.

The information in this chapter does not appear in journal articles, since most of it is implicit in the context of the study or it appears in other sections of the manuscript, such as the methods and discussion. It exists as a separate chapter in the thesis proposal to draw attention to components of the study that might otherwise be neglected or not fully appreciated by the student who is learning research skills. Hence, it is included to make sure the student author pays adequate attention to several important facets of the study.

## Purpose of the Study

This brief statement identifies the specific intention of the study. It should identify an exact problem to be studied. Commonly, this statement is difficult to write, because most students tend to be concerned with solving a major problem in their field which comprises many variables. A research problem is usually highly specific and addresses only one or two key factors involved in a given phenomenon. For example, a physical educator may have an interest in weight training and states the problem to be the determination of the best means of increasing muscular strength. Although this is an interesting topic, it is extremely broad. Numerous variables affect the acquisition of strength: frequency and intensity of training, volume of work per training session, work–rest ratio, type of apparatus used, diet, and so on. To carry out such a training study would require a large number of groups and subjects, making the project unrealistic.

It can be better understood now why most studies are limited to one or two variables. The novice researcher would be advised to select perhaps one variable for investigation. For example, comparing the effects of one, three, and five sets of weight training would be a far more manageable study than that previously given. Now three experimental groups plus a control group (a group not receiving the treatment or independent variable) would probably suffice to address the problem: Is there a significant difference in strength development when one, three, and five sets of selected weight-training exercises are compared? This graduate student will address a meaningful problem and be able to provide closer supervision of the training sessions as well as probably measure strength more accurately and reliably with fewer subjects. Also, the student may be able to carry out the study and graduate in a reasonable time!

So for these reasons, limit the purpose of the study. Do not attempt to answer numerous questions about the topic. Focus instead on the quality with which the study can be conducted. The quality of a study has little to do with the number of questions addressed. The following statement of the purpose of a study may be helpful. One purpose is clearly identified: "The purpose of this study will be to determine whether recreational activity and socioeconomic status are significantly related."

## Hypotheses

A hypothesis is a statement indicating the likely outcome of a study. It is often posed as a question. It can also be thought of as a prediction of findings based on the relevant literature. Hypotheses may be expressed several ways.

**Statistical Hypotheses: Null and Directional** **Statistical hypotheses** are stated in either a null form or a directional form. In the former form, no significant effect or relationship is anticipated. For example, using the example of body fatness and TV watching, the null hypothesis might be stated as "Body fatness and time spent watching TV will not be significantly related."

The directional hypothesis is stated so that a significant difference or relationship is predicted. In this case, TV watching would be projected to be significantly related to body fatness. Another example would be stating that practice with red playground balls will enhance catching and throwing skills in 8- to 10-year-old children more than practice with yellow playground balls.

Does it make a difference which way the hypothesis is stated? Most people new to research find it is easier to conceptualize the outcome of statistical analysis by using the null form. If statistical significance is found, the researcher readily can identify which experimental effect is superior or whether or not a real relationship exists. However, achieving statistical significance is more likely to occur when using the directional statement. This concept is more fully discussed in a later chapter. For now, it is probably easier to state hypotheses in the null or "no difference" format.

**Research Hypotheses** **Research hypotheses** are stated according to the results the researcher actually expects. They are written without symbols and might appear as follows: "Runners are more introverted than basketball players." Research hypotheses are used in this section of the research paper rather than statistical hypotheses. Statistical hypotheses are used to test the research hypothesis and are used in performing the statistical analysis of the data. Hypotheses are not always stated in journal articles because they are implied by the purpose of the study. Using the personality of runners and basketball players as an example, the purpose of the study would be to compare the degree of being an introvert in runners and basketball players. Logically, the research hypothesis states what the expected outcome is. The expected outcome is derived from knowledge of the related literature on the topic.

## Delimitations

Delimitations are the what, who, where, and when of the study. They summarize what is included in a study: the nature of the subjects, the location of the study, its duration, and variables studied. An example might be: "Eighty children aged 7 and 8 years enrolled at Rockbrook Elementary School in Omaha, Nebraska, will be subjects in a 12-week study in which throwing and catching skills with 9-inch rubber playground balls of three different colors will be compared." In journal articles, this information is covered in the methods section of the paper.

## Limitations

Limitations are events that may interfere with the results of a study and that the researcher cannot control. In the sample study on throwing and catching skills, other factors may affect learning as well as performance while testing subjects. The amount of practice outside the experimental procedure may affect skill level. Some youngsters may play on teams or informally with parents and siblings, whereas other children may engage in little or no outside activity using these skills. Performance during pre- and post-testing may be affected by children's emotions, such as performing in front of a stranger; attitudes such as "I hate ball games because I'm no good"; physical injury, and so on. Although some of these factors may be unknown to the researcher, the researcher is obligated to define any factors that are anticipated to affect the outcome.

A common limitation is the duration of the study. Short-term studies may be limited simply because some phenomena do not dramatically change in 10 or 12 weeks. Studies examining bone density alteration from exercise or diet should last many months because bone responds rather slowly to these stimuli. A 12-week study may conclude falsely that these variables have no effect on bone simply because of the overly short duration of the study.

Stating limitations in a distinct section of the proposal ensures that the student recognizes the possible influence of other variables. No study can perfectly control all factors in the environment, and therefore even the best-designed and best-planned studies have one or more limitations. In published articles, limitations are often mentioned in the discussion section or are implied.

## Definition of Terms

Certain terms, because they have multiple meanings, should be defined as they will be used in a particular study. For example, the word *health* is defined differently in the dictionary than in the professional field of health education. If health is assessed in a study, it should be defined **operationally** or **functionally** so that any reader of the paper understands the context to which it applies. The term *physical fitness* should be defined because it has different meanings, such as health-oriented fitness and athletic fitness. Definitions should adhere to what is commonly accepted and used in the professional literature.

Some terms are defined simply to assist committee members outside the discipline to understand the study. Many universities require that at least one thesis committee member be from outside the department. A professor with a doctor of philosophy degree in the psychology department may have difficulty understanding terms used in the allied health professions. Comprehension is facilitated by defining the words as used in the discipline.

## Significance of the Study

The significance of a study refers to its practical application in the discipline and perhaps to society in general. For example, if practice with red playground balls was found to enhance ball-handling skills more than practice with white and yellow balls, this information might be applied to other groups of children with similar characteristics. If TV watching was found to be related to body fatness, it might justify a study in which TV watching was experimentally controlled in a group of people to see if it reduced body fatness.

Significance of the study should not be confused with statistical significance. The latter deals with a statement of mathematical probability and is discussed in a later chapter dealing with statistics.

## CHAPTER 3: REVIEW OF LITERATURE

The review of the literature is written in the past tense because it deals with published work. A common format for its organization is three sections: introduction, body, and summary. The introduction is brief, indicating titles used for sections of the review and the inclusion of a summary. Therefore, the introduction informs the reader as to how the literature analysis is organized. A review of literature is not seen in journal articles as a section heading but instead is embedded within the introduction and discussion sections.

The body constitutes nearly all of the length of the review chapter. It is usually divided into several subsections. The most common misunderstanding of this chapter is that it is a series of paragraphs, each summarizing one study. This approach fails to collate the main themes about literature on the topic. It is easier to compose, for it requires no collation and comparison of findings across studies. However, this is exactly what the chapter is supposed to do, and quite honestly, it requires a bit of work. The task is to analyze the literature rather than to merely list results of separate studies.

 A review of literature should analyze and critique the findings across many studies on a given topic. It should provide more than a mere summarizing of the study and its results.

The task is more difficult if the student does not have in-depth knowledge of the topic. Faculty who publish on a regular basis, on the other hand, possess in-depth training in statistics, experimental design, and the subject matter in their field. Furthermore, they read research literature on a regular basis and have a good feel for its content. Obviously, one cannot expect a student to have this level of training, but the only way to learn to analyze literature is by doing so. Most professors adjust their level of expectation to coincide with the level of training of their students.

An understanding of literature analysis can be greatly enhanced by reading a review of the literature on any topic in a research publication. If you are able to obtain a review of the topic you are working with, so much the better. It will be noticed that the review is organized around concepts or themes rather than describing one study per paragraph. A review of literature, for example, on aerobic exercise training may be organized into headings including exercise intensity, duration, frequency, and mode of exercise. Several paragraphs under each topic depict the overall findings and cite individual studies to document the observations. For example, a sentence in one paragraph may be as follows: "Numerous studies have reported that the minimal exercise intensity that elicits an improvement in aerobic power is 50% of maximum oxygen uptake," and several key studies are cited to document the statement. Several of these cited studies can then be summarized regarding the characteristics of the subjects, their initial fitness level, age, and so on. A second paragraph might describe studies reporting other levels of exercise intensity. These studies should be analyzed to determine what they have in common, which helps to explain the different findings. Perhaps some of these studies observed a lower intensity to be effective in older and less fit subjects. Differences in training programs should be analyzed along with limitations, such as sample size, design, and methods. Note again that the literature is being analyzed rather than just summarized study by study. The term *review* perhaps connotes the wrong impression to students. Perhaps the term *critique* or *analysis* would better suggest the method to be used in writing this chapter.

The purpose of reviewing the literature is to develop an understanding of the state of knowledge on a topic. It includes not only the findings of many studies but also the methods used to study the problem. Consequently, you can learn much when reading the literature by carefully noting the instruments and procedures used to measure variables. There are often several means of assessing a variable, and the advantages and disadvantages of each should be examined.

A summary is the last component of the chapter. In long review chapters, summaries are sometimes written for each subsection as well.

## CHAPTER 4: PROCEDURES OR METHODS

The chapter on procedures or methods is analogous to a cookbook that provides precise details of how the study will be (proposal) or was (report) conducted. It describes the subjects, the means of collecting data, the treatment or intervention used if the study is experimental, and the statistical analysis. The purpose of describing the methods in such detail is to allow replication of the study by others, an essential step in research, and to enable others to judge how the methods may have affected the outcome of a study. For example, different means of measuring a variable may affect the scores, as might the procedures for administering a test or the means of statistically analyzing the data. The informed reader wishes to know these details so as to interpret the findings intelligently.

The methods chapter is written in the future tense for the proposal, since it is only a plan at that point and is subject to review and revision. Several components of this chapter may be thought of as **preliminary procedures** because they are steps to be accomplished before data are collected. Similarly, portions of the chapter dealing with data collection and statistical analysis are done while actually carrying out the study. They may be viewed as **operational procedures.**

## Subjects

This is a preliminary procedure identifying the source of subjects, criteria for being a subject, and the sampling technique used to obtain subjects. The source of the subjects may be a particular school or recreation setting, for example. **Inclusion criteria** are traits necessary for a person to be a subject. Criteria may include gender, age, medical or fitness status, or some special trait, such as being a female graduate student in recreation and leisure studies. For example, in many exercise training studies, subjects must be healthy and fit enough to participate in strenuous testing and training without risk to their health. These requirements must be clearly identified in this section.

The sampling procedure refers to the means of selecting people with the defined criteria at the given location. Random sampling means that anyone with the requisite criteria at a defined location is a possible subject. For example, every child at a school might be assigned a number with 100 numbers drawn out of a hat or from a table of random numbers. A number of sampling procedures exist, and the specific procedure used should be stated, because it affects the scores obtained. For example, the mean rate of school absenteeism from 100 randomly selected students would likely be different from the mean absenteeism rate of children with a chronic illness or from an unstable family. More details about sampling are covered in Chapter 7. Last, a statement should be made that approval from an institutional review board was received and that all subjects signed an informed consent document.

## Treatment or Experimental Design

Study design is an operational procedure that refers to the way the study will be or was conducted: how subjects are grouped (if appropriate) and the activity performed by the subjects. It is important to describe the experimental procedures in detail for two reasons. First, the results of the study depend on the treatment applied to the subjects, and second, other researchers may wish to replicate the study to determine whether similar results occur in other groups. They need detailed information to accomplish either of these functions. For example, if a recreator wished to measure the effects of high-risk outdoor activities on self-confidence, details regarding the exact activities used, their risk, involvement with other people, physical surrounding, number of activities used, and duration of the program must be known.

Similarly, if one is studying the effects of a health education unit on nutrition and its effects on eating habits at home, great detail describing the unit would be necessary: media used, duration, activities used in class, the number of teachers used, special training of teachers for the unit, collection of data describing food consumption, and so on. As a test to determine whether these details were adequately given, one can ask whether the study could be conducted identically by someone else with only the information provided.

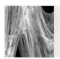 Why are the methods written in such great detail in a thesis or research paper?

## Data Collection

As with the previous section, considerable detail must be provided for possible replication and for full understanding of data collection. Details may include equipment or instruments used; validation of procedures; site of data collection; time of day; physiologic status such as fasting; omission of exercise the day before data collection; warm-up or practice trials; sequence of tests; and motivational strategies. For example, in an exercise physiology experiment, it would be necessary to explain the treadmill protocol used, including speed and duration of each stage, criteria for determining whether maximal oxygen uptake was achieved, and the like. The name and model number of the treadmill, gas analysis equipment or metabolic cart, and electrocardiograph are often given as well. If a practice trial was given to subjects running on the treadmill, this too should be noted.

In motor learning experiments involving use of novel tasks, such as juggling or balancing, the amount of practice should be controlled. If a number of different tests are administered, the sequence of tests should be explained, because fatigue, emotional changes, and learning from performing one task may affect performance on ensuing tests.

## Data or Statistical Analysis

Each statistical procedure used to analyze data is stated and the level of significance used. This section is usually brief. Here is an example: "Mean and standard deviation were calculated for each variable. A one-way analysis of variance (ANOVA) was used to compare the change in catching skill across the three groups. The .05 level of significance was used in all statistical analyses." Commonly used statistical procedures are not usually referenced, but unusual ones are to verify their use. The statistical software to be used should also be identified.

 **Summary**

The research proposal is a plan for research. It is divided into chapters that coincide with the steps in the scientific method. The introduction provides a justification for the study.

The problem chapter is a summary of the purpose, hypothesis, delimitations, limitations, definition of terms, and significance of the study. The review of literature is an analysis or critique of the pertinent published work, and the methods chapter details how the study will be conducted.

 ## Learning Activities

1. Have you accomplished the objectives stated at the beginning of the chapter? Reread the concepts you are uncertain about.
2. Visit your university library and examine a copy of a thesis written by a student in your discipline. Examine the contents of each chapter, the tense used within each chapter, format, and so on.
3. Attend a thesis colloquium presented by a graduate student in your discipline.
4. Discuss the values of writing a thesis with someone who has recently written one in your discipline.

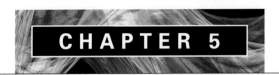

# CHAPTER 5

# Completing the Research Paper: Results, Discussion, Conclusion, and References

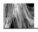

## KEY CONCEPTS

- Chapter 5: Results
- Chapter 6: Discussion
- Chapter 7: Summary and Conclusion
- References
- Appendix

## AFTER READING THIS CHAPTER YOU SHOULD BE ABLE TO:

- Explain how the results chapter is written.
- Explain how the discussion chapter is written.
- Write the references for a paper using an accepted format, such as American Psychological Association (APA).

The research proposal, being a plan for research, ends with the methods chapter. Once data have been collected and analyzed, the remainder of the research paper is written. This includes the results, discussion, conclusion, references, and appendix.

## CHAPTER 5: RESULTS

The results chapter is a brief statement of meaningful findings without an explanation. A logical place to begin is to state whether the hypothesis being tested was accepted or rejected. This is based on the results of an appropriate statistical procedure. Tables and figures (graphs) often supplement the narrative in this chapter. Numeric details are best depicted in tables and figures because they greatly simplify comprehension of large amounts of data. Attempting to read a mass of numbers in paragraph form is exceedingly difficult. Therefore, the text is best limited to identifying statistically significant

*Numeric details are best depicted in tables and figures, as they greatly simplify large amounts of data.*

findings and stating associated information, such as significance level. These details regarding statistics will make more sense after you have read the section in this text on statistics.

The results chapter should be brief because while the key findings are given, they are not interpreted. The latter is done in the discussion chapter.

## Tables

Tables are an effective means of presenting the results of a study because it is far easier to extract key information from a table than from text, particularly if many data are being summarized. An example of a table appears in Table 5-1. The guidelines of the American Psychological Association (APA) (2001) for the construction of tables will assist you in producing attractive and effective tables. These guidelines are as follows:

1. Place the title above the table.
2. Number tables consecutively.
3. Place a table in the text on the page immediately following where it is first mentioned. This format usually suffices for writing a thesis. However, when submitting a manuscript for publication, tables and figures are placed after the references.
4. Use horizontal lines to separate column headings from the body of the table, and place one at the bottom of the table.
5. Indicate units of measure for each variable in parentheses in the column head. Do not repeat the units of measure on each line.
6. Do not use vertical lines.
7. Report the sample sizes of each group in parentheses using $n$ to denote the sample size of each group. $N$ refers to the sample size for the entire study.

## CHAPTER 6: DISCUSSION

The discussion chapter is an explanation and interpretation of the results. It usually comprises the following topics, which may or may not be formatted as center or side

| TABLE 5-1. Physical Characteristics of Subjects ($N$ = 25) | | | |
| --- | --- | --- | --- |
| *Variable* | *Mean* | *SD* | *Range* |
| Age (yr) | 19.8 | 2.6 | 18.3–24.7 |
| Height (cm) | 164.5 | 7.8 | 156.5–174.0 |
| Weight (kg) | 62.2 | 5.1 | 54.0–66.7 |

headings: the main findings, comparison with the results of other studies, how the results relate to theory, limitations of the study, implications, and recommendations. Each of these are now explained.

The main findings regarding the hypotheses are typically restated in the beginning of the discussion. This information sets the stage for achieving the major purposes of the chapter, that is, to compare the results of the study with those of other studies, to relate the findings to theory, etc.

The results are compared with those of other studies, and relevant findings that may agree and disagree are cited. Then an analysis of the studies should be made to determine why the results agree or disagree. For example, some years ago several studies reported that elementary school-age children were unable to improve their maximum oxygen uptake with training. In writing the discussion for a paper with such a finding, the author would cite other studies with similar results and identify common factors in these studies, such as intensity, frequency, and duration of training. Similarly, studies that observed significant gains in maximum oxygen uptake are analyzed. Were subjects possibly more mature? Was maturity assessed in any of these studies? Was there a greater volume or intensity of training than in the studies not showing significant change? Analyzing differences in studies requires attention to detail and the ability to generalize. One should approach such analysis like a detective searching for clues.

In some cases, differences in results across studies have little to do with the experimental treatment used in the study but instead reflect differences in methods of measurement. For example, researchers who study the effects of various levels of physical activity on incidence of disease, body fatness, or cholesterol level commonly use a method that requires subjects to daily record the type and amount of physical activity. This method is limited by the memory and cooperation of the subject. A second technique uses the wearing of a motion sensor device that counts vertical or horizontal movements during the day. The latter probably is a more accurate way to quantify physical activity. Researchers who use the recall method may tend to find less impressive associations with cholesterol, cardiovascular disease, or fatness than those using a motion sensing device. Consequently, it is important to thoroughly analyze studies reporting different results, because an explanation should be offered as to why the differences may have occurred.

A second component of the discussion is **relating the results** to theory and accepted principles dealing with the topic. For example, if a study assessed personality traits of recreation administrators, these traits might logically be related to what is known in the psychological and sociological literature about personality development. Theory X might suggest that people who prefer working with others in an open, relatively unstructured environment rather than a more structured one have a common set of psychological traits. The researcher can compare the traits identified with those proposed by the theory to see how well the theory fits the subjects. Using another example, a researcher finds that abdominal girth is significantly related to mortality rate. The task confronted by the researcher is to attempt to identify some logical cause of the relationship. Perhaps it blends well with a theory that excessive body fat in this region results in more fat being carried in the blood to the liver, which increases cholesterol production from this added source of energy. In both cases, the researcher attempts to logically relate the results to theory. No means of proving the conjecture is available, because the results of the study offer only indirect support.

The attempt to explain a result logically when lacking definitive evidence is called **speculation.** It demands a good knowledge in one's general discipline and is an excellent brain teaser for most students, since it is a more complex intellectual task than writing most of the structured components of the research paper. It is important in reading articles to be able to distinguish between speculation and explanations directly supported by the results. Writers often use terms such as *may, possibly, could,* and *suggest* to indicate when they are speculating.

*Speculation is using logic to provide a plausible explanation for a result when definitive evidence is lacking.*

The danger in failing to recognize a statement that is speculation is that a reader may assume that it is actually a fact or finding. Readers of research need to make a clear distinction between fact and speculation.

A third component in the discussion is the **limitations of the study**. These extraneous or contaminating variables are ones that may not have been adequately controlled and may have had some effect on the outcome of a study. In the research proposal, these are covered in the problem chapter as well as the discussion. The reader is referred to that chapter for clarification if necessary. Common limitations are small number of subjects, use of a measuring instrument or method that is less than ideal, and short duration of a study. Sometimes limitations are not addressed directly, and the reader must inspect the study for possible flaws.

A fourth component in the discussion is implications. **Implications** refer to the possible application of the results. If a recreator finds in a study that injury rate of children on certain playground apparatus is significantly higher than on others, an implied application may be to alert school and recreation professionals about the finding so that they may modify the apparatus, warn children, or remove it from playgrounds. The application of research to the real world is the reason why most research is conducted, but great caution is needed to prevent it from being applied without justification. Typically, researchers must resist the tendency to apply the results of a single study to many other cases, because the situations may be markedly different. What happened in one environment with one group of people may not hold true for many other conditions. In the example of the playground study, perhaps the pieces of apparatus found to be dangerous were dangerous only because of the age of the children studied. Swinging ropes may tend to be more dangerous for very young children, whose upper body strength is limited or to heavier children with low strength related to body weight, or to playgrounds with inadequate depth of sand below the equipment, for example. Many factors may make the application specific, and if these factors do not exist, the generalization outside the study may be unjustified.

All those conducting research must learn to be very cautious in generalizing the results of their studies to other groups. It is human nature, perhaps, to want to generalize one's results to other people, but one study alone rarely is sound enough logic to extend the findings to other people. Before research results can be generalized, results must be replicated in other studies, and the results across the many studies must consistently demonstrate similar results. Consequently, the results of one study are valid only for the subjects who participated in the study.

 If dietitians observed in a study that people taking supplemental niacin reduced their LDL cholesterol by 10%, is it logical that everyone would experience the same effect? Should all people based on this evidence take a niacin supplement?

The issue of application of results of a study is known as **external validity**. It is covered in more depth in a later chapter. However, it is an important point, so here is a second example to consider. If a study found that visualization significantly aided the play of professional tennis players, is it justified to have complete novices use the technique? The results of a study pertain only to the subjects of the one study, and the only logical application is to others with as many similarities as possible to the subjects and conditions inherent in the original experiment, that is, other professional tennis players.

Lastly, recommendations are made in the discussion. This may be helpful to others who read the paper and may plan to carry out a study on the topic. Making recommendations also acknowledges that some insights have been developed about the research process in general as well as the state of knowledge on the topic. Therefore, it is worthwhile to include recommendations in a research paper or thesis. Typical recommendations include studying subjects with other traits (e.g., age, sex, fitness level, maturity level), considering alternative methods of measurement or experimental design, and citing the need for long-term or longitudinal study. In short, anything that may be helpful to other researchers is appropriate.

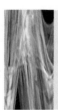 The purpose of the discussion chapter is to explain and interpret the findings of the study. Topics include restating the main findings, comparing results of the study with those of other studies, relating the results to theory, and explaining limitations, implications, and recommendations.

## CHAPTER 7: SUMMARY AND CONCLUSIONS

In journal articles, the summary and conclusions are given at the end of the discussion section. In the thesis, they typically are located in a short separate chapter. The summary is an overview of the need for the study, the statement of the problem, methods, and results. The conclusions are statements that are justified from the results. That is, they are not speculative comments. Researchers often use the words *justified* or *warranted* in their statement of the conclusions to make it obvious that they are data based and statistically tested, not speculations. One conclusion is usually written for each hypothesis tested. Below is a typical manner of stating a conclusion.

"The following conclusion is warranted from the results of this study: The use of visualization before competition enhances playing performance in professional tennis players." Note that no attempt is made to extend the findings to all levels of tennis players. Other studies would be needed to determine whether the same effect occurred in other tennis players.

## REFERENCES

References are sources actually cited or used in the preparation of a research paper. A bibliography cites literature for additional reading and should not be confused with the listing of references. Make sure that references cited in the text also appear in the list of references provided at the end of the paper. Listing references at the end of paper but not actually citing them within the body of the paper and vice versa is a common error, so it is wise to double-check.

### Reference Styles

A number of reference styles are seen in research publications. Every journal seems to have its own format. However, three basic styles of citation exist. The *name and year,* or *author–date,* style (e.g., Johnson and Kumquat, 2006) is the easiest to use because no numbering is required. If references are added or deleted as the paper is being prepared or revised, references do not have to be renumbered in the text. The disadvantage is that reading is made more laborious because a series of names and dates, which may be of little interest to many readers, must be gleaned. When references are cited several times in a paper, as is common in the introduction and discussion, the list of names can become lengthy and probably does slow the reader. To combat this problem, the phrase **et al.,** meaning *and others,* may be used in the text after the initial citation in which all of the authors' names are listed. For example, Johnson, Smith, and Kumquat (2006) is listed the first time the work is cited, but thereafter Johnson et al. (2006) is used.

The *alphabet–number* system numbers all references and lists them alphabetically. Only the number is given in the text, which aids reading and reduces the printing cost. For example, "The relationship of health knowledge and behavior is significant but explains only a small part of the variance in health behavior (11)." However, unless readers refer to the list of references, they are not informed of the date of the work, which sometimes is relevant.

The *order of citation* system is the third common style of listing references. Each citation is listed according to the sequence cited in the paper. Consequently, authors' names are not listed alphabetically. This system has the same advantages and disadvantages as the alphabet–number system, but many people like the names of authors appearing alphabetically.

## Components in the List of References

In addition to considering which reference citation style to use in the preparation of a thesis or research paper, you must also consider the format to use in listing the names of the authors, title of article, journal title, volume, and so on. Many styles or formats can be seen in journals, but APA style (5th edition, 2001) is described here because of its wide use in allied health professional journals and hence preference by many professors in these disciplines.

**Periodicals**  Example: McCall, L. T., & Washington, S. D. (1990). Differences in recreational patterns of the elderly living in retirement centers and privately. *Leisure Sciences,* 9, 167–171.

***Names***  The authors' names are given, with last name first followed by the initials. All authors are listed. Use an ampersand (&) before the name of the last author when there is more than one author.

***Date***  Give the date of publication in parentheses following the last author's name, and close with a period.

***Title of Article***  Give the title of the article, capitalizing only the first letter of the first word except for proper nouns and the first letter following a colon. Do not use quotation marks or underline or italicize the title of the article. Close with a period.

***Title of Journal***  State the full title of the journal and italicize it. Capitalize the first letter of key words. Italicize only the volume number, and do not include the word Vol. Give inclusive page numbers and end with a period. Use commas before and after the volume number.

**Books**  Example: Day, R. A. (1983). *How to write and publish a scientific paper.* Philadelphia: ISI Press.

***Author***  Use the same guidelines for periodicals. If the book is edited, place "Ed." or "Eds." in parentheses after the name of the last editor.

***Date***  Use the same guidelines for periodicals.

***Title of Book***  Capitalize only the first letter of the first word except for proper nouns and the first word after a colon. Italicize the title. Close with a period.

***Place of Publication***  Give the city and the state if the former is not well known.

***Publisher***  State the full name of the publisher, but omit details such as Inc., Co., and Company. Close with a period.

See the most recent *Publication Manual of the American Psychological Association* for more details on references.

## Location of the Citation in the Text

Place the citation at the point in the text to which it relates. This may be at the end of a sentence if only one point is made, but often the citation should be placed at a specific point in a sentence. For example: "Smaller values were reported in several investigations (Carson & Newman, 1989; Wellman & Denzi, 1991), but these values may reflect a lower baseline level (Beckman & Irish, 1992)." Here, the first two citations substantiate an observation, whereas the third refers to an explanation of the observation. Had all three citations been grouped together at the end of the sentence, one wouldn't know which references support each point. To avoid confusion, keep the citation close to the action. Also, when citing several studies within parentheses, sequence them alphabetically using the first author's last name.

## Accuracy

The accuracy of references, or more specifically the inaccuracy, has been highlighted in several publications. Among these was an analysis of 973 references in the 1988 and 1989 volumes of the *Research Quarterly for Exercise and Sport*. Some 47%, or 457, of the references contained at least one error. In all, 171 errors were found in the references. About 16% of errors were in titles and 13% were initials of authors (Stull, Christina, & Quinn, 1991). Similar analyses of other publications indicate error rates of 28% for the *American Journal of Epidemiology* and the *American Journal of Public Health*

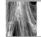 *Although checking the accuracy of references is a tedious task, it is the responsibility of all writers and researchers.*

(Eichorn & Yankauer, 1987) and 50% for the *Journal of the American Medical Association* (Goodrich & Roland, 1977), all prestigious publications.

The problem is obviously widespread, which should not condone the occurrence of errors but rather make all researchers, students and professors alike, take greater care in seeing that reference information is accurate. As suggested by one journal editor, researchers must check references against the original source rather than secondary sources and check for typographical errors (Yankauer, 1991). As explained in Chapter 3, primary rather than secondary references should be used to minimize transferring of information biased by opinion and possible misinterpretation, and now we can add a third reason: to ensure accuracy of references. Although checking the accuracy of references is hardly enjoyable, it is a responsibility of all writers and researchers. Failure to be accurate here may well suggest lack of accuracy in other facets of a paper or thesis.

## APPENDIX

An appendix is a supplementary item sometimes included in a proposal or paper for additional information, which may be helpful to some readers but not necessary to understand the paper. Items may include informed consent forms, correspondence, data collection forms, additional tables or figures, questionnaires or surveys used, and details of a measuring system. If one or more of these is included, each is listed as a separate appendix preceded by a page with its title, such as Appendix A, Informed Consent Form; Appendix B, Letter of Invitation to Parents.

## Summary

The results, discussion, and conclusion are not written until the research proposal has been approved and data collected and analyzed. The chapter on results states the basic findings and is typically accompanied by tables and possibly figures. The discussion is a comparison of the results of the current study with those of other findings and an integration of this new information with established theory and practice. The conclusion briefly states the major finding or findings of the study.

References may be listed within the text and at the end of the paper in several ways. An advantage of the author–date style is the ease in adding or deleting references. Far too commonly, errors appear in the references, demonstrating that care must be taken in accurately citing information from the primary rather than a secondary reference.

## Learning Activities

1. Have you accomplished the objectives stated at the beginning of the chapter? If not, reread the concepts you are uncertain about.
2. Examine a master's thesis or doctoral dissertation written by someone in your academic discipline. Note the format and content of the chapters on results, discussion, summary, and conclusion.
3. Examine a journal article in your discipline and note the format, length, and content of the results and discussion sections.
4. Attend a thesis colloquium defense of a graduate student in your department.

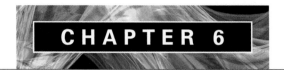

# CHAPTER 6

# Research Writing

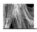

## KEY CONCEPTS

- Getting started
- Collating reference material and writing
- Tips for good writing
- Common faults in writing

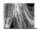

## AFTER READING THIS CHAPTER YOU SHOULD BE ABLE TO:

- Explain why several separate proofs of a paper should be made before submission.
- Define plagiarism and explain how to make decisions when some possibility for plagiarism exists.
- Explain why research writing should be brief and exact, and why clichés, jargon, and redundancy should be minimized.
- Properly use symbols, abbreviations, and numbers.
- Effectively use an accepted style guide.

Probably the most difficult part of writing for most people is simply **getting started**. Writer's block occurs even in veteran writers, so perhaps more than experience is needed to help get going. Let us share some observations based on our collective experiences with students as well as our own writing in hopes that we can facilitate not only getting started but getting the job done with quality and efficiency.

## GETTING STARTED

### Select a Topic

Select a topic that is of great interest to you. You will be spending considerable time in preparing it, so you may as well enjoy as much of it as possible. Pick a topic that relates to your field of study. It could be something dealing with teaching, such as curriculum, methods, or media; it could relate to some issue of healthcare, such as nutritional status in the elderly, osteoporosis, cardiovascular disease, or diabetes; it could deal with nutritional habits or the types of recreational activities people pursue. In short, pick something that will interest you and possibly even offer some professional benefit, such as information that may be used in your job. Helpful sources of ideas for research topics include classes, professors, journals, textbooks, presentations at professional meetings, and work experience.

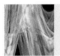 Select a topic that you are interested in; one that you will find stimulating to learn more about.

## Read About the Topic in a General Way

Do some general reading on the topic you have chosen. You will have ample time later to do some highly specific reading. A good place to start may be a recently published text from a course that you really enjoyed. What particular chapters interest you? Skim through one or two chapters, and within each specifically search for topics with controversy. Authors of textbooks often discuss controversial points. These topics obviously should be further researched, and it is possible that your proposal could be designed accordingly. Review articles are written by experts with knowledge and experience in research on a topic. Avail yourself of the writer's expertise, since it is free quality advice. Also, remember that any journal article typically contains the justification for the study in the introduction, whereas recommendations to other researchers are made in the discussion section. Both sections might identify rationales for a proposal.

Studies often necessitate replication to determine whether similar results are observed in subjects with other traits. This implies that a study in a journal could be modified by using different subjects or the same type of subjects but eliminating a limitation to the study you read. For example, a study may not have found significant results because the duration of the treatment or intervention was too short. Your proposal could thus repeat the study but run longer. This may be a legitimate rationale for doing a study. Replication is an excellent means of initiating oneself to research because a detailed plan from other studies is available from the onset.

## Consider the Feasibility of the Study

If your intention is to write a proposal for a class but not actually conduct the study and write a master's thesis, you do not have to be concerned with having access to sophisticated laboratory equipment or being able to obtain subjects with specific traits. One may assume that the necessary equipment and subjects are available to you. On the other hand, if you are planning on actually doing a thesis, you must be careful to plan a study that can reasonably be done given the limitations of time and the environment you are in. Does the institution where you are studying have the laboratory equipment you need? How accessible will the facility be for your needs? Will you need the assistance of trained personnel to collect data? If so, will you have to pay them out of your own pocket?

Can the study be conducted in a reasonable time to coincide with your graduation plans? All of these questions and others have to be addressed before you launch into a study. The professor teaching your research methods class is likely to be invaluable in answering some of the questions, and you may need to consult other faculty as well.

## Simplify the Study

Limit the complexity of the study. As discussed in Chapters 4 and 5, students often wish to take on far more than is reasonable. It is better to limit the study to one or two variables and to conduct the study well rather than to attempt to do too much, which may reduce the quality of the work as well as your level of satisfaction.

## Discuss Your Plans

Another useful way to help in getting started is to discuss your initial plans with the professor teaching the research methods class or some other professor with expertise in the topic of interest. Ask this person to respond to your initial plans for a proposal. He or she may even help you fine-tune the topic or develop it so that it is based on the latest research findings. Another possibility is that this professor has conducted research on the topic and has several useful suggestions concerning how your proposal might blend in with some of his or her work. Faculty in our department are accustomed to students in our research methods class knocking on their door to discuss plans for a proposal.

## Put It on Paper

Get something down on paper as soon as possible after having the research proposal explained in your research methods class. The longer you wait, the more difficult starting becomes, because more material is covered in class, a test may be forthcoming, and so on. We require the students in our research methods class to write a proposal, which is very common. Over many years we have learned that it is extremely helpful to have students submit a draft of the first several chapters early in the semester. An early start helps students find the rest of the semester's work more relevant, because many aspects of it are related to their own proposal. Also, receiving feedback early allows them to determine what they need to revise for the final copy to be acceptable. This submit–revise–resubmit cycle is exactly how research journals operate. So the student goes through the same procedures as faculty who publish.

## COLLATING REFERENCE MATERIAL AND WRITING

Writing ability is critical in the research process simply because the end product of most research is the written form. Similarly, for the student, the grade for writing a proposal is one important end product. One's ideas may be organized, logical, and meaningful, but unless the information is effectively expressed, the best ideas, plans, and logic may be lost along with the prospect of a reasonable grade or acceptance of an article for publication.

The remainder of this chapter is aimed at helping you to write effectively. Effective writing tends to give your work a positive "halo effect." It cannot replace good logic, organization, and content, but it certainly does not hurt.

## TIPS FOR GOOD WRITING

### Code and Organize Your References

Students typically photocopy a number of articles to use in writing a paper. Once the writer is sitting at the computer, the problem of actually knowing what to say is confronted. Two steps may be helpful in getting past this block. On the title page of each article copied, indicate which chapter or chapters in the proposal or thesis each article pertains to. For example, perhaps it relates to the introduction, methods, or discussion. Note this on each article so that it can easily be identified. Then collate the articles according to the section or chapter of the paper they pertain to.

### Develop an Outline

A good deal of outlining has already been done within the framework of each chapter of the proposal, but more extensive outlining is needed within certain sections or chapters, such as the introduction, review of literature, and discussion. To do this, one must begin reading the sections of the articles that apply. For example, if developing an outline for the introduction, read and highlight these articles and develop the outline as you go along, or you might try an initial outline something like this:

- What is known?
  Describe this state of knowledge and cite pertinent references.
- What is not known?
  Identify the shortcomings in the research citing related references.
- What is controversial?
  Mixed or antagonist findings are common in research. Describe the inconsistencies and cite references.
- What are limitations and recommendations of other studies?
  Point out the major flaws of other research as well as the suggestions of other authors.

These steps may greatly help get you started. However, a special tip may be useful for the introduction, review of literature, and discussion. The difficulty here is trying to collate and compare a number of studies. A useful technique is to make a table that includes the key elements needed (Table 6-1). The tabling method allows organizing and viewing the key elements of a number of studies simultaneously. It facilitates analysis of studies because they can be grouped according to findings, such as those reporting

| TABLE 6-1. Table Method of Summarizing Literature | | | | | |
|---|---|---|---|---|---|
| *Authors* | *Year* | *Subjects* | *Design* | *Results* | *Limitations* |
| Smith & Howard | 1988 | 110 children, K–3rd grade | PE curriculum: fitness vs traditional (games, skill, some fitness) | Fitness significantly greater than traditional on 3 of 5 fitness tests but no differences on social variables | Three teachers Study only 6 weeks long |

significant effects and those not reporting significant effects; characteristics of subjects; and limitations. Tables are sometimes used in review articles for the same reason: They can be used to help write a section of a paper to facilitate interpretation.

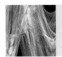 Read the introduction of a journal article in your field. Examine the logic used to justify the need for the study.

## Use a Dictionary

There is no excuse for misspelled words. Use the spell check on the software you are using.

## Use a Thesaurus

A thesaurus provides a list of synonyms. Most of us, if we were to examine the number of times we use some words, would be astounded at the frequency of use. Writing the introduction, review of literature, and discussion is particularly likely to cause the overuse of certain words, such as *studied, investigated, found,* and *concluded.* The software for most word processors contains a thesaurus, so when you are looking for a "new" word, a listing is made available on the screen. Use it.

Although a thesaurus is helpful to select alternative words, it should not be used to search for long, infrequently used, and not commonly understood words. This does not add to the quality or comprehensibility of a paper; rather it does just the opposite and should be avoided.

## Review the Paper Several Times

Some students may review or proof their papers only once before submitting them. One review is insufficient simply because there is too much to attend to. If striving for quality work, separate reviews, each with a single purpose, are helpful. First, review the paper for content, since this is the most important aspect of any paper. After making revisions, review just for grammar and repetitiveness of words. Then, review purely to make sure all necessary components have been included. Can you imagine the shock of a student when a paper is returned and the grade suffered because

 ***Review your paper several times before submitting it.***

a major section was omitted? This happens when one is disorganized and rushing to complete a paper in the last several days before a due date.

## Understand and Avoid Plagiarism at All Costs

Plagiarism is defined in *Merriam Webster's Collegiate Dictionary,* tenth edition, (1993) as "To steal and pass off (the ideas or words of another) as one's own." Note that the ideas and thoughts of others are included in the definition, so it is not merely limited to just their words. If the exact words are used, it is necessary to cite the reference and place the words in quotation marks (for short quotations) or to indent and single-space the words that are quoted (for quotations longer than 50 words). Both techniques vis-

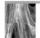 ***Plagiarism includes the words as well as the ideas of others.***

ually highlight the fact that the words and thoughts are not your own.

 ***When in doubt about citing a reference, cite it.***

A valid question about plagiarism arises when one considers whether or not nearly all information in a research paper is based on the thoughts and ideas of others and therefore should be referenced. An effective rule of thumb here is that if the idea or thought is known to you from past knowledge or experience or it is considered general knowledge, it does not need to be cited. This leaves much to the writer's sense of ethics, which usually suffices if the spirit behind the purpose of plagiarism is understood. However, realize that if others, such as the professor grading the paper or journal reviewer, disagree with you, you will be held accountable. In some cases, the penalty may be as severe as receiving a failing grade for a paper or even being dismissed from an institution.

Academicians take plagiarism extremely seriously. A student writing a paper has two options when confronted with the issue of referencing information: discuss it with your professor, if time permits, or simply reference the source. The worst that will happen if you make this decision is that you may have more references than perhaps needed. However, this is not usually a concern unless it becomes excessive. *So when in doubt, cite the reference.*

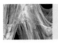 Cite the source when using the words or *ideas* of another person.

Most students are probably well aware of Internet sites that provide papers and essays on every topic imaginable. A few students might be tempted to use such Internet sources, but the flip side is that the Internet also makes it easier to catch them. For example, the search engine Google allows checking portions of a paper suspected of being taken from an Internet source to identify matches with actual published work.

## COMMON FAULTS IN WRITING

Writing is an art form with numerous rules, most of which we know intuitively from our daily reading and formal education. Although it is beyond the scope of this book to review the many rules of grammar and composition, we would like to share with you some of the most common mistakes in writing. If you are able to avoid most of these, your papers in graduate school will be much better.

### Verbose and Pedantic Style

**Verbosity** refers to being overly wordy, that is, beating around the bush. Many of us remember writing themes and papers that met a length requirement. This is commonly done to make sure that all students do some minimum of work that is believed to be conducive to achieving a learning objective. Although it is undoubtedly of some value, it may not be optimal in trying to produce the best quality of work, since it encourages padding and quantity, often at the expense of quality. Writing in research, however, emphasizes brevity and clarity. This saves time for readers and, by saving space, allows for publication of more studies in a given journal. Most research publications limit the length of submitted manuscripts to about 25 pages, including references, tables, and figures. In addition, the number of references is limited in some publications. Therefore, researchers tend to write succinctly rather than in a circuitous fashion. With practice, the ability to be brief and to the point is improved.

Some examples of wordiness appear in Table 6-2. Occasional use of the longer versions is not a major problem, but if your writing becomes saturated with extra words, at some point it begins to slow the reader unnecessarily.

**Pedantic** writing occurs when writers strive to show off their intellect by using uncommon words. One could say, "Deport to an environment conducive to academic endeavor," which more simply could be stated as "Study in a quiet place." Similarly, one could say, "Assume the supine position in a comforting manner for a period following

| TABLE 6-2. Examples of Wordiness | |
|---|---|
| *Wordy* | *Alternative* |
| Long period of time | Long time or long period |
| Month of June | June |
| At a rapid rate of speed | Fast |
| Decreased number of | Fewer |
| In close proximity to | Near |

neuromuscular activity" or "Take a rest after exercise." The object of writing in research is to communicate. The examples provided here are more a puzzle than an aid.

Do not confuse the use of scientific terminology with being pedantic. Terminology exists to give exact meaning to words. This enhances communication. The phrase "The respiratory exchange ratio exceeded 1.05 for all subjects" may appear to some as being pedantic, but to those trained in exercise physiology the terms are well known, easily understood, and specific.

 *Do not confuse the use of scientific terminology with being pedantic. Terminology of all disciplines is used to give exact meaning to words.*

Attempting to say it much differently would likely require more words, which may not be as well understood. For these reasons, all disciplines have their jargon.

## Clichés

Clichés are overused figures of speech that are best deleted. They do not enhance meaning but do add length to one's writing. Some common clichés are shown in Table 6-3.

## Subject–Verb Agreement

A sentence in which a singular subject is followed by a phrase in which the object is plural often tends to cause subject–verb disagreement. For example:

*Proper intake of essential nutrients (is, are) is vital to good health.*
**Answer:** "is" agrees with the subject, *intake.*
*Control of all variables in a study (is, are) important.*
**Answer:** "is" agrees with the subject, *control.*
*Each participant recorded (his or her, their) intake of all food and drink consumed for two weekdays and one day of a weekend.*
**Answer:** "his or her" agrees with the subject, *participant.*

| TABLE 6-3. Common Clichés | |
|---|---|
| *Cliché* | *Preferred* |
| First of all | First |
| A considerable amount of | Much |
| Last but not least | Last |
| At this particular time | Now |
| Accounted for by the fact | Because |
| It is suggested that | Possibly |

## Parallelism

Phrases in a sentence should use the same grammatical form. Here are several examples:

*The following were obtained from the subjects: medical history, height, and weight, and then we measured their blood pressure.*
**Corrected:** The following were obtained from the subjects: medical history, height, weight, and blood pressure.
*When teaching young children, wear a smile, be organized, have supplies ready, and if an emergency occurs you should have previously developed a plan.*
**Corrected:** When teaching young children, wear a smile, be organized, and have supplies and an emergency plan ready.

## Misused Commas

Commas should clarify meaning, but if improperly used they can change the meaning of a sentence. Examine these illustrations:

*The student, thinks the teacher, is a fool.*
**Meaning:** The student is thought to be a fool by the teacher.
*The student thinks the teacher is a fool.*
**Meaning:** The teacher is thought to be the fool.

The meanings are entirely changed by the insertion or absence of commas.

## Vogue Words

Vogue words enjoy short-term popularity. If they remain in common usage, they become clichés. Simplify communication by using simpler words. Some past examples of vogue words are *exacerbate, ameliorate, interface, expertise, via, vis-à-vis*.

## Redundancy

Repetitiveness adds length without meaning because both words mean the same. Here are some common examples: *basic essentials, refer back, viable alternative, authentic replica*.

## Jargon

Jargon is technical terminology often mixed with obscure long words. A few examples are borrowed from Day (1983). See if you can understand what is meant by each.

*It has been posited that a high degree of curiosity proved lethal to a feline.*
**Answer:** Curiosity killed the cat.

*From time immemorial, it has been known that the ingestion of an "apple" (i.e., the pome fruit of any tree of the genus Malus, said fruit being usually round in shape and red, yellow, or greenish in color) on a diurnal basis will with absolute certainty keep a primary member of the health care establishment absent from one's local environment.*

**Answer:** An apple a day keeps the doctor away.

*A sedimentary conglomerate in motion down a proclivity gains no addition of mossy material.*

**Answer:** A rolling stone gathers no moss.

## Symbols

Symbols are used in research to denote certain statistics and mathematical functions. Their main value is saving space on the printed page. Some of the rules for using symbols, which are not widely known, are described here.

1. Do not capitalize the letters unless the unit is derived from a person's name or you are using L for liter, which is done to avoid confusing it with the number 1.
2. Do not use a period after the letter and do not add an s to make it plural. There are exceptions to the s rule, however.
3. Leave a space between the symbol and number.

Examples of appropriate use of symbols:

> Cholesterol = 200 mg/dL
> Body weight = 82 kg

## Misuse of Words

Day (1983) describes several words commonly misused by writers. Notice how the meaning is altered in each example.

**Only** The word *only* can be positioned in several places in the following sentence. However, note the change in meaning depending on the location.

> I hit him in the eye only yesterday.
> I hit him in the only eye yesterday.
> I only hit him in the eye yesterday.

**It** If the antecedent (i.e., the word or thought being referred to) is not clear, the meaning can be changed. "Free information about venereal disease. To get *it*, call 555-7000." Problems with confusing antecedents commonly occur when a sentence refers to something in a previous sentence but two or more words could be the item being referred to. To avoid the problem, restate the word to which *it* refers: "Free information about venereal disease. To obtain the information, call 555-7000."

## Abbreviations

Abbreviations, as with symbols, are used to save space in writing, which in turn may facilitate reading. Writing the name of the professional organization, the American Alliance of Health, Physical Education, Recreation, and Dance, rather than using the abbreviation AAHPERD, becomes tedious for both the writer and reader. However, overuse of abbreviations, particularly if they are not commonly used, can be aggravating. Sometimes experimental groups in studies are abbreviated. For example, imagine a study in which four groups are compared based on their preference of recreational activities. One group might be abbreviated VO for those selecting vigorous outdoor activities; a second group is termed MO for moderate outdoor activity; a third group is termed SI because of their preference for social interaction while they recreate; and a fourth group is labeled SS for sedentary activities done alone or as a single. Although the abbreviations are logical when initially defined, they are not standard and require the reader to deal with four new abbreviations as they read the article. It frustrates most readers to have to refer several times to the spot where the abbreviations are initially defined. Consequently, minimize the use of uncommon abbreviations.

Define the abbreviation the first time you use it and note its abbreviation in parentheses. This includes the abstract, since the information here should be self-explanatory. Do not use an abbreviation in a title, because it may create problems for indexing and abstracting services and for information retrieval systems. Use only standard abbreviations, such as those listed in the *Council of Biology Editors Style Manual* (1978) or those in Système Internationale (SI) units.

## Tense

Tense can be a tricky issue in writing a research proposal. Some portions of the research proposal are written in the future tense because the research is in the planning stage and is yet to be carried out. For example, the second chapter of the proposal deals with the purpose, hypothesis, limitations, and so on, all of which deal with the future. The chapter on methods is also written in the future tense because it describes the plan for a study yet to be conducted. The review of literature is written in the past tense because published works are described. This means that in writing a proposal, the future, present, and past tenses will all be used depending on the chapter and situation. In writing the results and discussion chapters or sections of a research paper or thesis, the past tense should be used.

## Active versus Passive Voice

Researchers have generally used the passive voice (third person, i.e., he, she, they) in writing rather than the active voice (first person, i.e., I, we), perhaps trying to be modest. Consequently, in articles we typically read "it was found" or "Smith and Johnson reported" rather than "I" or "we." It is not wrong to use the active voice, and some experts recommend doing so because it is more direct and precise and less verbose (Day, 1983).

Some journals even encourage authors to use the active voice. However, because the issue is somewhat new and inconsistent, it would be wise to check with your professor.

## Unemotional Tone

Write in a somewhat detached, unemotional manner. You may not win a Pulitzer Prize using this style, but it helps objectivity. Superlatives and qualifiers, such as *extremely, unusually, very, considerably,* and *marked,* are best deleted, since they are inexact. Use less emotional words and let numerical values be interpreted by the reader.

## Numbers

The guideline used by the American Psychological Association (APA) is to use words to express values below 10 and numbers for values 10 through 99, that is, five subjects, 15 subjects. Numerals are also used for values below 10 if included in a list of numbers, some of which are greater than 10, such as 3 women, 56 men, and 78 children.

Use numbers whenever they immediately precede a unit of measure, for example 3 km, or when they are used in a statistical or mathematical sense, such as fractions and ratios, such as F ratio = 3.17, 2.5 times larger, 3:2 ratio. Lastly, use numbers when referring to time, age, dates, points on a scale, and amounts of money: 3 months, 5 years old, 5 on a scale of 1 to 7, and $5.

## User-Friendly References on Writing

Several excellent books on effective writing are surprisingly brief. They are filled with useful tips that we never learned before or have forgotten. Day's book is masterfully done because it is simply written, is fairly short (188 pages), and covers each segment of the research paper as well as information on manuscript submission, the review and publishing process, preparation of conference reports, and so on. Another valuable reference on writing is Strunk and White's *The Elements of Style.* This 92-page classic covers elementary rules of usage, principles of composition, misused words and terms, and style. It is filled with many useful examples of errors we all commonly make and see. The third reference that every graduate student should know is the American Psychological Association's *Publication Manual.* It covers every aspect of writing a paper that one might ever wish to know, and it is logically organized. Its coverage includes items listed in the two previous books but also includes great detail on headings, margins, numbers, tables, figures, references, and typing instructions. It is difficult to imagine anything relevant to writing that is not covered in this book.

 **Summary**

Good research writing is an art. To be a good artist or writer, one must practice. Write so that your work can be quickly and easily understood. No one enjoys being confused and lost halfway through a sentence or paragraph. A helpful tip to remember when writing is the KISS principle: Keep it simple, Stupid! When in doubt, shorten the length of sentences and paragraphs.

 **Learning Activities**

1. Have you accomplished the objectives stated at the beginning of the chapter? If not, reread the concepts you are uncertain about.
2. Read a research article and assess it for clarity, grammar, verbosity, active or passive voice, emotional tone, and so on.

# PART III

# Statistics

7. Basic Statistical Concepts

8. Central Tendency, Variability, and the Normal Curve

9. Probability and Hypothesis Testing

10. Relationships and Predictions

11. Comparison of Mean Scores

12. Selected Nonparametric Tests

# CHAPTER 7

# Basic Statistical Concepts

## KEY CONCEPTS

- Measurement scales: nominal, ordinal, absolute, interval, and ratio
- Parametric and nonparametric statistics
- Descriptive and inferential use of statistics
- Selected sampling procedures
- Computational tips and notations

## AFTER READING THIS CHAPTER YOU SHOULD BE ABLE TO:

- Identify data by their level of measurement.
- Differentiate between parametric and nonparametric statistics.
- Distinguish between descriptive and inferential use of statistics.
- Describe what populations and samples are.
- Describe several commonly used random sampling procedures.
- Perform simple statistical operations by identifying standard computational notation.

Statistics as a mathematical discipline is the study of the summary, analysis, and evaluation of data and is a most vital tool for research. The primary function of statistics is to reduce a large amount of data to a useful numerical value that represents a particular trait about the data. As previously mentioned, research is not based on making unsubstantiated guesses, hunches, or speculations. Most research decisions are based on the presentation of hard facts generated through the use of appropriate statistical techniques. Professionals in any field must have at least an elementary knowledge of statistics so that they can make judgments about the correct use and interpretations of statistical procedures. This is an essential skill whether producing or consuming research.

It has been our experience that the word *statistics* conjures considerable fear and anxiety in some students. Perhaps this is because they associate statistics with higher-order mathematics. However, we hope to dispel these negative feelings. First, from a mathematics standpoint, the statistical procedures presented in this text involve nothing more complicated than arithmetic. The operations consist of addition, subtraction, multiplication, division, and determining squares and square roots. Performing calculations from an equation is much like following directions on a road map. If one knows what the signs and symbols are, that person will have no problem getting to the destination. Solving equations is a matter of performing calculations to get to the end result. Nevertheless, as straightforward as this is, a modern researcher would be very unlikely to perform statistical computations by hand. There are numerous statistical software packages (e.g., Minitab, SPSS, Excel, SAS) that tremendously expedite and simplify data reduction and analysis. It can be argued that once someone understands the tenets of a statistic, particularly those related to its function and meaning, hand calculations are of little value. However, some initial number manipulation may be warranted to reach that level of comprehension.

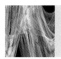 Most commonly used statistics do not require a background in mathematics.

Being a competent user of statistics doesn't mean that one must become a professional statistician. Most researchers are users of statistics, but are not mathematicians. They know what tool to select for the job, how to apply it, and how to interpret the results of its use. In everyday life, one can be an effective user of many tools without truly comprehending their underlying mechanics. How many pilots understand the elaborate engineering and mechanical operations of their aircraft? How many physicians understand the microelectronics of an electrocardiography machine? We all effectively operate and maintain sophisticated automobiles, but do we know how they work? One can effectively use statistics without understanding all of its intricacies.

Our philosophy should be apparent. Our emphasis is on presenting the basic theory, appropriate selection, application, and interpretation of statistical procedures commonly used in the allied health research. By reducing hand calculations and providing relevant examples of the use and interpretation of statistics, we hope to provide the basis for understanding common statistical procedures. Consequently, the reader should be more comfortable in reading professional literature and using it.

## MEASUREMENT SCALES

Consider what the number 23 means. For instance, the number 23 could be a famous ball player's uniform number or the rank of a student in a class of 500. The number 23 could depict the number of push-ups performed, the temperature in degrees Celsius, or the weight of an object in pounds. All of these representations of the number 23 typify a type of measurement that varies in terms of complexity. Scales of measurement allow us to know something about the intricacy of the numbers or data that are generated. It is important to know the scale of measurement because it directly affects our choice of the correct statistical procedure.

 It is important to know the scale of measurement because it in part determines selecting the correct statistic.

## Nominal Scale

Nominal (meaning *name*) scale measures are the most rudimentary, since they provide us only with information about a difference. Uniform number 15 is not the same as number 10; interstate highway 80 is different from route 29. These are examples of nominal values. Nominal scales are also associated with categorical data. Categories have to be defined so that they are mutually exclusive; an observation can belong in only one classification and not another. For instance, you could categorize athletic shoes as Nike, Adidas, or Reebok. The categories are mutually exclusive, since a shoe can't be both a Nike and an Adidas or Reebok. A number may be assigned to a given category, such as Nike = 1, for statistical analysis. A frequency count of observations in each category is made and used in a statistical analysis. If you walked through a fitness center and counted the varieties of shoes on people's feet, you might come up with something like Nike = 10, Adidas = 6, and Reebok = 4. These frequency counts may be used in a statistical analysis. Even though this measurement scale is basic, it is important because many types of data in the allied health professions meet only this level of precision.

## Ordinal Scale

Ordinal (meaning *order*) scale data demonstrate ranks, so they indicate difference and direction of difference. Thus, they provide more information than nominal data. Some-one who finishes second in a road race did better than someone who was third, and, of course, third place is better than fourth. What we don't know from rank data is the amount of difference between each, since there is no equality of units. For instance, the difference between second and third place may have been 0.5 seconds, and the difference between third and fourth is 30 seconds.

## Absolute Scale

When the number of events or observations is made to the whole unit, absolute scale measurement is the result. Examples are the number of campers using a state park on a weekend, the number of men participating in a stress management program, and the number of milligrams of sodium ingested each day. In any of these cases, it doesn't make sense to use decimals; there is no such thing as 10.2 campers. The frequency counts in our discussion of nominal level measurements are actually absolute scale: The assignment of a category is nominal, whereas the frequency count for the category is absolute.

Numerous research measurements are at this level of sophistication. Furthermore, absolute scale data may be analyzed statistically in ways that nominal and ordinal data can't. For instance, meaningful arithmetic averages may be computed for absolute level measurements and not for nominal and ordinal scales.

## Interval Scale

Interval (meaning *equal intervals*) scale data have all of the properties of ordinal measures plus equality of units. Therefore, we know that a temperature of 25°C is warmer than 20°C by 5° and a temperature of 5°C is 15° less than 20°C. Therefore, interval-level data inform us about difference, direction of difference, and amount of difference in equal units. Interval scales may also contain a zero point, which is called an **arbitrary zero**. Arbitrary zeros do not reflect the absence of the trait being measured. The following discussion helps to clarify this concept.

## Ratio Scale

Ratio (meaning numbers may be presented as ratios) scale measurement is the most complex because it has all of the elements of interval scale plus an absolute zero point. What is an absolute zero? It is not −273°C or at least not exactly. An absolute zero point on a scale represents the absence of the trait that the scale is measuring. Scales measuring variables such as weight, distance, and time all have meaningful absolute zero points. Zeros on interval scales are not absolute. For example, if it is 0°C, is there no temperature? There is, and it is quite cold. If someone can't do at least one pull-up, does that mean he or she has no upper body strength? Of course it doesn't.

Absolute zero points also allow us to make comparisons, such as 5 inches is half the distance of 10 inches and 60 seconds is three times as long as 20 seconds. Without an absolute zero or starting point, such comparisons are not valid. Does something that is 40°C have twice as much heat energy as something that is 20°C? The object is 20° warmer but not twice (100%) as warm. The reason is that the zero point on the Celsius scale is not an absolute zero. Since the true absolute zero point for temperature (i.e., absence of heat energy) is −273°C, 40°C = (273 + 40 = 313 degree points above absolute zero) and 20°C = (273 + 20 = 293 degree points above absolute zero). Therefore, 313/293 = 1.068; that is, 40°C is only 6.8% warmer than 20°C.

## PARAMETRIC AND NONPARAMETRIC STATISTICS

Statistical analyses can be classified as parametric or nonparametric types. Parametric statistics are used when the research data are interval or ratio scale and when the populations from which the observations were made are thought to be normally distributed. Interval and ratio data are considered measured or continuous. That implies that they can be measured with increasingly great precision. For example, distances can be measured to the closest inch, half-inch, quarter-inch, and so on, to a very small fraction. The level of precision is limited only by the sensitivity of the instrument being used.

Nonparametric statistics are used when data are nominal or ordinal level or when the populations from which the observations were made are thought not to be normally distributed. Sometimes these statistics are referred to as *distribution-free analyses*. We have mentioned that nominal and ordinal data are considered counted and ranked, respectively. They are also referred to as counted or discrete data because the observations are treated as whole values. For instance, when obtaining frequency counts for a divorced or not divorced classification, one can't have a count of 57.5 divorces because there is no such thing as half of a divorce. Also, absolute scale data, although technically discrete, are often analyzed using both parametric and nonparametric statistics.

Most data from laboratory based research are considered "hard data" because they are interval or ratio scale. They are "hard" in the sense that they are more objective and precise.

Parametric statistics are considered more powerful than their nonparametric counterparts because they are more likely to reject a false null hypothesis. (The null hypothesis is covered in more detail in Chapter 9.) However, when the criteria for the use of a parametric analysis can't be met, a nonparametric alternative must be used. Examples of statistics from both of these categories are given in later chapters. Finally, examples of measurement scales and their characteristics may be seen in Table 7-1.

## DESCRIPTIVE AND INFERENTIAL USE OF STATISTICS

Statistics may also be classified as descriptive or inferential, depending on their use. Descriptive use of statistics is used when measuring a trait or characteristic of a group without any intention to generalize that statistic beyond that group. The average 40-yard dash speed of a football team, the mean number of miles you drove your car per month this year, your grade point average, and the range of test scores on an exam are all examples of descriptive use of statistics.

**TABLE 7-1. Characteristics of Measurement Scales**

| Feature | Nominal | Ordinal | Absolute | Interval | Ratio |
|---|---|---|---|---|---|
| Difference | X | X | X | X | X |
| Direction of difference | | X | X | X | X |
| Equality of units | | | X | X | X |
| Continuous data | | | | X | X |
| Absolute zero | | | | | X |

Inferential use of statistics occurs when one makes generalizations or inferences from a smaller group to a larger group. What exactly does it mean to infer or generalize? An inference or a generalization is a type of prediction that is made by measuring a trait from a representative group and estimating what it would be in the larger group. The ability to infer is not so much based in the computation of the statistic but in the purpose for using it; that is, the researcher desires to make inferences. For inferences to be valid, it is critical that the subjects in the smaller group be good representatives of the larger group. An illustration should help.

Let's say that a health educator is interested in determining the cholesterol levels of the 10,000 students on a university campus so they can be compared with national norms. Does the researcher have to test all of the students to answer this question? No, thank goodness. This is because of the power to infer with statistics. The researcher obtains a random group of 100 subjects, for example, that make up a good model of the entire student body. (How this is done is discussed later.) She tests the subjects and determines their cholesterol levels. If the 100 subjects are representative of the entire student body, an inference may be made to estimate (usually with good accuracy) the typical cholesterol levels of all 10,000 students. This example shows that inferential statistics are one of the most valued tools of a researcher.

## SELECTED SAMPLING PROCEDURES

### Populations and Samples

In the previous example, we referred to large and small groups of subjects. These groups are more correctly called a population and a sample, respectively. A **population** is an all-inclusive group that is operationally defined by the researcher. These definitions may range from broad to specific descriptions. Based on the definition, membership in the population is mutually exclusive. That is, a subject is either in the population or not. Although we referred to the population as a large group, it may not be big at all. For instance, all university professors in a given discipline in the United States would define a fairly large population, but all university professors in the same discipline in the United States with annual incomes above $200,000 would probably be small. In short, a population's size is dictated by the researcher's definition of it. Also, it's easy to see by the definition whether one is included in the population. A trait or characteristic

*A population is an all-inclusive group. A sample is a subset of the population.*

of a population is known as a **parameter.** The Greek letter $\mu$ is the symbol representing a population parameter mean.

A **sample** is a representative subset of the population that contains the essential elements of that population. A trait or characteristic of a sample is known as a **statistic.** The letter M may be used to designate a sample mean. When researchers are interested in making inferences, they need a sample that is a good representation of the population. How does one obtain a good model sample? This can be done several ways.

## Random Samples

One of the principles of inferential statistics is that subjects are drawn from a population using a random selection technique. By definition, when random sampling is used, every constituent in the population has an equal probability of being selected for the sample. Random sampling is an impartial process that results in an unbiased sample of a population. An unbiased sample is one that is likely to be representative of the population, whereas a **biased sample** contains some type of systematic error and is not a good representation.

Random sampling can be accomplished many ways. One method is to use random numbers, which can be generated by computer or from statistical tables. If our cholesterol-testing health educator wanted to draw a random sample of 100 from the university population of 10,000, he first would require a list of all 10,000 students (perhaps use a registrar's list) and assign each a number from 1 to 10,000. Then he could use a computer to randomly select any 100 numbers from 1 to 10,000. The students matching the random numbers are in the sample. If the population is large and the process of assigning numbers to the entire population is performed by hand, this sampling procedure can be time consuming.

Another method that can be used especially when a population is large is called **systematic counting**. With this procedure, the researcher uses some type of list or inventory of subjects in a population, such as a phone book; a list of licensed drivers; or an index of registered voters. Suppose that we would like to form a random sample of 200 subjects and we have an alphabetical list of 30,000 drivers at our disposal. We could simply go down the list, selecting every 150th person. Of course whenever a list is used, the sample is biased by the trait used in making the list. For instance, if a telephone book is used, the sample is biased to people who have phones. Nonetheless, this is a commonly used sampling technique for broad-based public opinion surveys with the assumption that most people have telephones and therefore this list describes most people reasonably well.

The final procedure we describe is known as **stratified random sampling**. This method is used when the investigator has reason to believe that a population has distinct subgroups or strata and wants to have the appropriate representation from each. Using the example of the population of 10,000 university students, a conspicuous subgrouping could be freshmen, sophomores, juniors, and seniors. These students may be either male or female. After consulting with the registrar, the percentage of the population for each class level can be determined, as can the distribution of men and women. Table 7-2 illustrates the composition of a stratified random sample of 100 students for this university. Random sampling would be used to assign the requisite number of subjects into each stratum.

How different would our sample be if we used only the random numbers approach instead of stratification? This is difficult to say. Normally speaking, a very large random sample routinely contains representatives of all of the strata. The smaller the sample size, the more likely biased representation becomes even if random sampling is used. To that end, stratified random sampling offsets some of the potential for forming a biased sample and should be used when forming smaller samples.

| TABLE 7-2. A Stratified Random Sample | | |
|---|---|---|
| University population | $N = 10,000$ | |
| Percent men = 45 | Percent women = 55 | |
| Sample | n = 100 | |
| **Subset** | **Percent** | **Men/Women** |
| Freshmen | 29 | 13/16 |
| Sophomores | 26 | 12/14 |
| Juniors | 24 | 11/13 |
| Seniors | 21 | 9/12 |
| Total | | 45/55 |

Having said all of this about random sampling, one can appreciate that it is difficult to obtain a "true" random sample. It isn't very often that a researcher has access to or the freedom to manipulate all of the subjects in a population. For instance, what if someone were interested in studying the physical fitness levels of high school football players in the United States? That would be a massive population from which to draw a random sample and probably large portions of it would be inaccessible to the researcher. Or, if someone wanted to do school-based research, it would be difficult to randomly select students and place each one in classes in which different teaching methods were being studied. So in these types of cases the investigators use the best sampling technique they can. The reader then decides whether legitimate inferences or generalization can be made.

Often, researchers draw up specific delimitations for subjects and include any volunteer subject who meets that description. This isn't random sampling, and the ability to make generalizations may be limited. However, when random sampling from a population is not practical or possible, this is how samples may be obtained. For example, an athletic trainer may wish to study athletes with a history of hamstring or anterior cruciate (i.e., knee ligament) injury. Any conclusions drawn will obviously pertain only to the athletes in the study and those with similar traits (e.g., age, injury status, gender, sport). Such a sample is called a **convenience sample** because the subjects possessing the necessary trait or traits were readily available. Many studies in athletic training, nutrition, physical therapy, and the allied health professions in general use this approach.

How many subjects do we need in a sample to make accurate inferences? Generally speaking, a larger random sample is a better model of the population than a smaller one. There are equations to estimate the size of a sample based on an acceptable level of error defined by the researcher and the type of statistic used. Chapter 19 provides an equation for sample size and a discussion of this topic. Also, many statistical software packages have programs for calculating sample size. Norman and Streiner (1994) give a practical presentation of sample size.

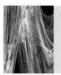 A person is overheard saying, "Nearly everyone thinks that American foreign policy is in trouble." How valid do you think this generalization is? What would need to be done to test whether or not the statement is true?

## Randomization into Groups

Once study subjects have been identified, the researcher may need to make decisions about group placement. The investigator should not allow subjects themselves to select their group, since this is a form of selection bias, which weakens the experiment. It is critical in some types of research that groups be equivalent at the onset of a study, and the best way to ensure this is to randomize the subjects into groups. Random numbers, blind draws of coded cards, and other such unbiased methods may be used. More is said about randomization of subjects in Chapter 15.

## SOME COMPUTATIONAL NOTATIONS AND TIPS

In our presentation of selected statistics, we provide some sample equations and problems. These problems may be solved with a computer or by hand or as a form of checking your work both ways. The emphasis that is placed on any of these approaches is at the discretion of your professor. To help understand statistical problem solving, some computational tips are given.

As has been said before, solving math problems is no different from reading a road map. If you know what the signs and symbols are, you'll have no problem getting to your destination. With equations it's just a matter of performing calculations to get to the end result. To help you remember the order of computations, some reminders that you probably learned in grade school are reviewed. "Please excuse my dear Aunt Sally" is the order of operations for *p*arentheses, *e*xponents, *m*ultiplication, *d*ivision, *a*ddition, and *s*ubtraction. Simply do the operations in parentheses first (start with the pair the farthest in, then work outward), followed by exponent operations, such as square or square root, then multiplication or division, and, last, addition or subtraction.

Statistical equations consist of some math symbols that you should be familiar with and a few that you may not know. X refers to the value of any variable in a distribution or column of scores. When a subscript appears with X (such as $X_1$), it refers to the position of the score in the distribution. Therefore, $X_3 = 57$ means the third score or variable in the distribution has the value 57. The symbol N or n refers to the total number of scores in a distribution. Technically, N denotes the size of a population, whereas n refers to the size of a sample. However, frequently N is simply used to denote the number of observations in a group whether it is a sample or a population. If $N = 20$, that means there are 20 scores in that distribution. If subscripts appear with N, it represents the number of scores in a certain group. For instance, $N_3 = 18$ means that there are 18 scores in

| **TABLE 7-3. Selected Statistical Symbols and Operations** |
|---|
| X (or Y): any variable |
| $\quad$ $X_3 = 8$: the third variable $= 8$ |
| $\quad$ $X^2 = 64$: the square of the variable $= 64$ |
| N: total number of observations in a group |
| $\quad$ $N_4 = 10$: the number of observations in group $4 = 10$ |
| $\quad$ $N^2 = 100$: the square of the N size $= 100$ |
| $\sum$: sum all of these variables |
| $\sum X$: sum all of the X variables |
| $\quad$ $\sum X = 1 + 2 + 3 + 4 = 10$ |
| $\sum X^2$: square all X variables, then sum |
| $\quad$ $\sum X^2 = 1 + 4 + 9 + 16 = 30$ |
| $\left(\sum X\right)^2$: sum all X variables, then square the sum |
| $\quad$ $\left(\sum X\right)^2 = (10)^2 = 100$ |

group 3. The symbols X and N both frequently appear with the exponent for squaring; for example, if $X = 12$, $X^2 = 144$, and if $N = 9$, $N^2 = 81$. What does $N_1^2 = 49$ mean? It means that the number of observations in group one squared, or $N_1^2 = 7^2 = 49$.

The symbol $\sum$ is the Greek capital letter sigma, which expresses addition. In some statistical texts, sigma may have extra notations, like subscripts and superscripts. They are used to indicate starting and stopping points of summing operations. We will not use these notations, however, so anytime you see $\sum X$ in an equation, assume that it means sum all of the variables in that column. Therefore, the sign $\sum X$ says to sum all of the variables in a distribution. So given the variables 1, 2, 3, 4, 5, then $\sum X = 15$. A summary of selected symbols and operations appears in Table 7-3.

Here are some review questions to test your mastery of the previously described points. Given the variables 1, 2, 3, 4, 5 then, $\sum X = 15$. What is $\sum X^2$? The order of operations says to do exponents first, then addition (remember, $\sum$ is the sign for summation or addition), so this expression tells one to square all of the X variables first and then sum them, so $\sum X^2$ is $1 + 4 + 9 + 16 + 25 = 55$. What does $(\sum X)^2$ equal? That expression is the sum all of the X variables, because it is in parentheses, squared. Therefore, $\left(\sum X\right)^2 = 15^2 = 225$.

All of this seems straightforward enough, and it is if you know the signs and the order of operations. There is a great deal of squaring and summing of variables in the computation of statistics, and you will see the operations of $\sum X^2$ and $(\sum X)^2$ many times again. These two operations are perhaps the most often mistaken for one another. In the examples above, $\sum X^2 = 55$ and $(\sum X)^2 = 225$, and as you are well aware, 55 doesn't equal 225. Confusing these operations (or any other for that matter) will lead to calculating the wrong statistical value and will start a domino effect ending with a headache. So if you are uncertain about these two statements, it would be helpful to review this last section before you go on.

## Summary

Statistics are probably the researcher's most important tool. Statistics may be classified as parametric or nonparametric and may be used for descriptive or inferential purposes. To make accurate inferences, a researcher needs a representative sample of a population, and the best way to establish a model sample is by random sampling. Professionals in HPER need at least an elementary knowledge of statistics so that they may make prudent decisions about the correct use and interpretations of statistical procedures. This is an essential skill whether they are producing or consuming research.

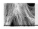
## Learning Activities

1. Have you accomplished the objectives stated at the beginning of the chapter? If not, go back and reread the concepts you're uncertain about. Also, ask your professor about these topics.
2. Read several selected research articles (perhaps focus on the methods section) to determine the following:
   - What type of sampling procedure was used?
   - Is the sample size adequate? How do the authors of the study justify the sample size used?
   - Did the researcher use statistics for descriptive or inferential purposes?
   - What scales of measurement were the data? Do the statistics used match the scale level of the data?

## Statistics Exercises

1. Indicate the level of measurement for the following:
   **a.** Driving on U. S. Highway 6.
   **b.** A runner's time of 18 minutes, 30 seconds in a road race.
   **c.** A student who is 27th in a class of 157 students.
   **d.** There are 44 women in a recreational golf league.
   **e.** The average daily temperature last March was 35°F.
   **f.** Locker number 16.
   **g.** A systolic blood pressure reading of 124 mm Hg.
   **h.** A score of 20 correct of 25 test items.
   **i.** A football lineman who weighs 275 lb.
   **j.** A swimmer finished third in a race.
   **k.** Eight pull-ups for a fitness test.
   **l.** Score of 70 in a golf tournament.

**2.** For the following data sets calculate $\sum X$, $\sum X^2$, $(\sum X)^2$.

| Group A | Group B | Group C |
|---------|---------|---------|
| 1 | 3 | 7 |
| 3 | 4 | 2 |
| 6 | 9 | 1 |
| 8 | 3 | 5 |
| 4 | 6 | 2 |
| 7 | 2 | 4 |

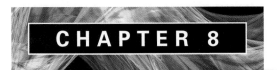

# CHAPTER 8

# Central Tendency, Variability, and the Normal Curve

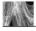

## KEY CONCEPTS

- Central tendency
- The mean
- The median
- The mode
- Variability
- Range
- Standard deviation
- Coefficient of variation
- Variance
- The normal curve
- Confidence intervals
- The $z$ score
- Nonnormal distributions and curves

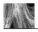

## AFTER READING THIS CHAPTER YOU SHOULD BE ABLE TO:

- Describe the characteristics of the normal curve and explain how it may be applied to sets of data.
- Calculate measures of central tendency and interpret the results.
- Calculate measures of variability and interpret the results.
- Calculate $z$ scores and interpret the results.
- Describe what nonnormal distributions are.

Measures of central tendency and variability are some of the most commonly used and important descriptive statistics. These statistics perhaps represent the most basic form of statistical analysis and are used in almost every form of research. These statistics are also the foundation of other higher-order techniques. The concept of the normal curve is the cornerstone of many statistical techniques. These concepts will be discussed in this chapter.

## CENTRAL TENDENCY

As mentioned previously, the general purpose of statistics is to reduce a large amount of data to one meaningful numerical value. In the case of measures of central tendency, that value is the one that best typifies or is the most representative of all of the scores in a distribution. Three measures of central tendency may be used: mean, median, and mode. Each will be described.

### The Mean

We are exposed to means or average values on a daily basis, and you have probably calculated a mean value numerous times in your life. The mean is simply the arithmetic average of a distribution of scores and is the most commonly used measure of central tendency. Customary symbols for the mean are $\mu$ for a population mean and $M$ for a sample mean. The equation for the mean is

$$M = \frac{\sum X}{N}$$

and given the values 1, 2, 3, 4, 5, the $M = 15/5 = 3$. The mean is used when the data are absolute, interval, or ratio level. The mean is usually regarded as the most reliable and meaningful measure of central tendency.

### The Median

The median is the midpoint in a distribution, where 50% of the scores lie above and 50% below. The symbol for the median is *MED;* in some cases the entire word is used. To determine the median of a distribution, the scores must be ranked from highest to lowest. With an odd number of scores, the median is the score that is the exact midpoint, and if there is an even number, the two middle scores are averaged.

Median for odd N: MED = 6, 7, 8, 9, 10 = 8

Median for even N: MED = 6, 7, 8, 9 = $\dfrac{(7 + 8)}{2}$ = 7.5

This approach is used only when there are not many tied scores. If there are several tied scores, another data analysis must be done, which is not presented here but is used in some statistical software. The median is the measure of choice when a distribution has a small N size and some atypical or outlying scores. Let's say that a physical education instructor has a group of students perform a push-up test for muscular endurance. In this

***The median is the measure of choice when a distribution has a small N size and some atypical or outlying scores.***

group, he has a junior Olympic gymnast who does unusually well. Compare the effect that this atypical score of 100 push-ups has on the mean and the median.

$$\text{Data: } 17, 19, 20, 22, 25, 27 \qquad \text{Data: } 17, 19, 20, 22, 25, 27, 100$$

$$M = \frac{130}{6} = 21.7 \qquad\qquad M = \frac{230}{7} = 32.9$$

$$MED = 21.0 \qquad\qquad MED = 22.0$$

You can see from this example that the atypical score of 100 push-ups inflated the mean value (actually the $\sum X$ component) and the median is not as much affected. In this case, the median is a better representation of the group's performance.

## The Mode

The mode is the crudest measure of central tendency and so is not used very often. The mode is the most frequent score in a distribution. It can be obtained by quick inspection of a ranked distribution. It may be that two scores occur most frequently. If this occurs, the distribution has two modes, or is **bimodal.** If three scores occur most frequently, the distribution is called **trimodal**.

$$\text{Data: } 10, 9, 9, 8, 7, 7, 7, 5, 3, 2$$
$$\text{Mode} = 7$$

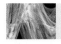 What are the three measures of central tendency?

## Application of Mean and Median

The primary use of the mean and the median is as an index of the most typical score in a distribution. These statistics also allow for the comparison of individual scores within the distribution ($M = 85$ was 10 points higher than a score $M = 75$) and to compare to like values between other distributions (group A $MED = 40$ vs group B $MED = 35$). We will be using these statistics frequently, since the mean is used extensively as a component in other parametric statistics, while the median appears in some nonparametric equations.

## MEASURES OF VARIABILITY

Measures of variability indicate the dispersion of scores in a distribution. These statistics provide information about how widely spread scores are and whether the scores are similar to one another. Most people focus on the mean or some measure of central tendency when examining data and tend to ignore the variability. Yet variability is often as important in the interpretation of data as is the mean. For example, if you were planning a trip to the mountains next summer, you may want to know what the average temperature is to guide you in selecting what clothing to bring. If the mean temperature is 74 degrees in July and you use this value as the sole basis for selecting your wardrobe, you might find yourself dressed inappropriately some days. If you knew the range of temperatures each day, this might be helpful. Suppose the range of temperatures each day was a low of 52 degrees and a high of 82 on average throughout the month. This knowledge may alter your planning since you realize that a jacket may be needed many mornings and evenings.

The most common measures of variability are range, standard deviation, and coefficient of variation. Each is now described.

## Range

The range measures just what its name implies, that is, the distance between the end points in a distribution. The range is determined by subtracting the low score from the high one in a distribution. Here is an example of a range calculation:

$$\text{Data: } 3, 4, 5, 6, 7, 8, 9$$
$$Range = \text{high score} - \text{low score}$$
$$Range = 9 - 3 = 6$$

Some statisticians use a variation of the first formula that adds a 1 to the difference in the high and low scores.

$$Range = (\text{high score} - \text{low score}) + 1$$
$$Range = (9 - 3) + 1 = 7$$

The addition of the 1 makes the calculated value inclusive of all of the scores in the distribution. In the example here, 7 different values occur between 3 and 9.

The range is a weak measure of variability because it is based on the extreme scores in a distribution and is determined by only two scores. Therefore, the range gives no information about the spread of all of the scores in the group. Sometimes the range is reported in a table by reporting the high and low scores. For example, if a range such as 25 is reported for a group of test scores, one knows nothing about the extreme scores. However, if the high and low scores, say 90 and 65, were reported instead, the information is more descriptive and the range can be easily calculated if desired.

## Standard Deviation

The standard deviation is the most frequently used measure of variability and is much stronger than the range. The standard deviation provides information on the average algebraic distance from the mean of each score in a distribution. The basis for computing a standard deviation is a **deviation score** ($x$), the difference from the mean of each score in the distribution ($x = X - M$). These differences are squared, summed, averaged, and unsquared to provide the standard deviation. The most common symbols for the standard deviation are $\sigma$ for population standard deviations and S and $SD$ for samples. One equation for $SD$ is based on computing a distribution mean:

$$SD = \sqrt{\frac{\sum X^2}{N} - M^2}$$

Another equation doesn't require a calculation of a mean:

$$SD = 1/N \sqrt{N\left(\sum X^2\right) - \left(\sum X\right)^2}$$

| TABLE 8-1. Example of Calculation of Standard Deviation | |
| --- | --- |
| X | X² |
| 1 | 1 |
| 2 | 4 |
| 4 | 16 |
| 6 | 36 |
| 8 | 64 |
| 9 | 81 |

$\sum X = 30 \quad (\sum X)^2 = (30)^2 = 900 \quad \sum X^2 = 202 \quad M = 5 \quad N = 6$

$SD = \sqrt{\dfrac{202}{6} - 5^2} = \sqrt{33.67 - 25} = 2.9$

$SD = 1/6\sqrt{6(202) - 900} = .167\sqrt{1212 - 900} = 2.9$

Table 8-1 shows examples of each formula. As can be seen from these examples, both equations give the same value, so it doesn't matter which you use. It is impossible to have a negative *SD* because squaring and square root processes yield only a positive number.

## Interpreting *SD*

How is *SD* interpreted? From the examples in Table 8-1, one can say that the scores in the distribution differ algebraically from the mean on the average 2.9 units. A larger *SD* means there is more variability in scores or they are spread out more, whereas a smaller one means that the scores are closer together or more similar. The *SD* from different distributions with scores reflecting the same variable may be compared only if they have the same *M* value. If group A has a *SD* of 10.5 and group B has a *SD* of 5.3 and they both have the same mean, then distribution A is more variable. The *SD* has many more applications in other statistics and concepts, which are discussed later.

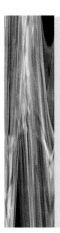

A person with diabetes strives to maintain blood glucose at average levels to minimize long-term health problems. If a patient's average blood glucose for a month is 100 mg/dL, can a nurse or physician assume that the patient is in good control? Without knowing how much fluctuation in blood glucose occurs around the mean of 100, one really doesn't know. If the *SD* in this time is calculated and found to be 40 mg/dL, a better judgment of degree of blood glucose control can be made. With a *SD* of 40, we know that the blood glucose values are varying widely so that a number of values are well above normal as well as below normal. This patient's data reveal the need for improved blood glucose control. Consequently, making a judgment solely on the mean may lead to a different conclusion than focusing on the mean as well as the SD.

## Coefficient of Variation

*SD*s cannot be used to compare the variability of two or more distributions whose measured means or variables are not the same. For instance, it wouldn't be logical to compare a *SD* of bowling scores to a *SD* from a statistics quiz. Under this condition the coefficient of variation (*CV*) is the statistic of choice. It represents the *SD* as a percentage of the **M**. The calculation of the *CV* is as follows:

$$CV = \left(\frac{SD}{M}\right) \times 100$$

Let's say an investigator measured the height of a sample of men and a sample of women and produced these findings: men, $M = 70$ inches, $SD = 5$; women, $M = 65$ inches, $SD = 3$. To determine which group of scores has more variability, *CV*s are computed as follows: men's $CV = (5/70) \times 100 = 7.1\%$, and women's $CV = (3/65) \times 100 = 4.6\%$. Since 7.1% is greater than 4.6%, there was more variability in the height scores for men than for women. Consequently, the *CV* allows comparing the variability of scores in different distributions.

## Variance

The square of a *SD* ($SD^2$) is the variance. Another measure of the variability of scores, variance is used extensively in the calculation of many other statistics. Consequently, it is a widely used term in statistics. However, variance is rarely used in place of the *SD* as a descriptor of a distribution's variability. This is because variance is expressed in squared units as opposed to the original units of the data.

 What are several ways to express the variation of scores in a distribution?

## THE NORMAL CURVE

The normal curve is a statistical and theoretical model that is used to visualize data, to interpret distributions of scores, and, most important, to make predictions and probability statements. The normal curve has several notable characteristics. The mean, median, and mode on the curve are identical and make up the vertical midpoint. The curve is perfectly symmetrical; that is, the halves are mirror images of one another. The right side of the curve is composed of positive values, or values above the mean, whereas the left side contains negative values, which are below the mean.

 *The normal curve is a statistical model that is used to visualize data, interpret distributions of scores, and make predictions and probability statements.*

Many data collected in research approximate the shape and characteristics of the normal curve. For example, if one were to measure a variable such as body weight in many subjects and make a frequency graph of the scores, the resulting figure would appear to be bell-shaped.

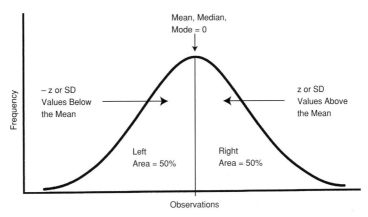

**Figure 8-1.** Features of the unit normal curve: perfect symmetry; mean, median, mode = 0; *SD* = 1; area = 1 (100%), or one square unit; 50% area to the right (+) and 50% area to left (−) of mean.

This bell-shaped figure represents the normal curve. Measurements of variables such as height, IQ, income, and strength result in a curve of the same shape. Figure 8-1 shows what the bell curve looks like. So assuming that the variable being measured approximates the normal curve, it can also be assumed that the variable will conform to the characteristics of the model curve. This concept can be seen in Figure 8-2, which features a bar graph with a superimposed normal curve of the heights of nearly 1000 subjects. Because many of the observations made in the allied health professions will approach characteristics of the normal curve, we may use the model to draw numerous statistical conclusions.

Many so-called normal curves are used to make statistical judgments, and the model that we will be discussing is referred to as the **unit normal curve.** The total area under

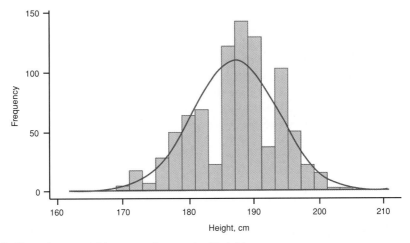

**Figure 8-2.** Normal curve and frequency bar graph of heights.

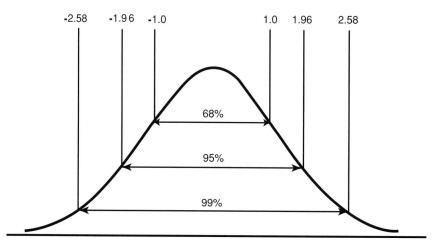

**Figure 8-3.** Selected areas of the normal curve.

the curve is equal to 1.0 (1 square unit; thus the name *unit* normal curve), or 100%. The unit normal curve has a mean, median, and mode that equal 0, and it is divided into *SD* units, which have a size equaling 1.0. These and other features may also be seen in Figure 8-1. As seen in Figure 8-3, approximately 68% of the area under the curve is between ±1.0 *SD* from the mean, about 95% of the area is between ±2 *SD*s (actually, 1.96 *SD*s) and close to 99% of the area is between ±3 *SD*s (actually, 2.58 *SD*s). Also notice in Figures 8–1 and 8–3 that the tails of the curve don't touch the baseline and would extend into infinity. This means technically that there is an infinite number of *SD*s on the curve. For instance, a billionaire may have an annual income that is 20 *SD*s above the mean of all those living in the same city. But since about 99% of the area can be accounted for within ±3 *SD*s, we don't get too concerned about the remaining 1% and how far from the mean these values are.

Of what value is knowing the characteristics of the normal curve? First of all, it is important to understand that references to a defined area under the curve actually account for the percent of the total scores in a distribution that are represented by that area. Applying the model on data from an actual distribution of scores allows one to make many statements about how the data are dispersed. The *M* and *SD* from a distribution may be substituted in the following equations to determine the 68%, 95%, and 99% values for that group of scores:

$$68\% = M \pm 1.0(SD)$$

$$95\% = M \pm 1.96(SD)$$

$$99\% = M \pm 2.58(SD)$$

In these equations *M* and *SD* are the mean and standard deviation of the distribution, whereas 1.0, 1.96, and 2.58 are the actual number of *SD* units above and below the mean that correspond with 68%, 95%, and 99% of the area under the curve, respectively. These intervals are also known as **confidence intervals,** of which more will be said later.

## Application of the Normal Curve

Let's say that a researcher has measured the body weight of 1000 young girls. The resulting distribution has a $M = 125$ lb and $SD = 5$. Therefore, the scores would be distributed in the following manner:

$$68\% = 125 \pm 1.0(5.0) = 120 \text{ to } 130.0 \text{ lb}$$

$$95\% = 125 \pm 1.96(5.0) = 115.2 \text{ to } 134.8 \text{ lb}$$

$$99\% = 125 \pm 2.58(5.0) = 112.1 \text{ to } 137.9 \text{ lb}$$

Many statistical statements can be made about this distribution. Below are some examples. Also, look at the figure associated with each statement. The shaded area depicts the percent of the scores referred to in the statement.

1. Of these scores, 68% are between 120 and 130 lb. How many actual scores does this represent? Since there are 1000 scores and 68% of them are between these values, 1000 (0.68) = 680 (Fig. 8-4).

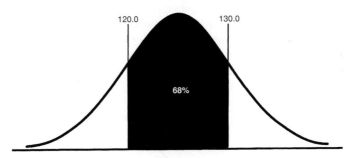

**Figure 8-4.**

2. Of these scores, 32% are either lower than 120 or higher than 130 lb. How many scores are there? There are 320 scores, since 1000 (0.32) = 320 (Fig. 8-5).

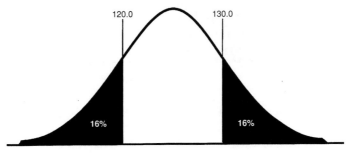

**Figure 8-5.**

**3.** What percent of the girls have body weight above 130 lb? Each half of the curve represents 50%, and one *SD* above the mean represents about 34% of the area. (34% + 34% = 68% for ±1 *SD*.) Therefore, we are interested only in the percent of the area above 1 *SD*: 50% − 34% = 16%. Now we can say that 160 women have body weight above 130 lb, since 1000 (0.16) = 160 (Fig. 8-6).

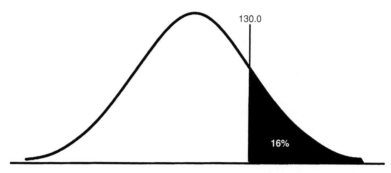

**Figure 8-6.**

**4.** What percent and number of these girls have body weight below 120 lb? The answer is identical with the one for question 3, 16% and 160, for the same reason. The only thing that is different is that now we are interested in the area under the curve that is below −1 *SD*. (Fig. 8-7). If you understand the logic in questions 1 through 4, the rest will be easy. We are solving for a portion of the area under the curve, and that can be done by simple deduction.

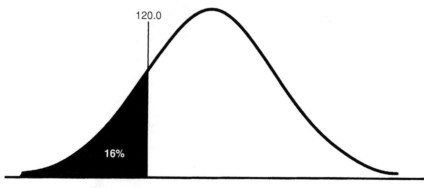

**Figure 8-7.**

**5.** What percent and number of these girls have body weight above 134.8 and below 115.2 lb? We are referring to 5% of the distribution, since 2.5% of the scores are above and 2.5% below these values. This represents 50 scores, since 1000 (.05) = 50 (Fig. 8-8).

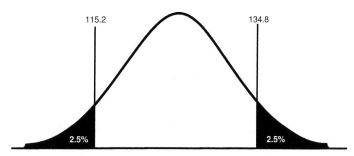

**Figure 8-8.**

6. What percent and number of the girls have body weight below 112.1 and above 137.9 lb? In this case we are interested in 1% of the scores, since 0.5% of the scores are above and 0.5% below these values. There are only 10 scores at these levels, since 1000 (0.01) = 10 (Fig. 8-9).

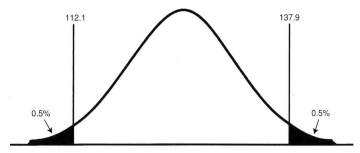

**Figure 8-9.**

7. Put on your thinking cap for this one! What percent and number of the women have body weight below 130 lb? The answers are 84% and 840 scores. The area in this case is all of the area below +1 *SD,* and since the area from the mean to +1 *SD* equals about 34% and the entire area on to the left of the mean is 50%, it follows that 50% + 34% = 84% (Fig. 8-10).

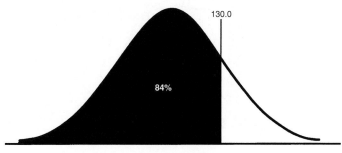

**Figure 8-10.**

8. What percent and number of the girls have body weight below 112.1 lb? We are referring to scores that are 2.58 *SD*s below the mean, which refers to 0.5% of the scores. There are only 5 scores in this category, since 1000 (0.005) = 5 (Fig. 8-11).

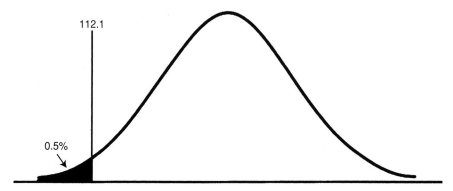

112.1

0.5%

**Figure 8-11.**

It is important to have a thorough understanding of the normal curve because its applications are vital to the study and use of statistics. You will see the 68%, 95%, and 99% confidence intervals and the corresponding *SD* units of 1.0, 1.96, and 2.58 are used frequently, so it is worthwhile to commit them to memory.

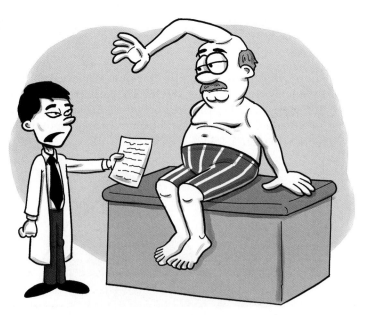

Mr. Smith, you're very normal: overweight, out of shape, and hypertensive.

## THE *Z* SCORE

The $z$ score is used to convert a raw score from a distribution into units of the normal curve called *SD* units. (The unit normal curve is sometimes referred to as the $z$ distribution). A $z$ score gives a raw score's distance from the mean in *SD* units. The equation for the $z$ score is

$$z = \frac{(X - M)}{SD}$$

where X is the raw score, *M* is the mean, and *SD* is the standard deviation of the distribution. Using $M = 25$ and $SD = 5$ from women's body fat data, what would be the $z$ scores for 18% and 35% body fat?

$$z = \frac{(18 - 25)}{5} = -1.4$$

and

$$z = \frac{(35 - 25)}{5} = 2.0$$

A positive $z$ score tells us how many *SD* units above the mean a score is, and a negative z score indicates the number of units below the mean. Recall that the mean of the unit normal curve or $z$ distribution is 0 and *SD* of 1. Therefore, a $z$ score of $-1.40$ means that 18% body fat is 1.40 *SD* units below the mean of 25, and a $z$ score of 2.0 means that body fat of 35% is 2.0 *SD* units above the mean. Thus, the $z$ score informs us of the exact position of the raw score in a distribution. What would be the typical range of $z$ scores? Since about 99% of scores in a distribution are within $\pm 3$ *SD*s, slightly more than 99% of $z$ scores will range between $-3.0$ and $+3.0$. Look at the $z$ distribution in Table A–6 in Appendix A to confirm this fact.

The $z$ score may also be used to compare raw scores from different distributions. When used in this manner, it may also be classified as a **standard score.** For instance, if someone had a score of 45 kg on a grip strength test and a score of 25 cm on a low back flexibility test, without any other statistical information we wouldn't know how good these performances were relative to the group or each other. Furthermore, comparing grip strength and flexibility scores in their original units would be like comparing apples and oranges. Given the following information, however, we may convert the scores into the same unit of measure (that is *SD* units, thus a standard score) by computing a z score for each and then make comparisons: Grip strength $M = 40.0$ kg, $SD = 3.0$, and flexibility $M = 30.0$ cm, $SD = 4.0$.

$$\text{Grip strength } z = \frac{(45 - 40)}{3} = 1.67$$

$$\text{Flexibility } z = \frac{(25 - 30)}{4} = -1.25$$

With the *z* score information, it can be concluded that a grip strength of 45 kg was 1.67 *SD* units above the mean and was a better score than a flexibility of 25 cm, which was 1.25 *SD* units below the mean.

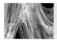    What does a positive z score indicate?

## Importance of Means and Standard Deviations

As you may now see, the *M* and *SD* provide considerable descriptive information about a distribution's scores. It is rare to read a research article and not find means and standard deviations reported. Therefore, a table that contains the *M* (or in some cases the *median*), *SD,* and *range* of key experimental variables is essential and should be part of any published or presented quantitative research.

## NONNORMAL DISTRIBUTIONS AND CURVES

Sometimes a distribution of scores will not fit the model of the normal curve. These atypical distributions are called **skewed,** and they result in curves that are **nonnormal,** particularly in shape. A skewed curve has a tail that represents few scores and is classified by the direction that the tail is pointing. A **positively skewed** curve has most of its scores depicted in the left, or lower value, side of the distribution with the tail pointing in the positive direction. A **negatively skewed** distribution is just the opposite, with most scores on the high-value side and the tail pointing left. Some of its features appear in Figure 8-12. A test that was very difficult would probably result in a positively skewed distribution and curve. For example, if a test developed for an advanced statistics course was given to an introductory class, the test scores would probably result in a positively skewed distribution. A negatively skewed curve is just the opposite, where most of the scores are on the right or higher-value side, with the tail pointing left. A distribution of grades given in graduate courses usually results in negatively skewed distribution, because graduate

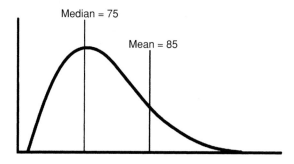

**Figure 8-12.** A positively skewed distribution: fewer high extreme scores, more lower scores; mean is greater than median (mean is pulled toward skewed end).

***Atypical distributions are called skewed; they result in curves that are not normal in shape or appearance.***

students typically perform at a high academic level, and few Ds or Fs are given. Annual incomes of residents living in Beverly Hills would result in a negative skew as well. A negatively skewed distribution appears in Figure 8-13.

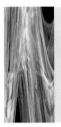 The words *positive* and *negative* can be misleading with some data because the words connote something good or bad, yet the opposite can occur as in the example of positive skew in the results of a class exam. So remember that the terms positive and negative skew refer only to the direction of the tail. Whether or not the data represent a good or bad thing can be judged only by context.

How is skewness determined? The amount and presence of skewness may be judged by eyeballing the shape of a curve of a distribution or by examining its measures of central tendency. As mentioned previously, the mean of a distribution is more affected by extreme scores than is the median. Therefore, in a positively skewed distribution with few high scores, the mean will be higher than the median. This positive skewness is depicted in Figure 8-12. The opposite is true in the negatively skewed distribution because the few scores are on the lower end of the distribution, which reduces the mean so that the mean is less than the median. This concept may be seen in Figure 8-13. An easy way to remember these concepts is to recall that the mean is pulled toward the tail in skewed distributions. A simple calculation for skewness is to subtract the median from the mean. The resulting difference, either positive or negative, indicates the type of skew. Although more elaborate equations may be used to determine the amount of skewness in a distribution, they are beyond the scope of this discussion. Also, you may recall from our discussion about means and medians that the median is less affected by skewness than the mean and is therefore the best measure of central tendency for skewed distributions.

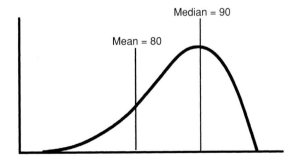

**Figure 8-13.** A negatively skewed distribution: fewer low extreme scores, more higher scores; mean is less than median (mean is pulled toward skewed end).

*The median is less affected by skewness than the mean and is the preferred measure of central tendency for non-normal distributions.*

Finally, when a distribution is markedly skewed, it won't accurately conform to the properties of the normal curve. Any application of the normal curve in this case may be suspect. In these cases, a special type of statistical analysis is used called *nonparametric analysis,* which is covered in a later chapter.

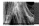

## Summary

Measures of central tendency are used to provide information about the most representative score in a distribution, with the mean and median being the most commonly used. Variability statistics are used to show the dispersion of scores in a distribution. The range and standard deviation are the most routinely used statistics for this purpose, with the standard deviation being the better of the two. The coefficient of variation may be used to examine variability in distributions that have different means or variables. The normal curve is an important statistical model that is used to visualize data, interpret distributions of scores, and make predictions and probability statements. A fundamental understanding of the normal curve and its applications is vital to the study and use of statistics. Positively and negatively skewed curves reflect distributions that don't conform to the normal curve model.

## Learning Activities

1. Have you accomplished the objectives stated at the beginning of the chapter? If not, go back and reread the concepts you're uncertain about. Also, ask your professor questions about these topics.
2. Create or ask your professor for some practice data sets. Perform calculations of the statistics presented in this chapter. You may do this by hand calculations, computer software or both.
3. Examine means and medians reported in some research articles. Determine whether data are skewed and defend your rationale.

## Statistics Exercises

| Body Fat, % | Income for Recreation, % | Stress Index |
|---|---|---|
| 13 | 10 | 7 |
| 8 | 15 | 8 |
| 5 | 12 | 12 |
| 11 | 9 | 15 |
| 6 | 10 | 6 |
| 7 | 20 | 9 |
| 9 | 11 | 5 |
| | 13 | 11 |
| | | 14 |

1. For the data sets above, compute the following:
   a. Mean and median
   b. Range, standard deviation, and coefficient of variation
   c. Confidence intervals of 68%, 95%, and 99%
2. Determine the area under the normal curve for the following $z$ scores:
   a. Above $z = 1.50$
   b. Below $z = -.25$
   c. Between $z = -.50$ and $z = .75$
   d. Above $z = 2.25$ and below $z = -1.45$
   e. Between $z = 1.00$ and $2.50$
3. Given the following test results, compute $z$ scores and report the **better** test score for each pair:

|  Health Test | Recreation Test |
|  :---: | :---: |
| $M = 75, SD = 7$ | $M = 50, SD = 4$ |

   a. Health score= 78, recreation score= 55.
   b. Health score= 85, recreation score= 59.
   c. Health score= 80, recreation score= 48.
   d. Health score= 65, recreation score= 45.
   e. Health score= 72, recreation score= 52.

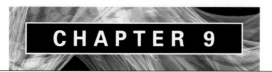

# CHAPTER 9

# Probability and Hypothesis Testing

## KEY CONCEPTS

- Theoretical probability
- Probability and the normal curve
- Hypothesis testing
- Sampling error
- Level of significance
- Type I and II errors
- Sampling distributions
- Critical statistics
- Calculated statistics
- Two-tailed hypothesis test
- One-tailed hypothesis test
- Practical versus statistical significance

## AFTER READING THIS CHAPTER YOU SHOULD BE ABLE TO:

- Define and provide examples of theoretical probability.
- Explain how probability statements are related to the normal curve.
- Describe all the components related to, and be able to conduct, a general hypothesis test.
- Differentiate between type I and type II errors.
- Explain the concept of statistical significance.

Hypothesis tests are perhaps the most important statistical procedures used by the researcher. These tests allow an investigator to make objective decisions about the outcome of a study. However, as important and useful as these procedures are, they do not provide absolute proof. All research decisions are made within a certain probability of being right or wrong. In this chapter, we discuss some of the elements of probability and general hypothesis testing.

## PROBABILITY

We are exposed to a variety of probability statements on a regular basis. "There is a 40% chance of rain today." "The odds are 75:1 that the Chicago Cubs will win the World

Series." "The odds of winning the lottery are 1 in 10 million." "A man between the ages of 55 and 65 has 1 in 100 chance of dying of heart disease." All of these are probability statements, which imply the likelihood or chance of a certain event occurring. As you can see, probability plays an informational role in many aspects of our lives.

Statistical decisions are not exact but are made with a certain probability or chance

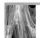

*Statistical decisions are not exact but are made with a certain probability or chance of being right or wrong.*

of being right or wrong. Therefore, a fundamental knowledge of probability is requisite for understanding many statistical tests.

## Theoretical Probability

Classical or theoretical probability is a traditional way of expressing the statistical likelihood of an event occurring and is the kind of probability with which we usually are the most familiar. Probability statements are commonly symbolized by using the lowercase italic letter $p$ and are expressed in proportions of 1. A probability of 1 is 100% certainty of an event occurring; conversely, a probability of 0 means there is no chance of an event occurring. Therefore, probability statements range from 0 to 1. Theoretical probability may be defined in words and mathematically as:

$p$ = the number of ways an event in question can occur divided by the number

of possible events

Several examples may illustrate probability statements. If one flips a coin, what is the probability that it will come up tails? Since there is only one tail on a coin, the number of ways it can happen is one, but the coin has a head and a tail, so there are two possible events. The probability of a tail appearing after a toss is $p = 1/2 = .50$, or 50%. What about the probability of rolling a single die and its coming up three? There is only one three and six possible events, so the probability is $p = 1/6 = .167$, or 16.7%. How about a roll that would produce either a two or a five? There are two ways the event can occur with six possible events, so $p = 2/6 = .333$, or 33.3%. What is the probability of pulling a jack from a deck of cards with a blind draw? There are four jacks and 52 cards in a deck, so there are 52 possible events. The probability would be $p = 4/52 = .077$, or 7.7%. How about pulling a red ace under the same conditions? That would be $p = 2/52 = .038$, or 3.8%. Theoretical probability is dealt with frequently in future chapters.

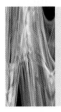

Many people seem not to understand the concept of probability. What else would explain why some people spend a portion of each paycheck hoping to win the Powerball lottery when the actual odds of winning are remarkably low? The same amount of money saved at 5% or 6% interest would earn them thousands of dollars over 20 or 30 years.

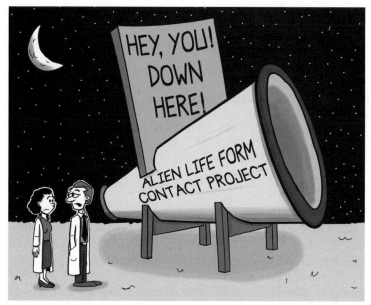

**"My grant funding was rather limited, but I have
an interesting hypothesis to test."**

## Probability and the Normal Curve

Recall that the applications of the normal curve include the ability to make predictions and probability statements. Making these determinations is straightforward because when we refer to a specified area under the curve, that area relates to a percent of a representative distribution. In the most simplistic sense, think of the number of observations in the given area or percent of the distribution in question as the number of ways the event can occur, and think of all of the observations in the distribution as the number of possible events.

A health educator is interested in determining the incidence of systolic hypertension in men aged 40 to 50 years in her community. The prevalence of hypertension is of interest to her for the programming and staffing of risk reduction programs and to compare the values with national averages. She obtains a random sample of 300 men in the community and measures their systolic blood pressure. She finds the $M = 125.0$ mm Hg (millimeters of mercury) and $SD = 15.0$. Based on previous discussion, confidence intervals for this distribution would be as follows:

$$68\% = 125.0 \pm 1(15.0) = 110 \text{ to } 140 \text{ mm Hg}$$

$$95\% = 125.0 \pm 1.96(15.0) = 95.6 \text{ to } 154.4 \text{ mm Hg}$$

$$99\% = 125.0 \pm 2.58(15.0) = 86.3 \text{ to } 163.7 \text{ mm Hg}$$

Imagine if we were to write the blood pressure readings for all 300 subjects on separate cards and put these in a basket. This is just another way of referring to all of the observations or the number of possible events. What is the event that we are talking about? It is the 40- to 50-year-old men's systolic blood pressure measurements. Now we will specify certain blood pressure measurements and make some probability statements. The figures related to each statement correspond to the areas under the normal curve for each probability.

What is the probability that any one subject selected at random would have a blood pressure reading between 110 and 140 mm Hg? Since 68% of the distribution has a blood pressure measure between those values, 68% of 300 subjects = 300(.68) = 204. So the number of ways the event, that is, systolic blood pressure, can occur is 204, and the number of possible events is 300 (all of the possible blood pressures). Therefore, $p = 204/300 = .68$. The logic for the remaining probabilities will follow the same pattern.

What would be the probability that any one subject selected at random would have a blood pressure reading *above* 140 mm Hg? Since 16% of the distribution is above 1 *SD* from the mean that represents 48 subjects: 300(.16) = 48. Therefore, $p = 48/300$ or .16.

What would be the probability that if any one subject were selected at random, they would have a blood pressure reading below about 96 mm Hg? Since only 2.5% of the distribution is below this level, $p = 7.5/300 = .025$.

Prediction statements that are based on probability and inference may also be made about the population that the subjects are representing. Since these 300 men were randomly selected, they probably are a good representation of 5000 such men in the community. Because of this, we may make fairly accurate generalizations from the sample. For instance, if 16% of the sample of 300 has a systolic blood pressure lower than 110 mm Hg, probably 16% of the population of 5000 also does. If this is true, how many men can we expect or predict (we are using these terms interchangeably) to be in the population? We would predict that there are 800 men, since $p = 800/5000 = .16$ and 16% of 5000 = 800. If blood pressure readings between 110 and 140 mm Hg typify men in this age group, how many men in the population can we expect to have readings in this range? We can expect 3400 men, since $p = 3400/5000 = .68$ and 68% of 5000 = 3400.

These examples of blood pressure were based on a calculation of probability. Actually, these problems can be solved by computing z scores, referring to the z distribution table and reading a probability directly from it. For instance, from our sample of 300 men whose mean systolic blood pressure is 125 with a SD of 15, the z score for a blood pressure of 110 mm Hg would be $z = (110 - 125)/15 = -1.0$, whereas a z score for 140 mm Hg would be $z = (140 - 125)/15 = 1.0$. Inspection of the z distribution table reveals that about 34% of the area under the curve is from the mean of 0 to a z score of 1.0; this is also true for $z = -1.0$. Therefore, 68% of the area under the curve is between z scores ±1.0. Identifying the area under the curve is the same as the probability of a z score occurring. Thus, the probability of any z score being between z scores of ±1.0 is .68. So the probability of any of the 300 men having a blood pressure between 110 and 140 mm Hg is $p = .68$. All of the other examples may be solved using this same approach.

Skill in playing poker is based largely on making use of probability theory. A good player is continually making decisions based on the probability that certain events might occur.

The normal curve can be used with both a sample distribution and a population. Furthermore, the $z$ distribution can be used to make probability statements by relating probabilities to areas under the curve. Also, it is apparent that probability and the ability to predict are related to one another. Subsequent chapters discuss prediction in more detail. As you might guess, normal curve concepts play an important role in these techniques.

## HYPOTHESIS TESTING

Recollect that the research hypothesis was discussed previously as a scientific hunch that the investigator has about the outcome of a study. Decisions to accept or reject the research hypothesis must be based on an objective and logical statistical process, which is generally known as hypothesis testing. The hypothesis test is a strict statistical process that is built on making probability statements for two possible states of actuality. Simply said, researchers use statistical tools to determine whether or not their guess about the anticipated results was correct. An appropriate statistic is selected and used to reflect a certain characteristic or event in the research. This objective piece of evidence is used to represent the event in question (e.g., a difference or a correlation) and is the prime ingredient in the hypothesis test.

The importance of understanding the nature, use, and interpretation of a hypothesis test in research must not be underestimated. Each of the statistics discussed in the remainder of the text has a hypothesis test associated with it. All hypothesis tests are based on the same logic, so an understanding of the basic steps and components, regardless of a specific statistic, is essential. The following discussion addresses the parts of a general hypothesis test.

### The Null and Alternative Hypotheses

The two states of reality that the hypothesis test is predicated on are known as the null and alternative hypotheses. They are sometimes referred to as **statistical hypotheses,** since statistical procedures are used to estimate whether they are true or not. It is important to emphasize at the start that the null and alternative hypotheses are merely statistical statements that are used in the hypothesis test, and they may or may not bear any resemblance to the research hypothesis. The investigator uses the results of the hypothesis test to draw conclusions about the validity of the research hypothesis. As we will soon see, these hypotheses are stated in such a way that one or the other *must* be true but not both.

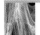 *Statistical hypotheses are used to estimate whether the research hypothesis is true.*

The **null hypothesis** ($H_0$) is traditionally defined as a statement of no difference or no relationship. This hypothesis may be written numerous ways, depending on the research condition and the statistical test. For instance, the null hypothesis for comparing two population means ($\mu$, pronounced mu) would be written $H_0$: $\mu_1 - \mu_2 = 0$ or its equivalent, $H_0$: $\mu_1 = \mu_2$. Both of these statements say the same thing; there *is no difference* between the two population means. In a hypothesis test, the null statement is assumed to be true until proved otherwise. As indicated, a null hypothesis may be stated many ways, and we will illustrate these as subsequent statistics are presented.

The **alternative hypothesis** ($H_A$) is the logical state of reality that must exist if the null hypothesis is not true. So in the example of comparing two population means, the null hypothesis stated that there was no difference between them. If this is not true, what has to be true? There is a difference between them. The alternative hypothesis in this case is written as $H_A$: $\mu_1 - \mu_2 \neq 0$, or $H_A$: $\mu_1 \neq \mu_2$, both of which say that there is a difference between population means. The alternative hypothesis provides no information about the amount of difference, and it doesn't have to, since it is just the logical option to the null.

## Sampling Error or a "Real" Difference or Relationship?

At the heart of the hypothesis test is the issue of whether an observed difference or a relationship is due to **sampling error.** Sampling error occurs when chance or random effects cause an event to occur in a manner different from what is expected. Sampling error is always present because there is always some probability or chance (even if it is remote) that any event will occur. Let's take an example of coin tossing to illustrate some concepts.

If a friend tosses a coin 10 times, what is the expected number of head and tail counts? Probability says that one would expect 5 head and 5 tail tosses. What if your friend came up with 4 heads and 6 tails? Would you be alarmed and think that he was using a rigged coin? You probably would not because it would not be unusual to have a 4:6 count. What made the tosses come up 4 and 6 instead of 5 and 5? Chance or sampling error is responsible.

 Why doesn't coin tossing always result in the expected outcome? How does the number of coin tosses influence the probability of an expected outcome?

If your friend continued with another set of 10 tosses and came up with a count of 3 tails and 7 heads, you say, "No big deal; it's sampling error," and you're right. What about a split of heads once and tails nine times? One would not expect this type of count to happen very frequently, but it can, and it's probably due to sampling error and not a fixed coin. What about 100 coin flips that came up heads once and tails 99 times; could sampling error have produced this? The answer is yes, but it would be a rare event, since the odds against this type of occurrence are 1 to 99. Even though there is a remote chance that sampling error could cause this to occur, a more likely explanation would be that there is something crooked going on!

There is an important point to all of this. Ultimately, the researcher has to make a decision whether sampling error is responsible for an event occurring. This is discussed shortly, but first we need to relate the concept of sampling error to the null hypothesis.

The null hypothesis is essentially a statement that sampling error or chance could cause the event in question to occur frequently. Remember that a statistic is a measure of the event in question. The alternative hypothesis, conversely, is a statement that the event in question could be caused by sampling error, but it is unlikely. If it is concluded that sampling error would rarely cause the event, it is probably due to something else such as the independent variable used in a study. We are calling this difference *real* (i.e., a real difference or a real relationship). For example, what if a 1% difference between two population means occurred, which in practical terms is quite small? Could we dismiss the 1% difference as sampling error, or does it represent a small but real difference between the two means? This is exactly the kind of decision that is made with a hypothesis test. The key to making this type of determination is deciding on a statistical reference point that defines the probability of an event in question occurring often vs. rarely due to sampling error.

## Level of Significance

The level of significance is the statistical reference point that is selected for the purpose of accepting or rejecting the null hypothesis. This level is set by the researcher and simply defines the probability of an event in question occurring often vs. rarely due to sampling error or chance. Figure 9-1 is a modification of one presented by Fox (1969). Examine it to see what this means. The probability that sampling error caused the event in question can range from $p = 0$ to $p = 1$, or from 0 to 100%. The researcher must decide on a point somewhere in that range that will functionally define whether an event may occur by chance often or rarely. What level would you feel comfortable with? If sampling error could produce an event up to 50% of the time, one would likely consider that as "often." What about 20% of the time? That's not very often. How about 5% of the time? Most would agree that 5% isn't very often, and 1% of the time is surely a rare event.

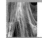 *The level of significance is the reference point that is selected for either accepting or rejecting the null hypothesis.* Remember that in principle this is up to the researcher to define, but we will soon see that most investigators by tradition and training typically use the 5% and 1% values for making statistical decisions.

So what does it mean if a researcher chooses a significance level at 5%, or $p = .05$, to test the null hypothesis? Essentially, the investigator is proposing that any event, as reflected by a statistic, that can occur by chance more often than 5% of the time is

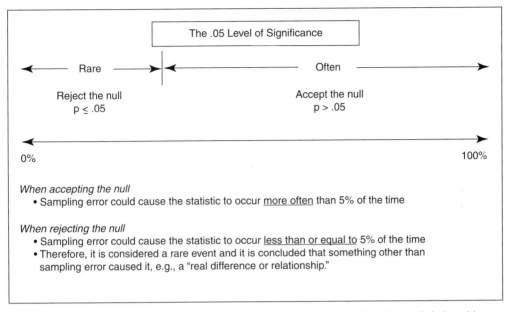

**Figure 9-1.** The probability that chance or sampling error alone could produce the statistic (result).

probably due to sampling error. If this occurs, the researcher accepts the null hypothesis. Conversely, if the statistic can occur by chance 5% of the time or less, it is rare and is probably not due to sampling error but to something real. In this case, the null hypothesis is rejected in favor of the alternative.

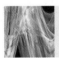 In research, is anything ever actually proved to the point of being 100% sure of a given finding?

## Type I and II Errors

The researcher needs to define an acceptable and reasonable level of significance to assist in making a sound statistical decision. How does the researcher decide on an acceptable level of significance? The primary factor is the willingness of the researcher to be wrong if incorrectly rejecting the null hypothesis. A **type I error** is made when the null hypothesis is rejected when it is actually true. In other words, the researcher has falsely concluded that a statistic was reflecting a real difference or relationship when it actually was sampling error. The probability of making a type I error is called the **alpha level,** or $\alpha$, which is in fact the level of significance we have been discussing all along. An

| TABLE 9-1. Decision Outcomes for Rejecting or Not Rejecting $H_0$ | | |
|---|---|---|
| **Decision** | **$H_0$ is actually true** | **$H_0$ is actually false** |
| Reject | Incorrect; type I error | Correct! |
| Accept | Correct! | Incorrect; type II error |

alpha level of .01 means that there is one chance in 100 of rejecting the null hypothesis when it is true. So if researchers want to reduce the likelihood of making a type I error, they just simply lower the alpha level perhaps from $p = .05$ to $p = .01$ or even $p = .001$.

In much of the research that is done in the allied health and other disciplines, alpha levels of .05 and .01 are commonly used. The reason for the use of these levels is probably bound in tradition and convenience, since most statistical tables are based on these levels. However, a researcher could justifiably use alpha levels of .075, .09, .025, and so on, if desired. Is there really much difference between the .05 and .06 levels of significance? This topic has been much discussed over the years and tradition seems to predominate in the use of .05 and .01, although a logical argument may question the use of these levels in all situations.

Lowering the alpha level to a more rigorous extent reduces the chance of making a type I error but increases the probability of making a **type II error.** A type II error is made when a false null hypothesis is accepted. The probability of making a type II error is called the **beta level,** or $\beta$. In this case, the researcher has falsely concluded that a statistic was due to sampling error and accepted the null hypothesis when it was a real event and the null hypothesis should have been rejected in favor of the alternative. The nature and calculation of beta are beyond the scope of this discussion. However, when researchers decrease the chance of making a type I error, they increase the probability of making a type II error and vice versa. Table 9-1, called a truth table, summarizes the correct and incorrect decisions related to rejecting or not rejecting the null hypothesis. Table 9-2 illustrates the effect on type I and II errors of raising and lowering the alpha above and below .05.

So if it's not possible to have an equally low probability of making both errors, which one is more important to avoid? The answer to this quandary is based on the type of research problem. For instance, a medical researcher who develops a new treatment

| TABLE 9-2. Effect of Alpha Level and Probability of Errors | | |
|---|---|---|
| **Alpha** | **Type I** | **Type II** |
| .01 | Decreased | Increased |
| .05 | — | — |
| .10 | Increased | Decreased |

The .05 level is a compromise between the pitfalls associated with .01 and .10.

that may revolutionize the management of an illness and replace a standard therapy must be very certain that the new approach is superior to the old one. Because of the potential impact on the field and the negative consequences of making a wrong decision, it is very important to take a conservative approach before claiming a difference. (Keep in mind that the outcome of only one study should never be a reason for dramatic change. Good science demands replication.) In this case, reducing the chance of making a type I error is more important, and making a type II error is more acceptable because this would suggest no change in medical treatment. This can be accomplished by the use of a more stringent alpha level, such as .01 or .001.

For less critical research decisions, decreasing the chance for a type II error is more appropriate. This can be accomplished by using a more liberal alpha level, say .10, which makes it easier to reject the null hypothesis. For example, a researcher in nursing wants to compare two hand soaps— both known from previous work to be effective—to see whether one is more effective in reducing infection in hospitalized patients. Does it really matter if it is concluded that one is better than the other if in fact there is little or no difference between them? Probably not, so in this case a type I error is more acceptable. In summation, it's the responsibility of the researcher to decide which error is the less important and to set the alpha level accordingly.

## Other Factors in Hypothesis Testing

In a hypothesis test, the researcher calculates an appropriate statistic and compares it with a value from a statistical table. There are many such tables, called **sampling distributions.** Basically, sampling distributions are probability tables that provide values for the chance occurrence of a particular statistic. The normal curve is actually based on a probability distribution called the $z$ distribution with the $z$ score as its statistic. We have already made several probability statements about this distribution, and here are a few more. The chance occurrence of a $z$ statistic with a value greater than $\pm1.96$ is $p = .05$, and greater than $\pm2.58$ is $p = .01$. Does this look familiar? The values $z = 1.96$ and $z = 2.58$ are actually significance or alpha levels for the chance occurrence of $z$ at the .05 and .01 levels, respectively. Sampling distributions for other statistics also have probability values that represent significance levels of .05, .01, and so on.

The investigator compares the **calculated statistic** based on the research data with one that is obtained from a sampling distribution at the desired alpha level. The statistic obtained from the sampling distribution is called a **critical statistic** or **value.** To determine the critical statistic, it is necessary to determine a quantity known as the **degrees of freedom.** Details for determining degrees of freedom for specific statistics are covered in subsequent chapters.

For example, if a significance level was set at .05 and a calculated statistic was greater than or equal to the critical value, the probability that sampling error could cause that statistic to occur would be less than or equal to .05, or $p \leq .05$. Since a statistic this size may rarely happen by chance (in this case 5% of the time or less), it is concluded that something other than sampling error probably caused it to occur, that is, something real. Of course, there is a small chance ($p \leq .05$) that the decision is wrong. On the other hand,

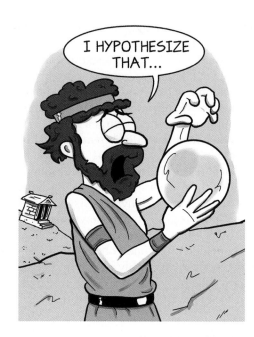

if the calculated statistic is less than the critical one, the probability that sampling error caused that statistic to occur is greater than .05, or $p > .05$. Since a statistic this size may happen often by chance— in this case more often than 5% of the time—we conclude that sampling error most likely caused it.

 ***If the calculated statistic is less than the critical statistic, the null hypothesis is accepted. However, if it is greater than or equal to the critical statistic, the null hypothesis is rejected.***

How does the investigator use this information? If the calculated statistic is less than the critical statistic, the researcher accepts the null hypothesis. However, if it is greater than or equal to the critical statistic, the null hypothesis is rejected. At this point the hypothesis test is complete, and the researcher is left with the task of interpreting the results and determining what it means in relation to the originally stated research hypothesis.

## Steps in the Hypothesis Test

Having discussed the components of a general hypothesis test, let's see how the process leads to a conclusion regarding the data. Follow the steps outlined in Table 9-3 to facilitate the process.

As an example, suppose a physical educator is interested in knowing whether there is a significant difference in the vertical jump height of college women's basketball (BB)

## TABLE 9-3. Steps in a Hypothesis Test

1. State the null and alternative hypotheses.

   $H_0: \mu_1 = \mu_2$ or $H_A: \mu_1 \neq \mu_2$
2. Set the level of significance (alpha).

   .05, .01, .001
3. Determine the appropriate statistic.

   Independent or correlated $t$, $r$, ANOVA, etc.
4. Calculate the degrees of freedom and determine the critical statistic value.
5. Place the critical values on a curve to determine the areas for "do not reject" and "reject".

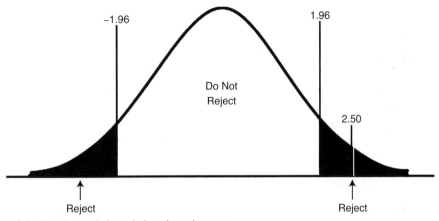

6. Calculate the statistic and place it on the curve.
7. Accept or reject the null hypothesis.
8. Draw statistical and research (practical) conclusions.

and volleyball (VB) players. The investigator's research hypothesis is that there will be no difference between the jump heights of the athletes from these two sports. The researcher obtains a random sample of 100 athletes from each sport and finds that the basketball players had a mean vertical jump of 27 inches, whereas the volleyball players had a mean of 25 inches. To determine if the 2-inch difference in jump height was due to sampling error or represented a real difference, she performs a hypothesis test. She starts off by stating the null and alternative hypotheses: $H_0: \mu_{BB} = \mu_{VB}$ and $H_A: \mu_{BB} \neq \mu_{VB}$. Remember that stating the null and alternative hypotheses may not reflect the original research hypothesis (i.e., what the researcher thinks will happen); they're simply tools used to test it. Also, recall that the null hypothesis is assumed to be true until proven otherwise and is the statement being tested with these procedures. She thinks the .05 level of significance is satisfactory for this research problem and uses that as the alpha level. The appropriate statistic in this case is called a $t$ statistic, and the $t$ sampling distribution is used to test it. (The $t$ statistic has not been discussed yet and is covered in a later chapter). Looking at the $t$ sampling distribution, she finds that the critical range of values of $t$ at the .05 level is $t = \pm 1.96$, then places those values on a model distribution and labels areas of "do not reject" and "reject." Those labels work like red and green lights and tell you what decision to make. Next, she calculates the $t$ statistic, determines that $t = 2.50$, and places it on the model distribution. Since the calculated $t = 2.50$ is greater than the critical value of $t = 1.96$ and falls in the reject area, the null hypothesis is rejected in favor of the alternative. She concludes that the 2-inch difference in vertical jump height is not due to sampling error but represents a real difference. Of course, there is a 5% chance that she is wrong, but a 95% chance she is correct. So her research hypothesis that there would be no difference in the vertical jump height is rejected. A summary of the steps in this hypothesis test appears in Table 9-4.

### TABLE 9-4. Summary of a Hypothesis Test Comparing Jump Height

1. State the null and alternative hypotheses.
   $H_0: \mu_{BB} = \mu_{VB}$
   $H_A: \mu_{BB} \neq \mu_{VB}$
2. Set the significance (alpha) level.
   .05
3. Determine the appropriate statistic.
   Independent $t$
4. Determine the critical statistic values.
   $t \pm 1.96$
5. Place the critical values on a curve and determine the areas of "do not reject" and "reject."

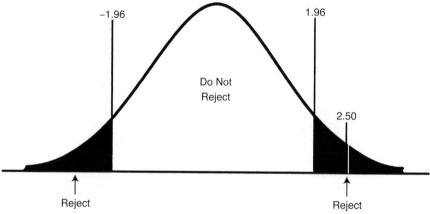

6. Calculate the statistic and place it on the curve.
   $t = 2.50$
7. Do not reject or reject the null hypothesis.
   Reject the null.
8. Draw a research conclusion.
   The 2-in. difference in vertical jump height is statistically significant.
   ($p \leq .05$).

## Two-Tailed versus One-Tailed Hypothesis Tests

In the previous example, critical values of *t* were ±1.96 and were placed on each end of the curve. In this case, that means that the area under the curve from the mean of zero to 1.96 is about 47.5%, with the remaining 2.5% outside of that value. This is also true for –1.96. Therefore, 95% of the sampling distributions values are in the range of ±1.96, and 5% of the values are outside those values, with 2.5% on each tail of the curve. Why is the probability divided that way? When a researcher cannot reasonably or logically hypothesize about the direction of the outcome of a study, a **two-tailed hypothesis test** should be used. In the jump height example, a two-tailed test was used because the researcher had no logical basis regarding which group was going to be better than the other because athletes in both sports lift weights, do jumping drills, and so on.

If an investigator has a strong sense about the direction of outcome in a study, a **one-tailed hypothesis test** may be used. Simply said, it is easier to reject the null hypothesis with a one-tailed test because all of the probability is shifted to one tail of the distribution. This allows for a smaller critical value, which means that the calculated statistic does not have to be as large for rejection of the null hypothesis. When a one-tailed test is used, the alternative hypothesis is actually the research hypothesis, since this is what the researcher thinks is going to happen. Perhaps an example will help.

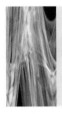

A dietitian wants to compare the intake of saturated, monounsaturated, and polyunsaturated fats in 10- to 12-year-old children in Spain and Portugal. Little previous research evidence is available. In comparing the two groups, should she use a one-tailed or a two-tailed hypothesis test? Defend your answer.

A wellness director for a company wants to determine whether a smoking cessation program is effective. It is unlikely for a smoking cessation program to cause subjects to increase their rate of smoking, and if the program is ineffective, smoking rates will probably stay about the same. The most likely outcome, if the program is effective, is that the smoking rates will decrease. This situation justifies the use of a one-tailed test. The investigator conducts the study and determines that there was a 20% reduction in smoking rates. He is now ready for the hypothesis test. This test is summarized in Table 9-5.

The null and alternative hypotheses are now stated directionally, with the null appearing as $H_0$: $\mu_{\text{Pre}} \leq \mu_{\text{Post}}$ and the alternative as $H_A$: $\mu_{\text{Pre}} > \mu_{\text{Post}}$. Note what these hypotheses are inferring. The null indicates that either there will be no difference between the pre-test and post-test means, suggesting that the program will not be effective, or there will be an increase in smoking rates, making the post-test mean larger than the pre-test mean, suggesting that the program increased smoking. The alternative hypothesis states that the pre-test values will be greater than the post-test values, or that smoking rates will decrease. This is probably what the researcher anticipates.

**TABLE 9-5. Summary of a One-Tailed Hypothesis Test on Smoking Cessation**

1. State the null and alternative hypotheses.
   $H_0: \mu_{Pre} \leq \mu_{Post}$
   $H_A: \mu_{Pre} > \mu_{Post}$
2. Set the significance (alpha) level.
   .05
3. Determine the appropriate statistic.
   Correlated $t$
4. Determine the critical statistic value.
   $t = 1.65$
5. Place the critical values on a curve and determine the areas of "do not reject" and "reject."

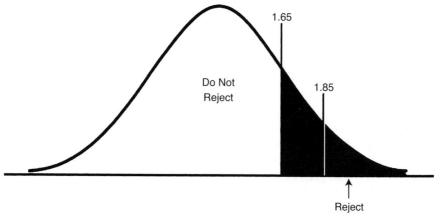

6. Calculate the statistic and place it on the curve.
   $t = 1.85$
7. Do not reject or reject the null hypothesis.
   Reject the null.
8. Draw a research conclusion.
   The 20% reduction in smoking rate is statistically significant
   ($p \leq .05$).

The correct statistic is the correlated $t$ (covered in a later chapter), and use of the $t$ distribution shows that the critical value for a one-tailed test is $t = 1.65$ at the .05 level. The calculated statistic is $t = 1.85$. These values are placed on the model distribution and labeled with areas of "reject" and "do not reject." It can be seen that the calculated $t = 1.85$ falls in the reject area, so the null hypothesis is rejected. Since the $t = 1.85$ may occur by chance or sampling error 5% of the time or less, it is concluded that the 20% reduction in smoking rates was real.

If the researcher had used a two-tailed test instead, the critical values would have been higher. In this example, the two-tailed critical values would have been $t = \pm 1.96$.

Since the calculated $t = 1.85$ does not exceed or is equal to $t = \pm 1.96$, the null hypothesis would *not* have been rejected and a different research conclusion would have been made. Therefore, when the investigator has a strong idea about the direction of outcome, a one-tailed test should be used. Examples of one-tailed tests will be presented in future chapters.

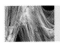 What is the advantage of using a one-tailed statistical hypothesis?

## INTERPRETATIONS AFTER THE HYPOTHESIS TEST

You may have read statistical analyses reported in a research journal that said something like "there was a significant difference between the two groups, $p \leq .01$" or "there was no significant difference between the two methods, $p > .05$." Two important points should be pointed out about these statements. The first deals with how the probability statements are made. When stating that a finding is statistically significant, the probability arrow that follows the $p$ level points in the less-than direction ($p <$). This statement means that the probability that sampling error could cause that statistic to occur would be less than or equal to the stated alpha level. Since a statistic this size may rarely happen by chance, it is concluded that something other than sampling error caused it to occur, that is, something real. However, when stating that a finding is not statistically significant, the direction of the probability arrow points in the greater-than direction ($p >$). The interpretation of that statement is that the probability that sampling error could cause that statistic to occur would be greater than the stated alpha level. Therefore, since a statistic this size may happen often by chance, it is concluded that sampling error caused it to occur.

The other point is that the significance level of statements of statistical significance must be reported. The consumer of research can't assume that all of the tests were done at the traditional .05 level. For example, an investigator may have set an alpha level of .10 for the hypothesis tests, which would take on a different interpretation than the .01 level. So remember that statistical significance is defined by the researcher's selection of whatever the probability level for alpha is. To that end, descriptors such as *highly significant* or *barely significant* should not be used when relating the results. Those terms are subjective and open to interpretation. One should simply report the alpha level and let the outcomes regarding probability of decision error speak for themselves.

### Practical versus Statistical Significance

The level of significance may have nothing to do with the magnitude or meaning of an observed effect. For instance, how meaningful would it be if an exercise physiologist showed a 2% change in serum cholesterol levels after a 6-month exercise program, even if that change was statistically significant at $p \leq .001$? While the researcher is 99.9% sure that the exercise program caused a reduction in total cholesterol, the 2% change probably has minimal effect on health. Consequently, when reading research, don't focus entirely on whether or not the statistic is significant, but if it is, then examine how large the effect is. With large sample sizes, the magnitude of change can be small but statistically significant. This concept is important in interpreting and reporting research and is discussed in later chapters.

 With large sample sizes, the magnitude of change can be quite small yet statistically significant. Hence, both significance and degree of change should be examined in research. They do not necessarily go hand in hand.

The hypothesis test is used to make a statistical decision, and once that is made, it is up to the researcher to draw the appropriate conclusions and interpretations about the results. In the example of the hypothesis test steps, it was concluded that basketball players had a 2-inch greater vertical jump height. What does that mean? Was a cause-and-effect relationship demonstrated? Does a 2-inch height difference have much practical meaning? What is this difference attributed to? How do these results compare with others that have been reported? All of these are questions that the researcher must answer.

Bear in mind that hypothesis tests are based on reasonable levels of probability of making good research decisions, but they don't provide unequivocal proof. It is tempting to overinterpret the results of analyses like these simply because they are a form of objective evidence. Hypothesis tests are highly valued tools of research but are only as effective as the person who uses them. Therefore, it is incumbent on the researcher to use hypothesis tests correctly and to interpret the results from them in a cautious and scholarly manner. Likewise, the well-educated reader has the responsibility to judge the extent that these criteria are met.

## PRACTICAL HYPOTHESIS TESTING

In the preceding pages, we have presented a formal method of hypothesis testing. However, experienced investigators rarely use this approach when interpreting research results. When given a computer printout of the data analysis, the researcher will probably examine it for the calculated statistic and the $p$ level of its occurrence to determine whether it is statistically significant. In the example of the vertical jump study, an alpha level of .05 was set, and a 2-inch difference in vertical jump height resulted in a calculated $t = 2.50$ (result on a computer printout). The computer printout also showed that the $p$ level of $t = 2.50$ was $p = .0367$. The researcher would examine this and conclude that since .0367 is less than .05, the null hypothesis can be rejected. In other words, $t = 2.50$ is statistically significant at the $p = .05$ level (actually at the .0367 level). Conversely, if $t = 1.40$ is reported to be at $p = .4520$, it would not be significant at the .05 level, since .4520 is greater than .05.

| Statistic | *p* Level | Alpha | Decision |
|-----------|-----------|-------|----------|
| *t* = 2.50 | .0367 | .05 | Since *p* .0367 is less than or equal to .05, *t* = 2.50 is statistically significant ($p \leq .05$), and the null hypothesis is rejected. |
| *t* = 1.40 | .4520 | .05 | Since *p* .4520 is greater than .05, *t* = 1.40 is not statistically significant ($p > .05$), and the null hypothesis is not rejected. |

**Figure 9-2.** A hypothetical computer output of data analysis.

Therefore, a simple way of interpreting a computer analysis or printout is to compare the *p* level of the calculated statistic to the predetermined alpha level. If it is less than or equal to that level, the null hypothesis may be rejected; that is, the results are significant at that alpha level (e.g., $p \leq .05$). If the calculated statistic's *p* level is greater than the alpha, the null hypothesis cannot be rejected (e.g., $p > .05$). Figure 9-2 shows a hypothetical computer output and interpretations of examples just given.

## Summary

Probability plays an important role in many research decisions. The normal curve and many sampling distributions are based on probability statements and are used extensively in hypothesis testing. The hypothesis test is a vital tool for making research decisions. When performing a hypothesis test, the researcher needs to consider the following: stating the null and alternative hypotheses, setting a level of significance in regard to making type I or II errors, selecting an appropriate statistic and sampling distribution, comparing a calculated statistic to a critical statistic, deciding whether to accept or reject the null hypothesis, and drawing a research conclusion. Since the hypothesis test doesn't provide absolute proof, the researcher has the ultimate responsibility of arriving at the appropriate conclusions.

## Learning Activities

1. Have you accomplished the objectives stated at the beginning of the chapter? If not, go back and reread the concepts you're uncertain about. Also, ask your professor questions about these topics.
2. Perform hypothesis tests for the examples given in the Statistics Exercises section.
3. Examine several research articles and determine the following:
   - Were two- or one-tailed statistical tests used? Explain the rationale for each in these studies.
   - What was the reported level of significance?

- Does the level of significance seem appropriate for the type of research that was done?
- Does a higher or lower alpha level seem justified?
- Was the beta level reported? If so, what was the level?

 **Statistics Exercises**

For the following research conditions perform a hypothesis test (show all major steps) and provide the appropriate research conclusion.

1. A health researcher compares a program of dieting (D) to a program of dieting and exercise (DE) on blood cholesterol levels. The DE group had a mean reduction in cholesterol 20% greater than the D group. This resulted in a calculated statistic of $t = 4.50$ with a critical statistic of $t \pm 2.30$ at $p = .05$. What do you conclude?

2. A recreation researcher wanted to compare the average percentage of income spent on leisure activities from families in Utah and Nebraska. The results showed that Utah families averaged 18% spent, whereas the Nebraska families averaged 12%. The calculated $t = 3.25$ with a critical $t \pm 2.65$ at $p = .05$. What do you conclude?

3. An exercise science researcher is interested in comparing running 4 days per week to 6 days per week for improving aerobic capacity. The result of the study was a 3% mean difference between the two groups favoring 6 days per week. This resulted in a calculated $t = 1.25$ with a critical $t \pm 2.45$ at $p = .05$. What do you conclude?

4. A health researcher wanted to compare biofeedback with a relaxation technique in reducing stress levels. At the conclusion of the study, the biofeedback group reduced stress levels 10%, whereas the relaxation group reduced stress by 12%. This resulted in a calculated $t = 1.85$ with a critical $t \pm 2.25$ at $p = .05$. What do you conclude?

5. A physical education researcher wanted to compare the results of percent body fat measures obtained by underwater weighing (UWW) and skinfolds (SK). The results showed a mean 3.1% fat overestimation by the SK. This resulted in a calculated $t = 7.95$ with a critical $t \pm 3.75$ at $p = .01$. What do you conclude?

# CHAPTER 10

# Relationships and Predictions

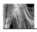

## KEY CONCEPTS

- Pearson correlation
- Simple linear regression
- Standard error of estimate
- Confidence intervals
- Multiple regression
- Multiple correlation
- Partial correlation
- Factor analysis

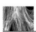

## AFTER READING THIS CHAPTER YOU SHOULD BE ABLE TO:

- Define and provide examples of each correlation-based statistic discussed.
- Differentiate between the strength of a relationship and the probability that it is real.
- Interpret correlations demonstrated in scattergrams as being positive or negative and high or low.
- Explain how the accuracy of a regression equation is determined and the factors that affect its accuracy.

Researchers and practitioners are often interested in studying the relationship between two or more variables. A swimming coach may be interested in the relationship between swimming performance and strength. A health researcher may wish to know how closely related eating habits and knowledge of nutrition are. A recreation professional may be interested in the relationship between income and percent of income expended on recreational pursuits. **Correlation** is the statistic that provides a quantitative means of expressing a relationship, and it is used widely in research.

Correlation is also used in prediction. For example, skinfold thickness can be used to predict the density of the body, which in turn is used to estimate body fatness. Universities use achievement tests and grade point average to predict success in graduate school. Buying and selling stocks is based on the prediction of prices. So prediction is commonly used in everyday life as well as in research.

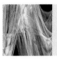

Correlation is used to express the degree that two variables are related. The relationship may be positive or negative.

## CONCEPTS IN CORRELATION

A **positive correlation** means that as the value for one variable becomes larger, the value for the other variable also *tends* to increase. Examples are age and height in children (as children increase in age, most but not all become taller), education level and income, height and weight, and saturated fat intake and incidence of cardiovascular disease. The word *tend* is important because as for the example with height and age, not every child 8 years old is expected to be taller than any 7-year-old child, and so on. Figure 10-1 is a graph or figure called a **scattergram** depicting the relationship between these two variables. With values for strength plotted on the vertical or Y-axis and values for age plotted on the horizontal or X-axis, pairs of scores (one for X and one for Y) are plotted graphically. When the plotted data run diagonally uphill from lower left to upper right, the correlation is positive. This indicates a trend for strength to increase with age. Note the exceptions to this trend, which indicate that the relationship is not perfect (see Fig. 10–1).

A **negative** or **inverse correlation** means that as the value for one variable increases, the value for the other variable *tends* to decrease. Examples of negative correlations are age of adults with strength (as adults grow older they usually lose strength), education level with smoking, and speed of sprinting 40 yards with percent body fat. Again the term *tend* is appropriate unless the correlation is perfect. For example, a few older adults may be stronger than some adults who are younger, which makes the relationship less than perfect. These exceptions can be seen in Figure 10-2. In negative correlations, the data run downhill from left to right.

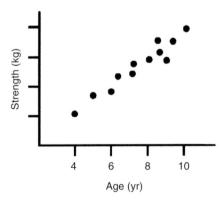

**Figure 10-1.** Relationship between strength and age in children.

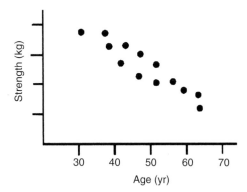

**Figure 10-2.** Relationship between strength and age in adults.

The size of correlations can also be estimated by the degree to which the data in a scattergram are clustered around a line running through them, called the **line of best fit** or **regression line.** Figures 10–1 and 10–2 show data closely clustered around an imaginary line of best fit. If the individual data points align themselves in a perfectly straight line, the correlation is perfect. The data in the two figures nearly form a straight line and therefore represent a high correlation. Figure 10-3 shows a positive moderate correlation, whereas Figure 10-4 illustrates a negative moderate correlation. Note the greater spread of data around the line of best fit in the latter two figures.

When data are weakly related or correlated, little or no apparent pattern is obvious. One would have difficulty judging whether the data are aligned in a positive or negative direction. Figure 10-5 shows a weak correlation.

## Scattergrams

Scattergrams are a useful way to depict data dealing with relationships. Some guidelines are presented here to facilitate producing them. Computer software is widely available to enhance the ease of producing good quality scattergrams.

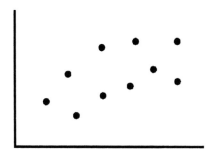

**Figure 10-3.** Moderate positive correlation.

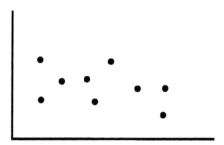

**Figure 10-4.** Moderate negative correlation.

1. Make the vertical (Y) axis three-fourths the length of the horizontal (X) axis. This allows a good spread of the data, which facilitates interpretation.
2. Place the title below the figure.
3. Label each axis and the unit of measure.
4. Provide a key or legend to identify symbols.
5. Consider using a break mark if not starting at zero. This eliminates having large portions of a figure void of any data. For example, if body weight is one variable, values for that axis would start a bit below the lightest weight plotted.

## Assumptions in Using Statistics

Use of the statistics in this chapter requires that data be absolute, interval, or ratio level. They must also be linearly related, be normally distributed, and have similar variances.

## PEARSON CORRELATION

The Pearson product moment coefficient of correlation, or Pearson $r$, is used to measure how well two variables are related to each other. Researchers use the Pearson $r$ to assess, for example, relationships between vertical jump and leg strength, cholesterol level and incidence of cardiovascular disease, score on a test in a health unit on nutrition and percent of calories consumed from fat.

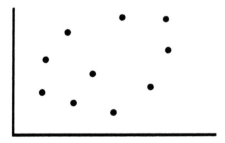

**Figure 10-5.** Weak positive correlation.

**TABLE 10-1. Calculation of Pearson *r***

| | Pull-ups | | | Push-ups | |
|---|---|---|---|---|---|
| Subject | X | Y | $X^2$ | $Y^2$ | XY |
| A | 8 | 17 | 64 | 289 | 136 |
| B | 5 | 12 | 25 | 144 | 60 |
| C | 7 | 11 | 49 | 121 | 77 |
| D | 12 | 26 | 144 | 676 | 312 |
| E | 2 | 4 | 4 | 16 | 8 |
| N = 5 | $\sum X = 34$ | $\sum Y = 70$ | $\sum X^2 = 286$ | $\sum Y^2 = 1246$ | $\sum XY = 593$ |

$$r = \frac{N \sum XY - (\sum X)(\sum Y)}{\sqrt{\left(N \sum X^2 - [\sum X]^2\right)\left(N \sum Y^2 - [\sum Y]^2\right)}}$$

$$r = \frac{5(593) - (34)(70)}{\sqrt{(5(286) - 34^2)(5(1246) - 70^2)}}$$

$$r = \frac{2965 - 2380}{\sqrt{(1430 - 1156)(6230 - 4900)}} = .969$$

The formula for calculating a Pearson *r* is

$$r = \frac{N \sum XY - (\sum X)(\sum Y)}{\sqrt{\left(N \sum X^2 - [\sum X]^2\right)\left(N \sum Y^2 - [\sum Y]^2\right)}}$$

The steps in a sample problem are summarized in Table 10-1. Here, a researcher wishes to measure the relationship between pull-ups and push-ups. The score for each variable is recorded under the X and Y columns. Either variable can be assigned as X or Y. The values are squared, summed, and cross-multiplied, with the appropriate values substituted in the equation. N refers to the number of pairs of observations or the number of subjects.

## Interpretation

The researcher usually wishes to know three things about a correlation: (1) whether it is significant, (2) whether it is positive or negative, and (3) how strong it is. If the relationship is real or significant, the second two questions must be addressed. If it is not significant, the latter two points are irrelevant.

**Significance** If a correlation is significantly different from zero, it indicates that it most likely exists and is not attributable to chance or sampling error. Correlation coefficients range from $-1$ to $+1$. The *r* of .969 is nearly a perfectly positive relationship. Examining Table A–4 in Appendix A (Critical Values of *r*), with degrees of freedom $(df) = N - 2$ or $5 - 2 = 3$, *r* must equal .878 or higher with a two-tailed test to be significant at the .05 level. The calculated *r* exceeds that amount and so is judged to be a real relationship. Thus, in

## TABLE 10-2. Steps in a Correlation Hypothesis Test

1. State the null and alternative hypotheses.
   $H_0: r = 0$
   $H_A: r \neq 0$
2. Set the significance (alpha) level.
   .05
3. Determine the appropriate statistic.
   Pearson $r$
4. Determine the critical statistic value.
   $r = \pm.878$
5. Place the critical values on a curve and determine the areas of "do not reject" and "reject."

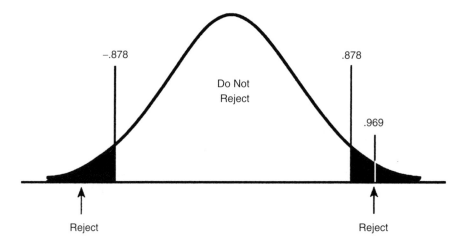

6. Calculate the statistic and place it on the curve.
   $r = .969$
7. Accept or reject the null hypothesis.
   The null hypothesis is rejected.
8. Draw a research conclusion.
   There is a significant relationship ($p \leq .05$) between pull-ups and pushups.

the sample problem, the null hypothesis, $r = 0$, is rejected, and the alternative hypothesis, $r \neq 0$, is accepted. Table 10-2 summarizes the steps in hypothesis testing for correlation. A computer printout of a correlation is typically used to determine whether a correlation is statistically significant. A typical computer printout with the interpretation of the information is shown in Figure 10-6. The interpretation here is that subjects performing well in the pull-up test tended to do well in push-ups, and subjects scoring low in one test tended to score low in the other. Thus, performance in the two tests is well related. The relationship is not perfect, however, because there are exceptions to this overall trend.

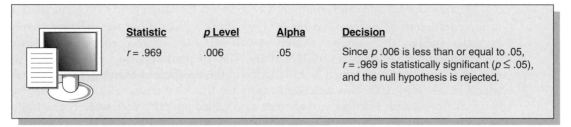

| Statistic | p Level | Alpha | Decision |
|---|---|---|---|
| r = .969 | .006 | .05 | Since p .006 is less than or equal to .05, r = .969 is statistically significant (p ≤ .05), and the null hypothesis is rejected. |

**Figure 10-6.** A typical computer printout showing a correlation.

When testing nondirectional hypotheses for correlation, a two-tailed test is used as was done in the sample problem for pull-ups and push-ups. Hypotheses are usually stated in the null form when the sign of the correlation to be determined is uncertain. However, when researchers are reasonably certain that most pairs of data will be positive or negative, they use a directional hypothesis. An example might be the relationship between height and weight. Overall, it would be strongly suspected before collecting data that the variables are positively related. Therefore the null hypothesis would be stated directionally: $r \leq 0$. The alternative hypothesis would be stated $r > 0$. Directional hypothesis testing allows use of the one-tailed column for critical values. This increases the likelihood of achieving significance, since the rejection area appears all on the positive end of the normal curve, which places the value closer to the middle. An example of an expected negative relationship would be incidence of cardiovascular disease and level of physical activity (i.e., as physical activity increases, the incidence of cardiovascular disease tends to decrease). Here also a directional hypothesis would be stated ($r \geq 0$; alternative hypothesis is $r < 0$) and a one-tailed test used.

**Positive or Negative Relationship** The sign indicates whether the correlation is positive or negative. The correlation calculated in the sample problem is positive, so we know that as performance measures in one variable increase, so do performance measures in the other variable.

**Strength** The strength of a correlation is entirely different from significance. It is commonly misinterpreted that significance denotes that a relationship is strong. One means of judging the strength of correlations is a subjective rating based only on the size of $r$. The ratings apply to both positive as well as negative correlations: .25 or lower is weak, .26 to .50 is moderate, .51 to .75 is fair, and .76 and above is high. The terms are limited in that what is weak or fair to one person may not be equally weak or fair to another. A common mistake in interpretation of correlations is that a negative $r$ implies a weak

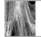

*The strength of a relationship is an entirely different quality from significance.*

relationship. This is not so, as is explained shortly. Terms such as weak, moderate, and fair are descriptive in a general way but lack precision. Therefore, they are best used to supplement more exact quantitative information.

The most meaningful and common way to assess the strength of $r$ is by calculation of the **coefficient of determination** ($r^2$), which is a measure of the variance shared by two variables. This variance shared by two variables is called **common variance** and represents what the two variables share. The calculation is easy: $r^2 \times 100$. The remaining variance is determined by calculation of the **coefficient of nondetermination,** which is $(1 - r^2) \times 100$. This represents variance that is unique to each variable and hence is not shared. For this reason, it is also called **specific variance.** These statistics indicate entirely different information from that provided by determining whether the $r$ is significant. The fact that an $r$ value is significant indicates only high confidence that a relationship exists; nothing is indicated about its strength. With a large N, a .20 correlation may be significant, yet the variance accounted for by the relationship is only 4% ($.20^2 \times 100 = 4$). Therefore, when correlations are presented in research, they should include information regarding both significance *and* strength.

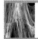

*Negative correlations do not imply weak relationships but simply the direction of the relationship.*

Negative correlations do not imply weak relationships, as is sometimes mistakenly thought. A negative number squared is positive, and therefore negative correlations can explain just as much variance as do positive correlations.

In our example, the $r$ between the pull-up and push-up scores was .969. The variance shared by or common to the variables is 94% ($.969^2 \times 100 = 94$). Consequently, the two variables have much in common. Theoretically, what might be some of the common factors? They may include upper body strength and local muscle endurance, total body weight, percent body fat, previous practice, and skill in the two tests, for example. The coefficient of nondetermination is 6% ($100\% - 94\% = 6\%$). Thus, 6% of the variance is not shared and is attributed to other factors. Sources of specific or unique variance in this example might include grip strength (more important in pull-ups than push-ups) and strength and local muscle endurance of the elbow flexors (more important in pull-ups) and elbow extensors (more important in push-ups). Figure 10-7 shows the degree of relationship by the degree of overlap of the two circles. The degree of overlap represents the variance common to both variables, whereas the portions of each circle not overlapping represent variance specific to each variable. This depiction is a useful conceptual aid called a **Venn diagram** (Fig. 10–7).

There is no universal standard for interpreting the size of the coefficients of determination and nondetermination. Researchers and readers of research must interpret the findings for themselves. In general, however, the more variance explained, the more meaningful the relationship.

## Cause-and-Effect Relationships

Researchers are often interested in determining whether one variable, such as an intervention, causes a change in a second variable. For example, medical researchers test the effectiveness of various drugs. By nature of the purpose and design of a study, some research attempts to establish cause and effect: variable A causes a change in

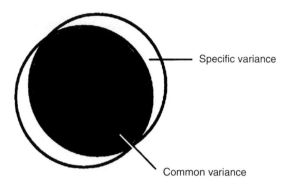

**Figure 10-7.** Percent common and specific variance.

variable B. Correlation by itself does not examine cause and effect. Yet the most common misconception about correlation is that a cause-and-effect relationship exists. Some variables may well have a cause-and-effect relationship, but a Pearson *r* by itself does not determine this. For example, decades ago, epidemiologists in a number of studies found high positive correlations between cholesterol level and incidence of cardiovascular disease. Yet they could not infer that high cholesterol caused cardiovascular disease. Only experimental studies in which intake of dietary fat is controlled can produce scientific evidence that excessive cholesterol in the diet or blood actually caused the disease. Because of this limitation in the use of correlation, it is often used as a preliminary stage of knowledge development. The study of lifestyle and disease by epidemiologists and health specialists often begins with examination of relationships between how people live and the incidence of disease.

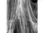 *The most common misconception about a correlation is that a cause-and-effect relationship exists.* Correlation is the statistic of choice because if significant and strong relationships are found, *then* experimental studies can be initiated to determine actual causes of disease.

So don't assume cause-and-effect relationships from correlation. Here are several examples of possible leaps in logic. A researcher found a significant $r = -.78$, between the amount of tea consumed in three countries and incidence of osteoporosis. It was concluded that the more tea one drank, the lower the incidence of osteoporosis. However, the correlation by itself does not mean the tea reduced osteoporosis; it may have been other health-related factors. For example, perhaps those who drank more tea also exercised more, so it may not have been the tea itself that caused the reduced osteoporosis.

Here's another example that demonstrates how illogical the assumption of cause and effect can be. An economist notes that as Halley's comet approached closer to earth over several weeks, inflation rose significantly and concluded that Halley's comet not only was causing inflation but predicted that as it passed by the earth and slowly burned itself out, inflation would gradually drop.

| TABLE 10-3. Correlation Matrix | | | | |
|---|:---:|:---:|:---:|:---:|
| *Variable* | *1* | *2* | *3* | *4* |
| 1. Height (cm) | — | .70 | .80 | .40 |
| 2. Weight (kg) | | — | .50 | .40 |
| 3. Leg length (cm) | | | — | .20 |
| 4. Wrist circumference (cm) | | | | — |

Here is one last example. A dermatologist noted that as more cases of severe sunburn occurred during an especially hot summer, the sales of ice cream also rose. It was concluded that ice cream increases susceptibility to sunburn and that fair-skinned people should eat ice cream in limited amounts.

## Correlation Matrix

A common method for reporting a number of correlations is by presentation in a table called a **correlation matrix.** Reading numerous correlation coefficients and the associated variables in paragraph form is tedious. A table greatly facilitates comprehension. Table 10-3 is an example of a correlation matrix. Each variable is numbered in column 1, and the same variables are listed as column headings by number. Either the row or column headings must be identified but not both, since each number represents the same variable. No value is given under column 1, row 1 because this value would represent the $r$ of height with itself, which, of course, would be 1.00. Therefore, the $r$ of each variable with itself is deleted in the table. The $r$ between any two variables is located where they intersect in the table. The $r$ between height and weight is .70; the $r$ between wrist circumference and weight is .40. Half of the values in the table appear to be missing. These values are not needed because the values to the left of an imaginary line running diagonally through the table are identical with the values already in the table. Thus, half of the table is a mirror image of the other half.

## Other Uses of Correlation

Pearson $r$ is used for several other purposes. Several of these are described here.

**Reliability** Reliability refers to the consistency of measurements. For example, in assessing nutritional status, subjects may be instructed to record all food and drink consumed for several days. The reliability of the measurement can be determined by assessing food intake a second occasion in the same subjects and performing a Pearson $r$ between the two measures. If protein intake is the variable of interest, then the $r$ between protein intake on each occasion is calculated. The higher the correlation is, the higher the reliability.

**Objectivity** Objectivity is the reliability or consistency of measurement between different test administrators. A high $r$ between two researchers measuring blood pressure in the same people indicates a good consistency in the measurements.

**Validity** Validity indicates how well a test measures what is intended to be tested. Researchers typically validate tests by correlating the results of a new test with the results obtained from the best accepted test, known as the gold standard. A high $r$ between the results of the two tests indicates a good level of agreement which validates the accuracy of the new test.

## PREDICTION: SIMPLE LINEAR REGRESSION

Most of us are involved at times with predictions. Acceptance into graduate school is often based on an achievement test score used to predict academic success. Fitness evaluations typically are based on field tests that predict the score you would have achieved on a more sophisticated test in a laboratory. Economists predict unemployment and business trends. **Simple linear regression** is used to make a prediction from a variable based on the correlation between two variables. It is the simplest form of prediction because only one predictor variable is used.

### Linear Regression Equation

The equation is based on the formula for a straight line ($Y' = bX + a$) and predicts a Y value from one value of X. Because a and b in the equation for a straight line must each be calculated, a one-step formula for simple linear regression is:

$$Y' = bX + A$$

where

$$Y' = \text{predicted score or dependent variable}$$
$$b = \text{slope of the regression line} = r(S_y/S_x)$$
$$a = \text{y intercept} = M_y - bM_x$$
$$X = \text{score for the independent variable}$$
$$M_y = \text{mean of Y scores}$$
$$M_x = \text{mean of X scores}$$
$$S_x = \text{SD of X scores}$$
$$S_y = \text{SD of Y scores}$$

The letter **b** stands for the slope or steepness of the regression line. It can be positive (line running uphill) or negative (running downhill). It represents the change in the

---

**TABLE 10-4. Simple Linear Regression Equation**

Bench press (Y): = 200 lb, $SD_y = 20$
Pushups (X): $M_x = 30$, $SD_x = 5$
Correlation: r = .80
$b = r (SD_y/SD_x) = .80 (20/5) = .80 (4) = 3.2$
$a = M_y - bM_x = 200 - 3.2 (30) = 200 - 96 = 104$
$Y = bX + a = 3.2X + 104$

---

Y variable for each unit change in X. If X increases one unit while Y increases four, the slope is four. The letter **a** represents the Y intercept, or point on the Y-axis where the regression line intersects (where X = 0). X represents the known value of the X variable used to predict Y; that is, you know the score for variable X and will use it to predict the Y score.

A sample problem appears in Table 10-4 in which a researcher wishes to predict the heaviest lift one can make in the bench press (Y). The independent or predictor variable (X) is the maximum number of push-ups one can do in 30 seconds.

This equation can be used to predict the maximum bench press lift for other participants from the same population. For example, suppose we wish to predict the maximum bench press for John Doe. He performs the 30-second push-up test and completes 25 repetitions; 25 is the X value used in the regression equation. His bench press maximum is estimated by substitution into the linear regression equation:

$$Y' = bX + a = 3.2(25) + 104 = 80 + 104 = 184 \text{ lb}$$

Therefore, John's estimated bench press is 184 lb. Such a prediction may be useful if a person cannot perform maximal lifting because of an injury or because the instructor didn't want to expose certain individuals to the risk of maximal lifting. Furthermore, a weight training instructor may wish to predict maximal scores simply to save time. Performance of a 30-second push-up test could be accomplished by an entire class in minutes, whereas strength in the bench press would require considerable time for thorough warm-up and gradually increasing loads up to maximum.

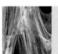
Simple linear regression is "simple" in that it uses only one independent or predictor variable.

## Line of Best Fit and Scattergram

A scattergram is often constructed via computer software to aid interpretation of the equation for the line of best fit. The points where each subject's pair of scores fall are plotted on a graph. This line of best fit passes through the mean of all of the X and Y scores. Figure 10-8 depicts the regression line for data on the 30-second push-up test and maximum bench press. The line of best fit can be used visually to predict any Y score by plotting the point on the regression line that intersects with the X score. The best

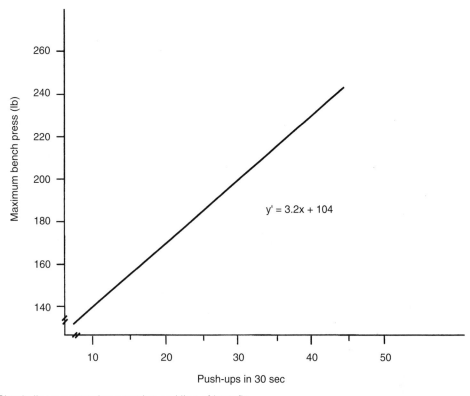

**Figure 10-8.** Simple linear regression equation and line of best fit.

predicted Y score is the value that intersects with the regression line at the same point as the associated X score.

The scattergram in Figure 10-9 depicts a line of best fit from the equation, $Y = -3X + 10$. Note that the slope is negative (a slope of $-3$ means a descent of $-3$ units for Y for each unit change of X), and that the line intersects the Y axis at positive 10.

## Accuracy of an Estimate

Although it is helpful to be able to predict something, the prediction is limited unless it is reasonably accurate. Nearly all prediction equations are in error to some extent unless they were generated from variables perfectly correlated. This is rarely if ever the case. The **standard error of estimate (*SEE*)** is the average error in a prediction equation. Statistically, it is the standard deviation of actual scores around the prediction line or the predicted Y value. The difference between each person's actual score and score predicted from the regression line is an estimation error, or a **residual.** The *SEE* quantifies the

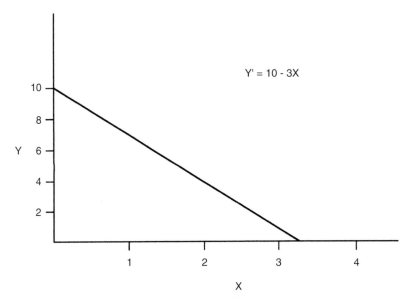

**Figure 10-9.** Simple linear regression equation and line of best fit.

size of this error and therefore is a measure of the accuracy of a prediction equation or prediction line. It is calculated as follows:

$$SEE = S_y\sqrt{1 - r^2}$$

A small *SEE*, which indicates greater accuracy of prediction, occurs when two variables are highly correlated with each other. Actually, if $r = 1.00$, there is no prediction error and the *SEE* = 0. One would not expect to obtain much accuracy in prediction if using finger length to predict bone density, because as far as we know the two variables are not related to each other. Thus, when examining scattergrams, unless the data are reasonably close to the regression line, the correlation is probably not particularly high, and one variable would not be a strong predictor of the other; that is, the *SEE* would be relatively large.

*The standard error of estimate (SEE) indicates the accuracy of a prediction equation.*

Typically, about 68% of predicted scores fall within 1 *SEE* of the prediction line; about 95% of scores lie within 1.96 *SEEs*, and nearly all scores fall within 2.58 *SEEs*. These represent the 68%, 95%, and 99% **confidence intervals,** respectively. For example, using data from the example on push-ups and bench press, the *SEE* equals

$$Sy\sqrt{1 - r^2} = 20\sqrt{1 - .80^2} = 20\,(.6) = 12\ \text{lb}$$

The confidence intervals for a predicted bench press score of 180 lb would be

$$68\% = 180 \pm 1(12) = 168\ \text{to}\ 192\ \text{lb}$$

$$95\% = 180 \pm 1.96(12) = 156.5 \text{ to } 203.5 \text{ lb}$$

$$99\% = 180 \pm 2.58(12) = 149 \text{ to } 211 \text{ lb}$$

Thus, we would expect about 68% of participants whose predicted score was 180 to be within one *SEE* or 12 lb of their actual value.

Researchers wishing to accurately predict a variable should strive to use variables as highly correlated as possible and to use a reasonably large sample size, since N size tends to improve the correlation and shrink the standard deviation of the Y variable. The combination of high $r$ and small standard deviation results in good predictive accuracy, or a low *SEE*.

A determinant of correlation and hence SEE is the concept known as **restricted range.** If one was trying to predict academic success in graduate school based on high school GPA, but the GPAs were all very high—say 3.60 to 4.00—then the correlation between GPA and academic success would also be small because there is so little variation in GPA. Hence, high school GPA would not be very effective in distinguishing academic success in graduate school. However, if GPA scores varied from 2.10 to 4.0, the correlation would be expected to be much higher, as would the ability to estimate academic success from GPA. To emphasize the point even further, if all the GPAs were identical in a subset of students, GPA would be of no help at all in predicting academic success. Therefore, the following principle may be stated: The size of a correlation and hence the accuracy of an estimate are both directly affected by the range of scores. Small or restricted range reduces the size of the correlation while a large range increases the correlation.

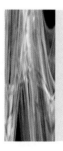

An athletic trainer wishes to determine whether hamstring flexibility can predict hamstring pulls in a group of athletes. Over 1 year, only two hamstring injuries occur in 50 athletes. Do you think the two variables will be significantly related? From these data, can the incidence of hamstring pulls be predicted very accurately? To effectively answer the research question, what would you advise the athletic trainer to do regarding the study?

When reading research that reports correlations, examine the range of the data to determine whether it explains in part how small or large the relationship is. For example, it is common to see values for Pearson $r$ that are high in one study but rather small in a different study. For example, the relationship between bone density and calcium intake in one study may be $r = .25$, whereas another study reports the $r$ to be .65. The difference may be explained partly by the fact that the calcium intake in the latter group was far larger than in the former group. The range is commonly reported in studies so become accustomed to noting it when interpreting the results of a study.

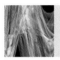 The size of a correlation is usually limited when the range of scores is very small. This also reduces the accuracy of prediction.

The size of the *SEE* should be a primary factor in deciding whether a prediction is accurate enough to use. Would you use an equation to predict cholesterol level if the *SEE* were 40 mg/100 mL? This would mean that about two-thirds of people tested would be within 40 units of their actual cholesterol or that the probability is .68 that the confidence interval contained the actual score. Some people may be as much as about 3 SEEs from the actual value, in which case the error would be 120 units! Because mean cholesterol values in the population are about 215 mg/100 mL, the predictive error associated with this equation would not allow its use. The point is that the size of the *SEE* should be considered in selection of measurements to use in the professional setting.

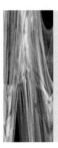 A group of researchers would like to determine if waist circumference is a good predictor of total daily physical activity in high school boys. If the range for waist circumference in the group studied is 28 to 32 inches, do you think that the predictive accuracy will be very high? What would likely happen to the correlation between the two variables and the SEE if more subjects were included in the study so that the range of values was 26 to 41 inches?

## PREDICTION: MULTIPLE REGRESSION

**Multiple regression** is a means of making a prediction from two or more independent or predictor variables. It is typically more accurate than simple linear regression because more information is used in making the prediction. Examples of multiple regression are predicting academic success from socioeconomic level, IQ, and score on a standardized test; predicting body fatness from skinfold thickness at three sites; and predicting participation in high-risk outdoor adventure activities from birth order, participation in interscholastic sport, and socioeconomic level.

 *Adding variables to a prediction equation tends to improve its accuracy.*

The concept of adding variables to improve prediction is intuitively logical. When a coach considers recruiting a football player, he undoubtedly uses more than one bit of information to predict the potential value of this player to the team. The coach may view game films from high school; request from the high school coach performance data, such as 40-yard dash time, strength, and agility; and even watch the player in a game. The sum of the information tends to allow the coach to more accurately predict whether a scholarship should be offered to the player than if only one piece of information is known.

The calculation of a multiple regression equation is an extension of the equation for a straight line or regression line:

$$Y' = a + bX_1 + bX_2 + bX_3...$$

For each predictor variable, a bX component is added to the equation. Each predictor variable contributes some information to the equation. Because the number of steps in the equation is proportional to the number of predictor variables, calculation of a multiple regression equation is rather lengthy. Because computer software allows one to derive an answer quickly, the mathematical steps are not shown here.

## Interpretation

The following is an example of a multiple regression equation used to predict the risk of coronary heart disease (CHD). CHD risk is the dependent variable or variable being predicted and four independent or predictor variables are used.

$$Y' = 35.0 + 1.0X_1 - .02X_2 + .10X_3 + .50X_4$$

where

$$Y' = \text{CHD risk score}$$

$$X_1 = \text{number of cigarettes smoke each day}$$

$$X_2 = \text{physical activity level each day}$$

$$X_3 = \text{stress rating}$$

$$X_4 = \text{waist circumference}$$

A computer program first correlates (Pearson $r$) each predictor or independent variable with CHD. Variables are selected to account for the most variance and in the sequence of the strongest to the weakest predictor. Therefore, in the CHD equation, smoking accounted for the most variance and waist circumference the least. As more variables are added to the prediction, more variance tends to be explained. The **multiple correlation, $R$,** is the correlation of two or more variables together with the dependent variable. The effect of each variable in explaining variance is often summarized in a table such as Table 10-5.

The $r$ between smoking and CHD was .50, which explained 25% of the variance in CHD ($.50^2 \times 100 = 25\%$). The addition of the second best predictor, physical activity level, increased the multiple $R$ to .60, which increased the explained variance to 36%. The third and fourth variable each increased the $R$ and explained a bit more variance. Realize that the improvement in explained variance is due to the pooled correlation of

| TABLE 10-5. Summary of Multiple Correlations of Variables with CHD | | |
|---|---|---|
| *Variable* | *R* | *R²* x 100 |
| Smoking | .50 | 25.0% |
| Physical activity | .60 | 36.0 |
| Stress | .65 | 42.2 |
| Abdominal girth | .68 | 46.2 |

CHD, coronary heart disease.

variables with CHD. Thus, in step two, smoking and physical activity *together* have an *R* of .60 with the criterion and *together* explain 36% of the variance in CHD.

An important question concerning prediction deals with the number of predictor variables. How many variables are needed to obtain a good prediction? Is there a point at which little or no improvement in predictive accuracy occurs by adding more variables to an equation? Researchers typically measure a number of factors that previous research indicates or suggests are good predictors. Others may be added because they logically appear to be related. The computer sorts through the individual Pearson correlations and develops an equation that explains the most variance. When no significant improvement in explaining variance is made by adding more variables, a predictive equation developed at this point is the best equation. Interestingly, the strongest predictors after the first one or two are usually not well correlated with the other predictors. This happens because they are measuring something unique or not measured by the other variables. Thus, it contributes something new in the way of variance, thereby enhancing the accuracy of prediction.

How many variables are needed to provide an accurate prediction? The best answer is that variables should be added until addition of more variables does not significantly contribute to the explanation of variance. The number of variables used is often limited by the number of subjects available. At least three or four subjects are needed per variable used in an equation for an equation to be reasonably accurate. Thus, if three predictor variables were used in an equation, at least 9 to 12 subjects would be required. A sample of about 10 to 20 subjects per variable provides even greater accuracy (Kerlinger & Pedhazar, 1973). It is common for journal reviewers to require this latter standard for studies using multiple regression. Great departure from this ratio tends to raise the correlation spuriously, which may falsely produce high multiple correlations. This is a common limitation seen in published literature. For this reason, researchers usually limit the number of predictor variables to those with some logical basis for inclusion.

The plus and minus signs in the equation denote whether the correlation between each predictor variable and the dependent variable was positive or negative. The positive signs before smoking, stress rating, and waist circumference indicate that each was positively associated with increased risk of CHD. The only negative correlation was with physical activity level, which is logical: as physical activity increased, risk of CHD decreased.

## Specificity of Prediction

The last point to be made in discussing prediction is that a prediction equation is sound or valid only for subjects with traits nearly identical with those of the subjects used in the development of an equation. This concept is expressed in the term **population specificity.** A good example deals with the many equations using skinfold thickness to estimate body fatness. Because many studies that developed equations were based on relatively small sample sizes of athletes of one gender in one sport in one small age range, perhaps as many as 100 prediction equations evolved. Each, however, was valid only for people with the identical sex, age range, and sport as those of the subjects in the original investigation. Each equation was thus population specific.

To develop prediction equations for a broader spectrum of the population, many more subjects with diversity of traits must be used. For example, a **general equation** to predict percent body fat from skinfold thickness in females in their mid teens to beyond age 60 was developed by Jackson, Pollock, and Ward (1980). They used several hundred female subjects in this age range with a wide variety of body fatness levels to formulate the equation.

An important criterion for making sound predictions is accurate measurement of the independent variable. If the accuracy of the value for an independent variable is inaccurate, one cannot expect the outcome of the prediction to be sound.

## PARTIAL CORRELATION

A partial correlation, $r_{12.3}$, determines the relationship between two variables, with the variance of a third variable removed, partialed out, or held constant. The subscripts 1 and 2 refer to the two variables of interest, and subscript 3 refers to the variable whose influence is to be controlled. The purpose is to derive a correlation that is more pure or less tainted than using Pearson $r$. Most phenomena studied by researchers are multifactorial in the sense that a number of factors are related to the variable of interest. A limitation of using a Pearson $r$ is that the influence of other variables can easily be overlooked. For example, suppose a researcher wishes to assess the relationship between time running the marathon and maximum oxygen uptake. However, the researcher realizes that body fatness probably has something to do with the relationship; that is, leaner people tend to have higher maximum oxygen uptakes and tend to run the marathon faster. Partial correlation can be used to remove the effect of body fatness on this relationship. This statistical adjustment usually reduces the Pearson $r$, because variance is removed. Therefore, partial correlations are usually smaller than Pearson correlations. The following values illustrate this effect.

$$\text{Pearson } r_{12} = .60, r^2_{12} \times 100 = 36\%$$

$$\text{Partial } r_{12.3} = .50, r^2_{12.3} \times 100 = 25\%$$

The correlation decreased, which also reduced the explained variance ($r^2$). However, the .25 partial $r$ provides a truer and hence better understanding of the actual relationship between the two variables than the Pearson $r$.

A good example of the use of partial correlation occurred some years ago with studies that found a significant correlation between coffee consumption and incidence of cardiovascular disease. However, when researchers in later studies used partial correlation to hold the effects of smoking constant, the relationship dwindled to insignificance. So it initially appeared that coffee drinking was harmful, but after researchers controlled for the smoking that characterized some of the coffee drinkers, the relationship was found to be weak.

Researchers sometimes wish to control the association of several variables on a relationship rather than just one. This is done using first, second, or even third-order partial correlation. The result is an especially clean correlation because the variance of other variables is adjusted for.

## FACTOR ANALYSIS

Factor analysis is a method using correlation to determine the commonality in a large number of measures. One application in the field of HPER is determination of the number and kinds of test items to use when a large number of possible tests are available. For example, hundreds of test items that measure physical fitness have been used by physical educators over the years. The problem for the practitioner in the school setting was knowing which tests to use. Fleishman (1969) used factor analysis to identify different components of fitness. The procedure involved correlating all of the tests with each other. Those that were highly intercorrelated were analyzed to determine what they had in common. By noting the common feature, he could use a descriptive word or term to describe a cluster of tests. Thus evolved three areas of strength he termed explosive strength (e.g., short sprints, hops, jumps, ball throws), static strength (e.g., isometric contractions using strength measuring devices called dynamometers), and dynamic strength (e.g., pull-ups, push-ups, rope climb, dips on parallel bars). Because the tests within one cluster were well intercorrelated, a practitioner might select just one or two tests within each cluster or factor rather than using a much larger number in a haphazard manner of selection. Thus, one test from each cluster would measure a different type of strength. The same procedure was used to develop groups of tests measuring such factors as local muscle endurance, cardiovascular endurance, and flexibility.

A **factor** is a group of measures that hypothetically have something in common. Factors of human intelligence often include verbal ability, quantitative ability, abstract reasoning, spatial perceptiveness, and so on. Recreation behavior could similarly be classified using factor analysis with the result that a number of separate distinct entities might exist, such as intellectual pursuits, activities that promote physical development, activities involving social interaction, and stress reduction.

## TABLE 10-6. Summary of Correlation-Based Statistics

| *Statistic* | *Symbol* | *Key Word and Concept* |
|---|---|---|
| Pearson *r* | $r$ | Relationship between two variables |
| Partial *r* | $r_{12 \cdot 3}$ | Relationship between two variables with variance of a third variable "removed" or "controlled for" |
| Multiple correlation | $R_{1 \cdot 234}$ | Relationship of one variable with several others "combined" or "pooled" |
| Simple linear regression | $Y = bX + a$ | Prediction based on one independent variable |
| Multiple regression | $Y = b_1 X_1 \pm b_2 X_2 + a$ | Prediction from > 1 variable |
| Coefficient of determination | $r^2 \times 100$ | Variance common to two variables |
| Coefficient of nondetermination | $1 - (r^2 \times 100)$ | Variance not common to two variables; specific variance |

## Summary

The Pearson *r* correlation coefficient is used to determine the relationship between two variables. The relationship is evaluated by determining whether it is statistically significant or real as well as its strength. Care must be taken not to infer that significant relationships are causal: they may or may not be, and only experimental research can confirm cause. Pearson *r* is the basis for prediction based on one independent variable (simple linear regression) or two or more independent variables (multiple regression). The accuracy of a prediction equation is expressed by *SEE* (standard error of estimate). Correlations can also be made between several pooled variables (multiple correlation) and with the variance of a third variable removed (partial correlation). Finally, correlation is used in factor analysis to determine similarities among various tests or measures. A summary of correlation based statistics appears in Table 10-6.

## Learning Activities

1. If an *r* is significant at the .05 level, exactly what does this mean?
2. How is the strength of an *r* determined? Explain.
3. Why might two variables be significantly related yet not be strongly related?
4. Give an example in which it might be logical to think that correlation means a cause–effect relationship exists.
5. The *r* between IQ and GPA is studied in two samples. One sample consists of all 1000 students in a high school, and the other is 200 National Merit Scholarship winners.
   **a.** In which sample would you expect to find a higher *r*?
   **b.** In which sample would IQ likely be a better predictor of smoking behavior?

   **c.** When reading studies reporting correlations why should you note characteristics of the sample?

**6.** Define:
   **a.** Simple linear regression
   **b.** Multiple regression
   **c.** Partial correlation

**7.** Sketch a line of best fit or regression line with a:
   **a.** Positive slope
   **b.** Negative slope

**8.** Draw a regression line for:
   **a.** $Y' = 3 + 2\,X$
   **b.** $Y' = 7 - 3\,X$

**9.** Sketch a scattergram for a perfect correlation.

**10.** Sketch a scattergram for a:
   **a.** Positive $r$
   **b.** Negative $r$
   **c.** Small $r$

**11.** Write the symbol for each statistic:
   **a.** Pearson correlation
   **b.** Multiple correlation
   **c.** Partial correlation

**12. a.** As more variables are added to a multiple regression equation, does $R$ tend to increase or decrease?
   **b.** Give an example of this.

**13. a.** What does $R_{1 \cdot 234} = .69$ mean?
   **b.** How much variance is explained by variables 2, 3, and 4?
   **c.** How much variance is not explained by these variables?

**14. a.** Explain what $r_{12 \cdot 3}$ means.
   **b.** What is this statistic called?
   **c.** Give an example where this statistic might be used.

**15.** Does a negative $r$ mean the relationship is weak?

 **Statistics Exercises**

**1.** A health official wished to know the relationship between health care cost per family member per year and years of education. Using the following data, calculate a Pearson $r$ between the two variables. Determine whether or not the $r$ is significant at the .05 level, and the percent common and specific variance.

| Health Care Cost per Family Member | Years of Education |
|---|---|
| $1200 | 13 |
| 1400 | 14 |
| 900 | 11 |
| 1100 | 12 |
| 1500 | 17 |
| 1400 | 14 |
| 1100 | 16 |
| 1300 | 15 |
| 1700 | 19 |
| 1500 | 16 |

2. A physical education teacher administered a trunk curl test to a group of students and wanted to know how reliable the scores were. Calculate a Pearson $r$ to express reliability. What do you conclude?

| Test 1 | Test 2 |
|---|---|
| 24 | 23 |
| 23 | 23 |
| 22 | 20 |
| 22 | 25 |
| 19 | 18 |
| 17 | 19 |
| 17 | 18 |
| 17 | 16 |
| 16 | 20 |

3. A recreation director examined the relationship between the number of summers children attended an outdoor adventure camp and their grade point average. Calculate a Pearson $r$ to determine whether the relationship was significant ($p = .05$) and calculate the percent explained variance.

| Number of Summers | Grade Point Average |
|---|---|
| 2 | 3.11 |
| 1 | 3.87 |
| 4 | 2.95 |
| 2 | 3.10 |
| 3 | 3.02 |
| 4 | 2.75 |
| 3 | 2.86 |
| 3 | 3.00 |

4. The following data were collected by an exercise physiologist who wanted to derive a simple test not requiring laboratory equipment to predict overall body strength. The following data were collected:

| Grip Strength (kg) X | Overall Strength (kg) Y |
|:---:|:---:|
| 13 | 43 |
| 16 | 44 |
| 17 | 45 |
| 13 | 41 |
| 18 | 40 |
| 15 | 43 |
| 14 | 46 |
| 10 | 38 |
| 9 | 37 |
| 10 | 36 |

   **a.** Calculate the linear regression equation.
   **b.** Calculate the standard error of estimate.
   **c.** Calculate the predicted score if grip strength (X) = 13 kg.

5. A physical educator conducted a study examining the relationship between $VO_{2max}$ (Y) and 1.5 mile run times (X). A statistical analysis resulted in the following: $M_y = 45$ mL/kg/minute, $M_x = 12$ minutes, $S_y = 4.0$, $S_x = 3.0$, $r = -.85$.
   **a.** Calculate the linear regression equation and *SEE*.
   **b.** Calculate the predicted $VO_{2max}$ (Y′) and 68% confidence interval if the run time was 11 minutes (X).

6. A park official studied the relationship between the number of people who used the lake area of a park (Y) and the number who used a certain trail (X). Data revealed that $M_y = 400$ people, $M_x = 140$ people, $S_y = 80$, $S_x = 30$, and $r = .70$.
   **a.** Calculate the linear regression equation and *SEE*.
   **b.** Calculate the predicted use of the lake area (Y′) and 95% confidence interval if the use of the trail (X) was 160 people.

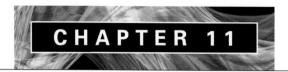

# CHAPTER 11

# Comparing Mean Scores

## KEY CONCEPTS

- Statistical assumptions
- Correlated or dependent *t* test
- Independent *t* test
- Omega squared
- One-way ANOVA
- Multiple comparison test
- Randomized blocks ANOVA
- Factorial or two-way ANOVA
- Interaction
- ANOVA with repeated measures
- Order effect
- Analysis of covariance
- Covariate

## AFTER READING THIS CHAPTER YOU SHOULD BE ABLE TO:

- Calculate and interpret a dependent and independent *t* ratio, determine whether it is significant, and interpret the result.
- Calculate and interpret omega squared.
- Define each statistic covered in this chapter and describe when it is used.
- Interpret summary of ANOVA tables and determine whether the *F* ratio is significant.
- Explain when and why multiple comparison tests are used and how the results may be expressed.
- Explain interaction and graph the results of a study where interaction is significant.
- State examples of an order effect.
- Explain several reasons initial mean scores of groups may not be equal.

Professionals in HPER using research often wish to assess the effect of more than one level of an independent or experimental variable on a dependent variable or to determine the effect of more than one independent variable. Performance on the dependent variable is measured before and after a treatment period, and the change in performance for each group is compared. When only two mean scores are compared (and the data are absolute, interval, or ratio), a type of *t* test is used for the comparisons. If more than two mean scores are compared, the most common type of statistic used is **analysis of variance,** or **ANOVA.** Each of these statistics is covered in this chapter.

## STATISTICAL ASSUMPTIONS

Before using a statistical test, a researcher should examine the criteria for using the test. The criteria for using any type of *t* test or ANOVA are as follows:

1. Data are drawn from normally distributed populations.
2. Data represent random samples from the population.
3. Variance in each group is similar. If variance in one group greatly exceeds that of another group, the within-group variance or denominator of a *t* or *F* ratio is inflated. As will be seen,

$$t \text{ and } F = \frac{\text{variance between groups}}{\text{variance within groups}}$$

Therefore, inequality of within-group variance reduces the *t* or *F* ratio, which in turn reduces the likelihood of significant differences occurring between the means of two or more groups.
4. Data are absolute, interval, or ratio. The data should be continuous and have equal intervals.

Some assumptions do not have to be strictly met. Kerlinger (1964) supports the opinion of others that the normality and equality of variance criteria are probably overrated. Furthermore, he advocates that unless there is good reason to believe that the data are not normal or do not have equal variance, it is not recommended to use a nonparametric test rather than a parametric one, such as a *t* test or ANOVA. Nonparametric tests are less powerful, meaning that attaining significance is more difficult. Therefore, whenever possible, parametric tests should be used. As can be seen, determination as to whether a given set of data meet these criteria is somewhat subjective. A novice researcher would be wise to discuss the issue with an experienced investigator.

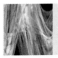 Before using a statistical test, first determine if the criteria are reasonably met.

## CORRELATED OR DEPENDENT *t* TESTS

The purpose of the correlated or dependent *t* test is to compare two mean scores that are related. The analysis typically involves pre-test and post-test data within one group or comparison of two groups matched on a key trait. In either case, the scores are related or correlated. Examples where correlated *t* would be used are comparisons made within one group of subjects such as change in body weight before and after 10 weeks of walking and resting blood pressure before and after a month of meditation. The formula to calculate a correlated *t* test is as follows:

$$t = \frac{\Sigma D/N}{1/N\sqrt{[N\Sigma D^2 - (\Sigma D)^2]/(N-1)}}$$

where

$D$ = the difference in the pre and post score for each subject
$N$ = number of subjects

For example, suppose a coach wished to determine whether shooting free throws in basketball 30 minutes a day twice a week improves free-throw shooting skill after 4 weeks. There are 10 subjects, each with a pre- and post-test score. The steps used to calculate the *t* ratio are summarized in Table 11-1.

The *df* is $N - 1$. Therefore, $df = 10 - 1 = 9$. Consult Table A–4 in Appendix A for the critical values of *t* to determine whether the *t* ratio is significant using a one-tailed

## TABLE 11-1. Calculation of Dependent *t* Test

| Subject | Pre-test | Post-test | D | D² |
|---------|----------|-----------|-----|-----|
| 1 | 19 | 20 | 1 | 1 |
| 2 | 17 | 15 | −2 | 4 |
| 3 | 19 | 20 | 1 | 1 |
| 4 | 14 | 16 | 2 | 4 |
| 5 | 13 | 17 | 4 | 16 |
| 6 | 16 | 16 | 0 | 0 |
| 7 | 16 | 15 | −1 | 1 |
| 8 | 17 | 18 | 1 | 1 |
| 9 | 17 | 19 | 2 | 4 |
| 10 | 14 | 17 | 3 | 9 |
| Σ | 162 | 173 | 11 | 41 |
| M | 16.2 | 17.3 | | |

$$t = \frac{\Sigma D/N}{1/N\sqrt{[(N(\Sigma D^2) - (\Sigma D)^2]/N - 1}}$$

$$t = \frac{11/10}{1/10\sqrt{[10(41) - (11)^2]/10 - 1}}$$

$$t = \frac{11/10}{.10\sqrt{(289/9)}} = \frac{1.10}{5.67} = 1.94$$

$df = 10 - 1 = 9.$

$t(9) = 1.94$, $p \le .05$ for a one-tailed-test.

## TABLE 11-2. Hypothesis Testing For Dependent *t* Test

1. State the null and alternative hypotheses.
   $H_0$: $\mu_{pre} \geq \mu_{post}$
   $H_A$: $\mu_{pre} < \mu_{post}$
2. Set the significance (alpha) level.
   .05
3. Determine the appropriate statistic.
   Dependent *t* test.
4. Determine the critical statistical value.
   The critical value for a one-tailed test with 9 *df* is 1.833.
5. Place the critical value on a curve and determine the values of "do not reject" and "reject."
6. Calculate the dependent *t* ratio and place it on the curve.
   $t = 1.94$

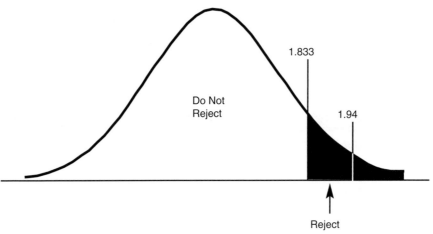

7. Accept or reject the null hypothesis.
   The null hypothesis is rejected.
8. Draw a conclusion.
   It is concluded that free throw performance did improve significantly, $p \leq .05$.

test. A one-tailed test was selected because the direction of change is obvious: free-throw skill should improve with practice and the question really is a matter of how much. The critical $t = 1.833$, so the $t$ ratio 1.94 is significant at the .05 level, and it is concluded that practice improved free throw performance. Table 11-2 summarizes the steps in hypothesis testing for this experiment. A sample computer printout of the correlated $t$ test with an interpretation of the results appears in Figure 11-1.

## Interpretation

Researchers using correlated $t$ tests often are sure that the direction of change will represent improvement in the test measured. In the study described here, it is assumed

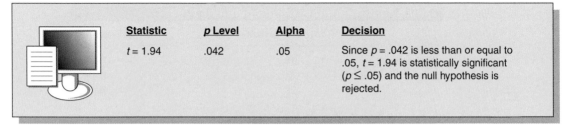

| Statistic | *p* Level | Alpha | Decision |
|-----------|-----------|-------|----------|
| *t* = 1.94 | .042 | .05 | Since *p* = .042 is less than or equal to .05, *t* = 1.94 is statistically significant ($p \leq .05$) and the null hypothesis is rejected. |

**Figure 11-1.** A sample computer printout of the correlated *t* test and results.

that free-throw practice will improve skill, but it is unknown how much. In such a case, one would logically use directional hypothesis testing. Thus, the hypothesis to be tested is $H_0$: $\mu_{\text{pre}} \geq \mu_{\text{post}}$. If this hypothesis is rejected, the alternative hypothesis is accepted: $H_A$: $\mu_{\text{pre}} < \mu_{\text{post}}$. Directional hypothesis testing allows use of the one-tailed column, which increases the likelihood of achieving significance. Therefore, it is to the researcher's advantage to use directional testing when the direction of change is obvious.

*Directional hypothesis testing allows use of the one-tailed column, which increases the likelihood of achieving significance.*

Other examples of obvious direction change are comparison of weight loss in a control group versus a jogging group and reduction in serum cholesterol in nonexercisers versus regular exercisers.

A second useful tool in interpreting the result of statistical tests is to determine the magnitude of change as a result of a treatment. This can be done by calculating the percent change in pre-test to post-test mean scores. In the example here, $M_1$ and $M_2$ represent the means for the pre and post conditions, respectively, and the percent change equals

$$= \left( \frac{M_2 - M_1}{M_1} \right) \times 100$$

$$= \left( \frac{17.3 - 16.2}{16.2} \right) \times 100$$

$$= (1.1/16.2) \times 100 = 6.8\%$$

Thus, performance improved 6.8%. With other statistics, formulas are available to calculate the percent of variance or change due to the experimental variable, which most readers of research are concerned with. A technique to do this is not available for correlated *t* test, so the magnitude of the independent variable can be simply expressed by percent change.

## INDEPENDENT *t* TEST

The independent *t* test determines whether the means from two separate groups are significantly different. An example of such research, assuming that one experimental

### TABLE 11-3. Summary of Independent *t* Test

| | Football Players | Wrestlers |
|---|:---:|:---:|
| *M* % body fat | 13 | 9 |
| *SD* | 3 | 2 |
| *N* | 20 | 20 |

$$t = \frac{M_1 - M_2}{\sqrt{\left[\dfrac{(N_1 - 1)S_1^2 + (N_2 - 1)S_2^2}{N_1 + N_2 - 2}\right]\left[\dfrac{N_1 + N_2}{N_1 N_2}\right]}}$$

$$t = \frac{13 - 9}{\sqrt{\left[\dfrac{(19)3^2 + (19)2^2}{20 + 20 - 2}\right]\left[\dfrac{20 + 20}{(20)(20)}\right]}} = \frac{4}{\sqrt{.65}} = 4.96$$

$df = (N_1 + N_2) - 2 = (20 + 20) - 2 = 38.$

$t(38) = 4.96, p \leq .05.$

group and a control group are involved in the design of each study, would be the effect of videotape feedback versus no videotape feedback on acquisition of a novel skill. Another example would be the difference in dollars spent on recreation in coastal versus noncoastal states. The formula to calculate an independent *t* test is as follows:

$$t = \frac{M_1 - M_2}{\sqrt{\left[\dfrac{(N_1 - 1)S_1^2 + (N_2 - 1)S_2^2}{N_1 + N_2 - 2}\right]\left[\dfrac{N_1 + N_2}{N_1 N_2}\right]}}$$

Suppose a researcher wanted to compare the percent body fat between wrestlers and football players. Twenty athletes from each sport are randomly sampled. The means were 9 and 13%, respectively. A summary of the calculations appears in Table 11-3.

After calculating the *t* ratio, refer to Table A–4 in Appendix A to determine whether the *t* ratio of 4.96 is significant. Because there are two independent groups in this comparison, $df = (N_1 + N_2) - 2$ or $(20 + 20) - 2 = 38$. Table A–4 does not indicate a critical value for exactly 38 *df*. In such a case, one may use the next lowest value in the table, which is 30. This is acceptable because the critical values change only slightly. The critical value for 30 *df* at the .05 level using a two-tailed test is 2.042, whereas for 40 *df* it is 2.021. The *t* ratio is significant not only at the .05 level but also at the .01 level (critical value = 2.750). Therefore, we are at least 95% confident (alpha of .05) that the difference in percent body fat between the two groups is real, whereas there is only a 5% probability that the difference is due to chance or sampling error. With an alpha level of .01, we are 99% confident that a real difference exists, whereas only a 1% likelihood exists that the difference is due to chance or sampling error. The null hypothesis is therefore rejected and the alternative hypothesis accepted. A sample computer printout of the test with an interpretation appears in Figure 11-2.

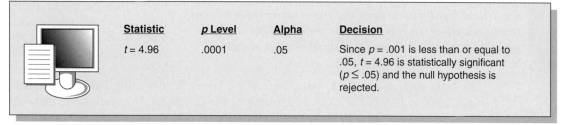

| Statistic | p Level | Alpha | Decision |
|-----------|---------|-------|----------|
| t = 4.96 | .0001 | .05 | Since p = .001 is less than or equal to .05, t = 4.96 is statistically significant (p ≤ .05) and the null hypothesis is rejected. |

**Figure 11-2.** Sample computer printout of independent *t* test.

## Omega Squared

While a high level of confidence exists that the difference between the two groups used in the example is significant, how much of the difference can actually be attributed to the participation in the two sports? This information is just as important as knowing whether or not significance occurs. Remember that with the Pearson $r$, $r^2$ was used to determine the variance common to two variables. Thus, $r^2$ was used as a measure of the strength of the correlation. Similarly, a procedure is needed to determine the strength or magnitude of the difference in the mean scores. The statistic that does this is known as omega squared ($\Omega^2$) (Tolson, 1980). The formula is as follows:

$$\Omega^2 = \frac{t^2 - 1}{t^2 + N_1 + N_2 - 1} \times 100$$

Table 11-4 summarizes the steps in calculating omega squared.

The answer, 36.0%, means that 36% of the variance or difference in percent body fat between the two groups is due to the effect of the variable examined, that is, being a wrestler or a football player, while the rest of the difference is caused by other factors.

Two statistics are needed to analyze the results of the study: an independent *t* test to determine whether there is a difference in the means and omega squared to measure the size or magnitude of the difference.

*Knowing how much of the difference that occurs in two groups is due to the independent variable is just as important as knowing if the difference is statistically significant.*

Surprisingly, omega squared is not as widely used as one would think. Significance does not necessarily infer a large difference. As sample size increases, smaller *t*

## TABLE 11-4. Summary of Omega Squared

$$\Omega^2 = \frac{t^2 - 1}{t^2 + N_1 + N_2 - 1} \times 100 = \frac{4.96^2 - 1}{4.96^2 + 20 + 20 - 1} \times 100$$

$$\Omega^2 = \frac{23.6}{65.6} \times 100 = .36 \times 100 = 36\%$$

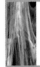
*Statistical significance does not necessarily infer a large treatment effect. In reporting the results of research, significance as well as magnitude of change should be expressed.*

ratios may be found significant. For example, if $N = 122$, a $t$ ratio of 1.980 is significant at the .05 level with a two-tailed test.

In Table A–4, Appendix A, note that with a larger $N$, a smaller $t$ ratio is required for significance. If $N = 12$, 2.228 is significant. The difference in mean scores between two groups may not have to be large to be significant and consequently, the magnitude of the difference should be expressed when interpreting the results of a study. When testing the effectiveness of new medications, pharmaceutical companies that sponsor research use very large sample sizes to boost the probability that significant differences will be found. If a medication is found to be significantly better than another, we have confidence that the difference is probably real. However, the size of the difference should always be addressed. A difference could be real statistically without having a great effect on people's health. In short, such a finding indicates that the effect is likely real but the *size* of the effect is small.

Suppose an expensive piece of exercise equipment used to develop strength is found to be significantly better ($p \leq .001$) than the standard barbell. Should commercial fitness centers and weight trainers necessarily switch to the new piece of equipment? If the mean difference in strength development is 3% across a number of basic exercises, does a change of this magnitude justify the purchase or use of the new equipment? For serious weight trainers and competitive lifters, the small difference may justify a switch, but the average fitness enthusiast may not think the small difference makes a change worthwhile.

## ANALYSIS OF VARIANCE

Analysis of variance (ANOVA) is used to compare more than two mean scores. Several types of ANOVA are discussed in the remainder of this chapter.

### One-Way ANOVA

The purpose of one-way ANOVA is to compare two or more means on one dependent variable. Examples of using one-way ANOVA are comparing the effect of three ball colors on ball-catching skill. Another is a comparison of the effect of lecture, small-group discussion, and role playing on health behavior. Comparing the groups in pairs, that is, group 1 with group 2, group 1 with group 3, and so on, with a number of independent $t$ tests is invalid, because it violates an assumption regarding the alpha level. An alpha level of .05 means that there is a 1 in 20 probability that a difference could be due to chance if the groups compared are independent and random. In this case, the groups are not independent because each group is compared more than once with every other group. ANOVA allows making any number of group comparisons without violating the alpha level. This topic is discussed in more detail later.

| TABLE 11-5. Summary of One-Way ANOVA | | | | |
|---|---|---|---|---|
| **Source of Variance** | **SS** | **df** | **MS** | **F Ratio** |
| Treatment or between groups | 100 | 2 | 50 | 12.5* |
| Error or within groups | 80 | 20 | 4 | |
| Total | 180 | 22 | | |

*$p \leq .01$.

Calculation of ANOVA involves a number of steps. Computer software to calculate ANOVA is widely available, and therefore it is not covered here.

The results of an ANOVA are often summarized in a table such as Table 11-5. Each subject's score is squared, and the sum of the squared values is used in several steps to determine the **sum of squares (SS)** for **treatment** or **between-group variance, error or within-group variance,** and **total variance.** Then each SS is divided by the appropriate number of *df* to calculate the **mean square (MS)** for treatment and error variance. Thus, a mean square is a measure of variance. The *df* are determined as follows:

$$\text{Treatment } df = k - 1, \text{ where k = the number of groups}$$

$$k = 3 \text{ so treatment } df = 2.$$

$$\text{Error } df = N - k$$

where

$N$ = the total number of subjects in the study.
$N = 23$ and k = 3, so error $df = 23 - 3 = 20$.
Total $df = N - 1$
$N = 23$, so total $df = 23 - 1 = 22$.

A large *F* ratio indicates that a good portion of the variance is due to the actual difference in mean scores, whereas chance and sampling error are secondary sources in causing the mean scores to vary. Conversely, if the *F* ratio is less than 1.00, less than half of the variance is due to the treatment. If *F* is 1.00, the treatment and error have an equal effect in causing scores to vary. For example, an *F* ratio of 5.0 means treatment variance was five times error variance. *F* ratios less than 1.00 are never significant, because they imply that the effect of error exceeded the effect of the treatment in causing mean scores to vary.

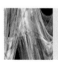

One-way ANOVA compares more than two groups on one independent variable.

The *F* ratio is the statistic calculated in ANOVA. It represents the ratio between variance due to the treatment or experimental variable and the variance due to error, the latter representing chance and sampling error. Thus, mathematically the *F* ratio may be expressed as follows:

$$F = \frac{\text{treatment or between-group variance}}{\text{error or within-group variance}}$$

The *F* ratio is calculated by dividing treatment *MS* by error *MS*. Even without calculating the *F* ratio, we know that the treatment *MS* greatly exceeds the error *MS* in the sample problem, which indicates that *F* will be well over 1.00. The larger the *F* ratio, the greater the proportion of total variance due to the treatment. Therefore, there is a greater probability that *F* will be significant.

*The larger the F ratio, the greater the proportion of total variance due to the treatment and therefore the greater the probability that F will be significant.*

The sample problem here is a comparison of one, two, and three sets of weight training on strength development. The null hypothesis in a study comparing three group means is stated as follows: $H_0: \mu_1 = \mu_2 = \mu_3$. The alternative hypothesis is $H_A: \mu_1 \neq \mu_2 \neq \mu_3$.

To determine significance, consult Table A–5 in Appendix A with 2 and 20 *df*, the *df* associated with the treatment and error *MS*, respectively. First, locate the *df* for the greater *MS* on the horizontal axis. In our example, the *MS* for treatment is larger than the *MS* for error, and the associated *df* is 2, on the horizontal axis. Then find the *df* for the smaller *MS* error, which is 20, on the vertical axis. The *F* ratio for significance at the .05 level is 3.49 and 5.85 for the .05 and .01 levels, respectively. The .05 level is the first value given at each *df*, and the second value, which appears in bold, represents the .01 level. Consequently, the *F* ratio 12.50 is significant at the .01 level. A sample computer printout of the test with an interpretation is provided in Figure 11-3.

The significant *F* means that the null hypothesis is rejected and the alternative hypothesis is accepted. We are 99% confident that a real difference exists among one, two, and three sets in building strength.

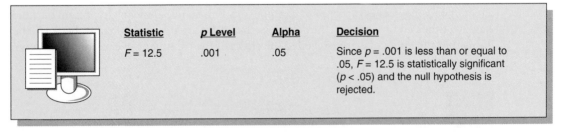

| Statistic | *p* Level | Alpha | Decision |
|---|---|---|---|
| $F = 12.5$ | .001 | .05 | Since $p = .001$ is less than or equal to .05, $F = 12.5$ is statistically significant ($p < .05$) and the null hypothesis is rejected. |

**Figure 11-3.** Sample computer printout of one-way ANOVA.

## Post Hoc Tests

A question arises, however. Which of the means are significantly different from each other? The significant *F* indicates only that at least one pair of means is truly different (the largest and the smallest means are the obvious choices), but it does not indicate whether other differences exist. All three means could be different or perhaps only one pair of means. Therefore, a second statistical test is required to identify which means are different when *F* is significant. Several terms are used to describe the second test: **follow-up, multiple comparison, post hoc,** and **a posteriori.** Implicit in each of these terms is the fact that they are used after an initial test to determine the *F* ratio. Thus, a follow-up test follows the ANOVA; a multiple comparison test compares each group mean with every other group mean; and post hoc and a posteriori both imply a test done after the fact or after the *F* test.

Several post hoc tests are available. They perform the same function as a *t* test in comparing each group with every other group and do so while maintaining alpha at the desired level, which is usually .05. They provide similar but not identical results. The tests vary in their likelihood of producing a significant difference. Liberal tests are more likely to yield significance than conservative or stringent tests. Several of these tests are listed in sequence from very liberal to very conservative (Winer, 1962): *Duncan Multiple Range, Newman-Keuls, Fisher's Least Significant Difference, Tukey's Honestly Significant Difference (HSD),* and *Scheffe.* Thus, use of the Duncan Multiple Range test would more likely produce significant differences when pairs of means are compared. The

*A second statistical procedure known as a post hoc test is needed to determine which groups are significantly different from each other.*

Scheffe test would be least likely to yield significance.

Does it make a difference which test is selected? Is it unfair to use the most liberal test? The decision lies with the researcher but should be experimentally defensible. For example, if the study dealt with medications for patients with AIDS, researchers may be wary of proclaiming that one medication is more likely than others to be effective unless they made it as difficult as possible for significance to be detected. In such a case, the Scheffe test would be justified and the researchers could claim that statistical decisions were made to minimize the chance of type I error (falsely rejecting the null hypothesis).

Most research in HPER and most academic disciplines does not address issues of life and death. If a researcher in our disciplines chose a Duncan Multiple Range multiple comparison test and significant results were obtained but they would not have been with the conservative Scheffe test, the effect would probably not be great. As a matter of fact, researchers are rarely if ever questioned about the rationale for selecting a particular post hoc test. Most researchers probably select the test that is most likely to support their hypothesis. The actual differences among the tests are small anyway.

**Limitations of the *t* Test as a Post Hoc Test**  Why cannot independent *t* tests be used to make group-by-group comparisons? The *t* test is appropriate *only* for comparing two means on a single dependent variable. If the group training with one set is compared with the groups using two and three sets, the chance of falsely finding significant differences or making a type I error is increased. If a statistic is significant at the .05 level, the probability that it is not significant is 5%. One can be only 95% confident when $\alpha = .05$. With two $t$ tests used with the same dependent variable, the chance of finding significance by chance alone increases to 10%. If three $t$ tests were used, as would be the case here, the probability of type I error rises to 15%. Obviously, this poses a problem, because although more significant findings would tend to occur, the researcher would lose confidence that any one finding is true. The multiple comparison tests avoid this problem because the calculated statistic takes the number of comparisons into account. Thus, no sacrifice in confidence of the findings occurs, and the chance of making decision errors is not affected.

**Reporting Results of Post Hoc Tests**    The results of a multiple comparison test are expressed in several ways. If only three mean scores are compared, the results may be explained in a sentence or two, such as "Three sets was found to be significantly greater than either one or two sets, but no difference was observed between one and two sets." However, as more means are compared, results become more difficult to understand because a large number of comparisons are made. To facilitate communicating the results with a large number of comparisons, the information is often presented in a table. Table 11-6 is based on imaginary data but demonstrates how this can be done. Imagine that five groups for number of sets was used in a study rather than three: one set, two sets,...up to five sets. This technique is known as the **underlining method**. Group means are arranged according to the size of the gains made in strength measured in kilograms from small to large. Lines appear below means that are *not* significantly different. Therefore, means not underlined by the same line are significantly different. In the example, the mean gains for groups 1 and 2 are not significantly different, whereas the scores for groups 3, 4, and 5 are significantly higher than those of both groups 1 and 2. Groups 3, 4, and 5 are not significantly different from each other.

A **matrix** is a second means of indicating results from a number of comparisons. A sample is given in Table 11-7. A matrix is a table read the same as a correlation matrix covered earlier. The mean differences between groups are noted in the table, and an asterisk denotes a significant difference. The significance or $p$ level indicated by an asterisk is given in a table footnote.

| **TABLE 11-6. Reporting Results of Multiple Comparisons: The Underline Method** | | | | |
|---|---|---|---|---|
| *1 Sets* | *2 Sets* | *3 Sets* | *4 Sets* | *5 Sets* |
| 10.2 | 11.8 | 15.1 | 15.9 | 16.4 |

Scores represent gains in strength in kilograms (kg). Means underlined together are not significantly different from each other.

| TABLE 11-7. Reporting Results of Multiple Comparisons: The Matrix Method | | | | |
|---|---|---|---|---|
| *Group* | *2* | *3* | *4* | *5* |
| 1 | 1.6 | 4.9* | 5.7* | 6.2* |
| 2 | | 3.3* | 4.1* | 4.6* |
| 3 | | | 0.8 | 1.3 |
| 4 | | | | 0.5 |

Values represent mean differences between groups in strength improvement (kg).
$*p \leq .05$.

Most people find reading a table faster and easier than trying to extract the same information from a paragraph. Both tables provide the key results in abbreviated form.

**Magnitude of the Treatment Effect** If a $t$ test is significant, it means that one has considerable confidence that a difference is likely to be real rather than due to chance, sampling error, or measurement error. However, this finding provides no quantitative analysis regarding how much of the variance or difference is due to the experimental variable. One means of estimating the difference is by calculating the proportion of the total variance that is explained by treatment variance. A more precise means of determining percent of variance due to the treatment variable is omega squared ($\Omega^2$) (Tolson, 1980). The formula is a variation of the one used for $t$ test:

$$\Omega^2 = \frac{F(k-1) - (k-1)}{F(k-1) + (N-k) + 1} \times 100$$

where

$F = F$ ratio
$k$ = number of groups
$N$ = total number of subjects in all groups

Using the values from the ANOVA summary table (Table 11-5), $F = 12.5$, $k = 3$, and $N = 23$. Therefore,

$$\Omega^2 = \frac{12.5(2) - 2}{12.5(2) + (23-3) + 1} \times 100 = \frac{23}{46} \times 100 = .50 \times 100 = 50\%$$

A value of 50 means that 50% of the variance in mean scores is accounted for by the treatment or experimental variable, whereas the remaining 50% of the variance is due to other factors. Estimation of omega squared by dividing treatment variance by total variance equals 55.6% ($100/180 = 55.6\%$). Here the estimate agreed well with the calculated omega squared value. The estimation technique is simple and can often be done even without a calculator. This simple tool may be useful when reading journal articles that do not report omega squared. The insightful reader can easily calculate or even roughly estimate the percent variance due to the treatment if a summary ANOVA table is included.

Statistics can be significant without explaining a high percentage of the variance. Too often students and researchers indicate which comparisons are significantly different but then provide no information as the size of the treatment effect or the variance that is explained by the independent variable. Most of us are just as concerned with the latter as we are the former.

## Randomized-Blocks ANOVA

Randomized-blocks ANOVA is used to equate groups on the basis of pre-test data. The procedure reduces the error mean square, which increases the *F* ratio and the likelihood of significance. Using the example cited for the one-way ANOVA, that is, comparing three strength training programs, a researcher will carry out the same study using the **blocking procedure**.

Subjects are ranked according to performance on the dependent variable. If more than one dependent variable exists, which normally is the case, the most important variable that theoretically may affect the results of the study is selected. For example, if a researcher wished to study strength development, pre-test performance on the dependent variable strength may be used to equalize the groups.

Next, a procedure known as blocking is done. The procedure is similar to choosing sides before playing a game. If three groups are to be formed, the three subjects having

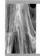

*Blocking is the process of randomly assigning subjects based on their rank on one or more key dependent variables to make groups as equal as possible.*

the best total or sum of the three lifts (e.g., bench press, leg press, biceps curl) are assigned block 1. These three subjects are each randomly assigned to one of the three groups.

The next block of three strongest subjects (block 2) is also each randomly assigned to a group. The blocking and random assignment continue until all subjects have been placed in a group. The process of randomly assigning subjects based on their rank on one or more key dependent variables makes the groups initially as equal as possible.

**Interpretation**  A summary table for a randomized-blocks ANOVA is identical with that of the simple one-way ANOVA except that one additional source of variance is accounted for. Table 11-8 illustrates a summary of a randomized-blocks ANOVA.

The variance due to blocking was more than 10% of the total variance ($16/150 \times 100 = 10.7\%$). Had blocking not been used, the error or within-groups variance would have been enlarged by 16. This would have resulted in a smaller *F* ratio, since *F* equals treatment variance divided by error variance. With 2 and 16 *df* for the greater and lesser mean square, respectively, *F* is significant at the .01 level. The null hypothesis is rejected and the alternative hypothesis accepted. We can be 99% confident that there is a real difference in mean scores. To identify which means are different, a multiple comparison test is used. A sample computer printout with interpretation appears in Figure 11-4.

| TABLE 11-8. Summary of Randomized Blocks ANOVA | | | | |
|---|---|---|---|---|
| **Source of Variance** | **SS** | **df** | **MS** | **F Ratio** |
| Treatment or between-groups variance | 70 | 2 | 35 | 8.75* |
| Blocks | 16 | 8 | | |
| Error or within-group variance | 64 | 16 | 4 | |
| Total | 150 | 26 | | |

*$p \leq .01$ level.

How much of the variance in the dependent variable can be attributed to the treatment or experimental variable? As a quick estimate, treatment variance divided by total variance equals 70/150 = 46.7%. Therefore, approximately 47% of the variance is due to the experimental variable. This quick calculation is a practical and easy technique to use when reading journal articles that do not report this important interpretation. The computation of omega squared equals 43.7% for these data, illustrating that the estimation method is accurate.

## Factorial or Two-Way ANOVA

Two-way ANOVA is used to examine the effect of two independent variables on a dependent variable. As with any ANOVA, more than two groups are compared. Two-way ANOVA provides a realistic analysis because rarely, if ever, does one independent variable completely determine the change in a dependent variable. Most likely human behaviors that are studied in HPER are multifactorial in nature. By studying the effects of two independent variables on a given behavior, the researcher is able to more comprehensively assess behavior change. Examples of research with two independent variables include comparing the effects of two types of feedback and age on dental care (type of feedback and age are the independent variables, and dental care is the dependent variable) and comparing two exercise intensities and two training durations on swim performance (exercise intensity and duration are each independent variables, and swim performance is the dependent variable).

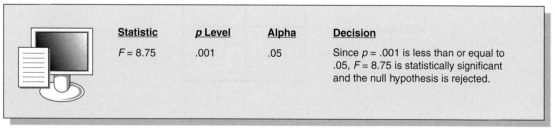

| Statistic | p Level | Alpha | Decision |
|---|---|---|---|
| F = 8.75 | .001 | .05 | Since p = .001 is less than or equal to .05, F = 8.75 is statistically significant and the null hypothesis is rejected. |

**Figure 11-4.** Sample computer printout of randomized-blocks.

Although either of the above studies could be analyzed with a one-way ANOVA on each independent variable, the combined or synergistic effects of the two independent variables working together could not be assessed. In many professional situations, we do not limit our choices to a single factor. For example, when teachers select textbooks, they probably consider many factors, such as age of the children, reading level, socioeconomic status, and psychological maturity. Two-way ANOVAs permit studying the integra-

 *The integrated or synergistic effect of two or more variables on the dependent variable is called interaction.*

ted effect of different variables on some type of behavior. In research, this is termed **interaction.**

A two-way ANOVA research design allows asking at least two questions: (1) Does each independent variable have a significant effect? (2) Do the independent variables interact? These two-way or two-factor designs permit a more complete research design and assessment of the effects of two or more independent variables than studies examining a single independent variable. Consequently, more findings and conclusions can be drawn.

Suppose a researcher wishes to study the effects of exercise intensity and exercise duration on swim performance. The independent variables are intensity of exercise during training, expressed as a percent of maximum heart rate, and duration of exercise in minutes at target heart rate. The dependent variable is swim performance as measured by the time to cover a given distance. It is helpful to sketch the design of a factorial study, as it aids understanding how many levels of each independent variable are used and the number of groups needed to carry out a study. The study here is depicted in Figure 11-5. There are two levels of each independent variable in this study: 20 and 30 minutes for duration and 70% and 80% for intensity. The effect of each independent variable with the influence of the other independent removed is also known as a **main effect.** It assesses the effect of one independent variable with the effect of the other independent variable

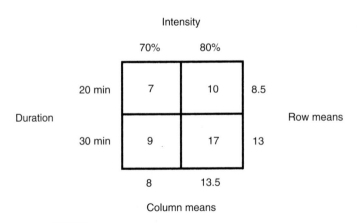

**Figure 11-5.** Summary of a two-way ANOVA.

held constant. Thus, the study is investigating two main effects and the possible inter-action of the main effects on swim performance. The type of factorial ANOVA used to examine the results of a study with two main effects or independent variables is called a **two-way ANOVA.** If three main effects or independent variables are studied, a three-way ANOVA would be used, and so on.

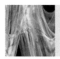 A two-way ANOVA measures the separate effect of two independent variables on behavior as well as their combined effect or interaction.

The sketch indicates the number of groups to be used in this study. There are four boxes in the table, and each depicts one group. Therefore, two groups swim for 20 min-utes, one at 70% of maximum heart rate and one at 80%; the other two groups swim for 30 minutes, one at 70% and one at 80%. Because two levels are found for each indepen-dent variable, this could be called a **2 × 2 ANOVA** and **design.** It is called a 2 × 3 ANOVA and design if there are three levels of one of the independent variables, for example, if a 40-minute level was added. Three hypotheses are tested in a two-way ANOVA. One examines the main effect duration (H$_0$: 20 minutes = 30 minutes; H$_A$: 20 minutes ≠ 30 minutes); a second tests the main effect intensity (H$_0$: 70% = 80%; H$_A$: 70% ≠ 80%); and the third tests the interaction between the main effects: H$_0$: $\mu_1 = \mu_2 = \mu_3 = \mu_4$; H$_A$: at least two of the groups are different.

The main effects are tested by comparing the two row means and the two column means. The row means for improvement in swim performance, 8.5 and 13 seconds, rep-resent the average improvement in performance for the two levels of exercise duration. Thus, the mean of 8.5 seconds is the average improvement for the groups exercising for 20 minutes. This mean is compared to the mean for the two groups exercising for 30 minutes, which is 13 seconds. An $F$ ratio is calculated and compared with the critical value for $F$ to determine whether the $F$ ratio for row means is significant. In Table 11-9, the $F$ ratio for the rows, representing duration, is 12.0 with 1 and 16 $df$. This ratio is significant both at the .05 and .01 levels with tabled values of 4.49 and 8.53, respectively.

| **TABLE 11-9. Summary of Two-Way ANOVA** | | | | |
|---|---|---|---|---|
| *Source of Variance* | *SS* | *df* | *MS* | *F Ratio* |
| Intensity (column) | 600 | 1 | 600 | 12.0† |
| Duration (row) | 600 | 1 | 600 | 12.0† |
| Interaction | 200 | 1 | 200 | 4.0* |
| Error | 800 | 16 | 50 | |
| Total | 2200 | 19 | | |

\* $p \leq$ .05 level.
† $p \leq$ .01 level.

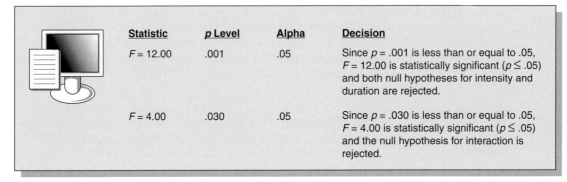

| Statistic | *p* Level | Alpha | Decision |
|---|---|---|---|
| *F* = 12.00 | .001 | .05 | Since *p* = .001 is less than or equal to .05, *F* = 12.00 is statistically significant (*p* ≤ .05) and both null hypotheses for intensity and duration are rejected. |
| *F* = 4.00 | .030 | .05 | Since *p* = .030 is less than or equal to .05, *F* = 4.00 is statistically significant (*p* ≤ .05) and the null hypothesis for interaction is rejected. |

**Figure 11-6.** Sample computer printout of a two-way ANOVA.

Similarly, an *F* ratio is calculated for the main effect intensity. The mean of column 1 averaged across both durations is 8 seconds. The mean gain in column 2, averaged across the two groups exercising for 20 and 30 minutes, is 13.5 seconds. This ANOVA thus compares the mean gains of 8 and 13.5 seconds. The resulting *F* ratio for the main effect intensity is compared with the tabled value to determine whether the difference is significant. The *F* ratio of 12.0 with 1 and 16 *df* is significant at .05 and .01. A sample computer printout of the two-way ANOVA with interpretation appears in Figure 11-6.

A summary table of the two-way ANOVA (Table 11-9) shows that it is identical to the one-way ANOVA table except that it includes a second main effect and interaction as sources of variance. The table indicates that both independent variables or main effects were significant. Because there are only two levels of each variable, a follow-up test is not needed. We know that the larger row or column mean is significantly greater than the smaller one. So we reject the null hypothesis for intensity and accept that training at 80% of maximum heart rate is superior to training at 70%. We also reject the null hypothesis for duration and accept the alternative hypothesis that 30 minutes is superior to 20 minutes of training.

The table also indicates that interaction between the two main effects was significant. Interaction means that some combination of the two variables elicited a particularly strong effect on performance. The improvement in swim performance for the two groups training at 70% are fairly similar, 7 and 9 seconds. However, a greater disparity in results occurred in the groups training at 80%, 10 and 17 seconds. A multiple comparison test is used to compare the four cell means. Let us assume a Newman-Keuls multiple comparison test is used. The results are depicted here using the underlining method.

| *20 min at 70%* | *30 min at 70%* | *20 min at 80%* | *30 min at 80%* |
|---|---|---|---|
| 7 | 9 | 10 | 17 |

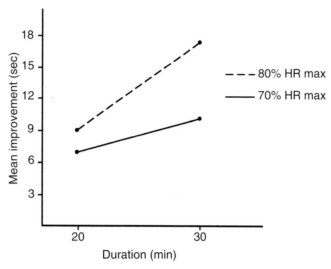

**Figure 11-7.** Interaction of exercise intensity and duration.

The table indicates that the group improving by 17 seconds gained significantly more than the groups improving by 7, 9, and 10 seconds and that the differences of 7, 9, and 10 were not significantly different from each other. Thus, 30 minutes of training at 80% maximum heart rate is an especially effective combination of the variables studied. The existence of an especially effective combination of independent variables illustrates interaction.

When significant interaction occurs, plotting the results greatly aids interpretation, and a figure normally accompanies the text. Figure 11-7 illustrates significant interaction of the results discussed. When interaction is significant, the lines are not parallel. Significant departure from parallel means that a greater effect on the dependent variable occurs with a particular combination of variables. If the lines are nearly parallel, no special or disproportionate effect occurs under any of the combinations examined in the study.

Interpretation of the results of factorial studies should not be limited to the main effects, because an erroneous conclusion might be drawn. In some studies, neither main effect is significant but interaction is. In such cases, one should not conclude that the independent variables do not affect the dependent variable. The results mean that the independent variables acting alone may not, but acting together, they do. In reality, few things in life depend solely on one factor. Rather,

*In some studies neither main effect is significant but interaction is. However, one should not conclude that the independent variables do not affect the dependent variable.*

combinations of variables determine the outcome. Consequently, it is important to analyze the effects of interaction.

**Other Types of Factorial ANOVA**   If the effects of three independent variables are studied, the result is a three-way ANOVA. For example, if two curricula (first independent variable) in health education are compared in three grade levels (second independent variable) in low and middle socioeconomic levels (third independent variable), the result is a three-way ANOVA or, more specifically, a 2 × 3 × 2 factorial ANOVA. Such designs require a large number of subjects, and interpretation is complex. Studies examining the effect of more than three independent variables are not frequently used in HPER.

## ANOVA with Repeated Measures

A repeated-measures design means that the same subjects are tested several times for a measure of an independent variable. Use of the same subjects reduces the problem of obtaining an adequate number of subjects, and for this reason alone it is a widely used design in HPER. The procedure also reduces the component of error variance due to differences among individual subjects, which increases the likelihood of detecting significant differences. Repeated-measures ANOVA is also frequently used to assess changes in a variable over time, such as variation in cholesterol with aging or changes in locomotor skills at different levels of maturity. Another example is measuring reaction time in the same subjects at three levels of arousal. Repeated-measures designs may use any number of independent variables and so may use one-way ANOVA, two-way ANOVA, and so on. Table 11-10 is an example of a summary of a repeated measures ANOVA.

Subjects in repeated measures studies should be exposed to each independent variable on a random basis to prevent an **order effect.** An order effect is a change in behavior resulting from the sequence of activities in a study. For example, if all subjects were observed doing the activities listed for a social contact study in the order given, subjects may become better acquainted and more familiar with each other as they proceed from the first to the last activity. This can increase the number of social contacts made. If the activities are randomly sequenced for each subject, the effects of order are eliminated.

### TABLE 11-10. Summary of Repeated Measures One-Way ANOVA

| Source of Variance | SS | df | MS | F Ratio |
|---|---|---|---|---|
| Between subjects | 760 | 4 | 190 | 5.9* |
| Within subjects | 480 | 15 | 32 | |
| Treatments | 360 | 3 | 120 | 12.0* |
| Error | 120 | 12 | 10 | |
| Total | 1720 | 19 | | |

* $p \leq .05$.

Other examples of order effects include fatigue, boredom, and discomfort on one test affecting performance on ensuing tests.

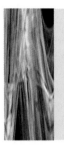

A study reports using 15 subjects in a study comparing the effect of various durations of warm-up on running performance. Thus, on different days all subjects warm-up for 5, 10, or 15 minutes and then run a mile as fast as possible. This is an example of a repeated-measures design and a one-way ANOVA would be used to compare mean run times associated with each warm-up duration. The sequence of the warm-ups is randomized for each subject to prevent an order effect.

## ANALYSIS OF COVARIANCE

Analysis of covariance (**ANCOVA**) is a special version of ANOVA that statistically adjusts the means of groups when they may be different at the onset of a study. This occurs frequently in research. Adjustment for differences makes comparisons more valid because the degree of change in studies is often related to the initial score. For example, if the mean sprint speed of professional football players is compared with the mean of college students who are not athletes and enrolled in a track and field class, a sizable difference can be expected. Suppose both groups train to improve sprint speed. The professional athletes will probably show little or no progress, whereas the college students are likely to demonstrate a significant training effect. ANCOVA, by adjusting initial sprint times, provides a better comparison than a *t* test or one-way ANOVA. The variable adjusted is termed the **covariate.** The pre-test score for the dependent variable often serves as the covariate. Table 11-11 is an example of a summary of ANCOVA.

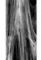
*Adjustment for initial differences in groups using AN-COVA makes comparison of groups more valid because the degree of change is often affected by the initial scores of the subjects.*

Sometimes random assignment is difficult, and therefore initial group scores may be different. For example, a health researcher may wish to have different classes remain intact as each class receives some treatment in a study. In comparing teaching techniques, it is easier to have each class exposed to a specific treatment than randomly assign each

| TABLE 11-11. Summary of ANCOVA | | | | |
|---|---|---|---|---|
| *Source of Variance* | *Adj. SS* | *df* | *Adj. MS* | *F Ratio* |
| Between | 550 | 2 | 275 | 10.08* |
| Within | 300 | 11 | 27.3 | |
| Total | 850 | 13 | | |

* $p \leq .01$.

student to a class receiving a treatment. The latter would disrupt a school schedule and be difficult to carry out. Research in the field or clinical setting frequently precludes random assignment, which makes ANCOVA the preferred statistical tool. Research comparing the response to training of males and females often is corrected for basic gender difference, such as percent body fat, weight, and height, using ANCOVA.

Sometimes differences in initial mean scores occur because subjects drop out of a study. They may have been equal at first but not at the end of a study. ANCOVA can be used to equalize the groups by adjusting the pre-test score (covariate).

ANCOVA is also used to remove the effect of an extraneous variable on a dependent variable. For example, in a study assessing the effect of diet on cholesterol level in men and women, women's values may be different because of the difference in body composition, that is, higher percent fat and lower percent muscle. The differences in body composition can be controlled using ANCOVA, thus eliminating an extraneous variable. Multiple regression can also be used, with several extraneous variables simultaneously used as covariates.

## Summary

Much research involves comparison of mean scores. When only two means are compared, either a correlated *t* test (pre- and post-differences within one group) or independent *t* test (two groups) is used. ANOVA is used to compare more than two mean scores. A one-way ANOVA examines the effect of one independent variable, whereas a two-way ANOVA determines the effect of two independent variables. Several levels of an independent variable are often compared in studies so that a two-way ANOVA may also be termed a 2 × 3 ANOVA if two and three levels, respectively, of each independent variable exist. The combined effect or interaction of two independent variables can be assessed with factorial ANOVAs. If mean scores of a dependent variable are different at the onset of a study, ANCOVA may be used to adjust the means, thereby providing a more valid

### TABLE 11-12. Summary of Tests Comparing Group Means

| *Statistic* | *Key Word/Concept(s)* |
| --- | --- |
| Correlated *t* | Same group pre- and post |
| Independent *t* | Two different groups |
| 1-way ANOVA | 1 independent variable; post hoc test if significant *F* ratio |
| 2-way ANOVA or factorial ANOVA | 2 independent variables; post hoc test if significant *F* ratio Interaction between variables Example: 2 X 2 |
| 3-way ANOVA | 3 independent variables; post hoc test if significant *F* ratio Interaction among variables Example: 2 X 3 X 2 |
| Randomized blocks ANOVA | Block to equalize group means at onset |
| ANCOVA | 1 or more independent variables Statistically "adjusts" or equalizes groups |
| Omega squared | Percent variance explained by independent variable |

comparison of a treatment effect. A summary of tests used to compare mean scores appears in Table 11-12.

Criteria called assumptions must be satisfied in selecting an appropriate statistical test. They are based primarily on type of data and the normality and variance of data. Although nearly all studies report whether significant results occurred, often information regarding the magnitude of the results is omitted. The size of the treatment effect is a vital concern in any study and should be quantified in some way, such as omega squared.

## Learning Activities

Name the appropriate statistic for comparing mean scores for each situation.

1. Did a significant decrease in body weight occur in a group of subjects as a result of training?
2. Three types of feedback are compared as to the effectiveness on motor learning.
3. A physical education instructor wished to determine whether students from her fourth-hour class of high school sophomores were as strong as her seventh-hour class of juniors.
4. After randomly assigning subjects to groups, an investigator compares mean initial scores and finds that one group has significantly higher LDL cholesterol levels than the other two groups. At the completion of the intervention, the investigator selects a statistical analysis that accounts for the initial difference in scores, thus allowing a valid comparison of changes in LDL cholesterol in the three groups.
5. Explain how one might use blocking based on anxiety scores in a study comparing the effectiveness of three stress reduction techniques.
6. A researcher has compared three levels of caffeine to determine whether it enhances the ability to run a series of sprints with a short recovery between each. Results of a repeated-measures one-way ANOVA indicate a significant $F$ ratio for the main effect.
   a. What statistical test will identify what groups are different form each other?
   b. How might the magnitude of differences in mean times be expressed?
7. Twelve subjects run a 1-mile race on three different days at three varying paces: even, fast start-slow finish, and slow start-fast finish.
   a. What is the type of design called?
   b. What statistic would determine whether there is any difference in the three mile run times?
   c. How should one determine the sequence of the three runs?
8. A study is conducted on the effects of weight training on bone mineral density and leg strength. The independent variable is the frequency of lifting: 2, 3, and 4 days per week.
   a. How many ANOVAs are needed for the study?
   b. What type of ANOVA would be used?

## Statistics Exercises

1. A health researcher examined the influence of a stress management program on diastolic blood pressure.
   Initial scores, mm Hg: 120, 124, 132, 148, 160, 144, 124, 136
   Post-scores, mm Hg: 120, 118, 118, 140, 124, 140, 124, 126
   **a.** Calculate a two-tailed correlated *t* test.
   **b.** Did the program significantly (*p* <.05) reduce systolic blood pressure?
2. A recreation researcher compared the expenditures for families over a year for outdoor recreational activities in several Sun Belt states with several states bordering Canada.
   Sun Belt states ($): 300, 450, 600, 400, 200, 350
   States bordering Canada ($): 200, 250, 400, 300, 350, 350
   **a.** Calculate an independent *t* test.
   **b.** Is the difference significant at the .05 level?
3. A fitness director for a company compared the sit and reach flexibility of men and women in an adult fitness program.
   Flexibility for women, cm: 7, 3, 4, 9, 2, 8, 10, 5, 12, 13
   Flexibility for men, cm: 2, 3, 9, 4, 1, 3, 6, 2
   **a.** Calculate an independent *t* test to determine whether a significant difference at the .05 level existed.
   **b.** What conclusion can be made?
   **c.** Calculate omega squared and interpret its meaning in this study.
4. A recreation researcher found that entry level salaries of professionals in recreation were significantly higher than those of police officers. The independent *t* test was 3.6, and the sample sizes were 200 and 100, respectively.
   **a.** Calculate omega squared.
   **b.** Interpret your finding.
5. You are interested in comparing percent body fat for a select group of junior Olympic female volleyball players and swimmers. Calculate an independent *t* test to determine whether a significant difference exists at the .05 level.
   Percent fat for volleyball: 11, 15, 17, 16, 13, 14, 12, 9, 10
   Percent fat for swimmers: 21, 19, 18, 22, 17, 16, 20
6. Three groups of female athletes are compared by $VO_{2max}$ (mL/kg/minute): track, n = 4, *M* = 61.0; basketball, n = 5, *M* = 45.0; volleyball, n = 7, *M* = 46.0.

   | Source | SS | df | MS | F |
   |---|---|---|---|---|
   | Between | 725 | | | |
   | Within | 150 | | | |
   | Total | | | | |

   **a.** Complete the rest of the ANOVA summary table.
   **b.** Is the *F* ratio significant at the .05 level?
   **c.** If it is significant, what does this mean?

      **d.** If it is significant, what is the next step in the data analysis?

      **e.** Calculate omega squared and interpret the value.

**7.** The effect of different levels of estrogen replacement therapy on bone mineral content is compared in three groups of subjects. Each group consists of 50 subjects ($N = 150$). The following ANOVA table appears in a journal article summarizing the results.

| Source | SS | df | MS | F |
|--------|-----|-----|-------|-------|
| Between | 100 | 2 | 50.00 | 92.59 |
| Within | 80 | 147 | .54 | |
| Total | 180 | 149 | | |

      **a.** Is the $F$ ratio significant at the .05 level?

      **b.** Interpret the finding.

      **c.** If $F$ is significant, what is the next step in the data analysis?

      **d.** Calculate omega squared and interpret the value.

# CHAPTER 12

# Selected Nonparametric Statistics

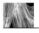

## KEY CONCEPTS

- Empirical probabilities
- One-way chi square
- Two-way chi square
- Cramer's phi coefficient
- Spearman $r$
- Mann-Whitney $U$
- Wilcoxon matched pairs
- Kruskal-Wallis one-way ANOVA
- Friedman's ANOVA

## AFTER READING THIS CHAPTER YOU SHOULD BE ABLE TO:

- Calculate, interpret, and know when to use a one-way chi square.
- Calculate, interpret, and know when to use a two-way chi square.
- Calculate, interpret, and know when to use a Cramer's phi.
- Calculate, interpret, and know when to use a Spearman $r$.
- Identify research situations that require the use of a nonparametric test and know which one to use.

The statistics presented thus far in this text are those used only for data that are absolute, interval, and ratio level. For most parametric statistics, nonparametric alternatives must be used when data are only nominal or ordinal or when the assumptions underlying the parametric tests can't be met. Sometimes these tests are also preferred for analyzing small sets of data with no normality. Overall, nonparametric tests are not as powerful as parametric ones. **Power** is the ability to reject a null hypothesis when one should, that is, when it is false. A wide variety of nonparametric statistics may be used. Several of the most commonly used ones are presented here.

## CHI SQUARE

The chi square analysis ($\chi^2$, pronounced "ki" as in "kind") is one of the most commonly used nonparametric tests and is used for frequency counts. Frequency counts may be the number of boys and girls on a playground, the number of votes cast in an election, the number of Hondas in a parking lot, and so on. With a chi square analysis, observations are made and counted in only one category. In this way, the observations are said to be *independent* of one another. The premise underlying the $\chi^2$ analysis is a comparison of what is expected to occur (theoretical probability) with what is observed (empirical probability).

*The premise behind chi square analysis is a comparison of the frequency expected to occur versus the frequency actually observed.*

**Empirical probabilities** are derived from observations of certain events. Projections of future events are based on the frequency of occurrence. For example, a recreation center director has observed and counted the number of men and women who entered the facility in a day and found that 200 men and 100 women entered the building. Based on these *empirical* observations, what would be the probability that the next person who entered the center would be a man? The empirical probability would be $p = 200/300 = .67$, since 200 of the 300 participants in the past observations were men. The empirical probability of a woman entering the facility would be $p = 100/300 = .33$. Of course, the theoretical probability of either a man or a woman entering is $p = 1/2 = .50$. The chi square analysis, then, is a test to determine whether there is significant deviation from what is theoretically expected. This statistic has several applications, which are discussed in this chapter.

### One-Way Chi Square

The one-way chi square is used to determine whether there is a significant difference between the frequency of observed and expected (theoretical) observations in two or more categories. The equation for a one-way chi square appears as:

$$\chi^2 = \sum \left[ \frac{(O - E)^2}{E} \right]$$

where O is the observed frequency and E is the expected frequency of a given category. Suppose that an outdoor recreation director polled 100 people to determine whether they would partake in the high-risk leisure activity of bungee cord jumping. Because of the recent popularity of this type of activity, he feels that many more people will want to try it than not. The categories in this case are yes and no responses. The expected or theoretical frequency is 50 yes and 50 no answers. Because there are only two choices to select from, one would expect a probability of $p = .50$ of selecting one answer or the other. The recreation director determined that the answers were actually 20 yes and 80 no responses. The following question now needs to be examined: is a 20/80 observed frequency significantly different from a 50/50 expected frequency? To answer this question,

| TABLE 12-1. Chi Square Analysis for Bungee Cord Jumping | | | | | |
|---|---|---|---|---|---|
| *Category* | *O* | *E* | *O – E* | *(O – E)²* | *(O – E)²/E* |
| Yes | 20 | 50 | −30 | 900 | 18.0 |
| No | 80 | 50 | 30 | 900 | 18.0 |
| Totals | 100 | 100 | | | $\chi^2 = 36.0$ |

O, observed frequencies; E, expected frequencies.

a one-way chi square analysis is performed. A summary of the analysis appears in Table 12-1.

## Interpretation of Chi Square

In any chi square analysis, the totals for the observed and expected frequencies must be equal. With the $\chi^2$ value of 36.0, a hypothesis test is performed. The steps in this test are summarized in Table 12-2. The null hypothesis for a chi square analysis is stated as $H_0$: $O = E$, which means that there is no real difference in the observed and expected frequencies and that any observed difference is to be attributed to sampling error. Conversely, the alternative hypothesis is $H_A$: $O \neq E$, that there is a significant difference between the observed and expected frequencies. Therefore, sampling error rarely produces a statistic that large, so something other than sampling error probably caused it. The critical chi square is referenced from Table A-1 under the appropriate alpha level and degrees of freedom. The degrees of freedom for a one-way chi square are $r - 1$, where $r$ is the number of categories. The chi square sampling distribution is one-tailed, since it contains only positive values, just like the $F$ distribution. For this example, there is one degree of freedom (2 categories −1 = 1), and at the .05 level the critical chi square is 3.84. The calculated chi square of 36.0 is greater than 3.84; therefore, we conclude that there is a significant difference between what was observed and what was expected. So the hypothesis of more people wanting to try bungee cord jumping is not supported. Figure 12-1 shows a hypothetical computer printout.

Another example of using chi square is a university wellness center director who wants to determine the number of users of a campus exercise facility. She thinks that there may be fewer freshmen than seniors using the complex and if so she may need to promote the wellness center to freshman more effectively. Data on use of the fitness center are collected for a week with the following results for 400 participants in four categories. A summary of this analysis appears in Table 12-3.

The degrees of freedom would be four categories (freshmen, sophomores, juniors, and seniors) −1 = 3, and the critical value at the .05 level would be 7.82. Since the calculated chi square of 7.50 is less than the critical value of 7.82, the null hypothesis is accepted, and it is concluded that there is no significant difference between what was observed and what was expected. Therefore, it is concluded that participation numbers

## TABLE 12-2. Summary of a Chi Square Hypothesis Test for Bungee-cord Jumping

1. State the null and alternative hypotheses.

   $H_0: O = E$

   $H_A: O \neq E$
2. Set the significance (alpha) level.

   .05
3. Determine the appropriate statistic.

   chi square
4. Determine the critical statistic value.

   $\chi^2 = 3.84$
5. Place the critical values on a curve and determine the areas of "do not reject" and "reject."

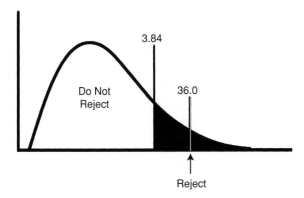

6. Calculate the statistic and place it on the curve.

   $\chi^2 = 36.0$
7. Do not reject or reject the null hypothesis.

   Reject the null.
8. Draw a research conclusion.

There is a significant difference ($p \leq .05$) between what was observed and what was expected. Therefore, more people than expected did not want to try bungee-cord jumping.

| Statistic | p Level | Alpha | Decision |
|---|---|---|---|
| $X^2 = 36.0$ | .0001 | .05 | Since $p = .0001$ is less than or equal to .05, $X^2 = 36.0$ is statistically significant ($p \leq .05$) and the null hypothesis is rejected. |

**Figure 12-1.** A sample computer printout of a chi-square analysis.

| TABLE 12-3. Chi Square Analysis for Wellness Center Users | | | | | |
|---|---|---|---|---|---|
| *Category* | *O* | *E* | *O − E* | *(O − E)²* | *(O − E)²ᐟᴱ* |
| Freshmen | 105 | 100 | 5 | 25 | 0.25 |
| Sophomores | 90 | 100 | −10 | 100 | 1.00 |
| Juniors | 85 | 100 | −15 | 225 | 2.25 |
| Seniors | 120 | 100 | 20 | 400 | 4.00 |
| Totals | 400 | 400 | | | $\chi^2 = 7.50^*$ |

O, observed frequencies; E, expected frequencies.
* $p > .05$

are similar for all four categories. Sampling error likely explained whatever differences that occurred.

Further interpretation of the chi square analysis is made possible by examination of the summary (the $[O − E]^2/E$ column) to determine which category or categories make the greatest or least contribution to the total chi square. In this way, the investigator may identify the category or categories that contribute the least or most to the research question.

## Goodness of Fit Application

Another application of the one-way chi square is to determine the **goodness of fit** of a set of data. Goodness of fit is actually a comparison of an observed set of data with expected values derived from some preexisting group of observations. Let's look at an example. A health educator reads a government report that shows typical cholesterol levels of adults in the United States. The document indicates that 30% of the population has low readings, 40% have average scores, and 30% have high values. A large-scale cholesterol screening was recently done in the health educator's community, and he wants to know how well his town's values compare with those in the government report. He thinks many people in his town have healthy lifestyles and that they should have significantly better readings than the population at large. Cholesterol values for 500 people were used in the analysis and placed into three categories. Table 12-4 contains a summary.

| TABLE 12-4. Chi Square Analysis of Cholesterol Levels | | | | | |
|---|---|---|---|---|---|
| *Category* | *O* | *E* | *O − E* | *(O − E)²* | *(O − E)²ᐟᴱ* |
| Low (30%) | 200 | 150 | 50 | 2500 | 16.7 |
| Average (40%) | 225 | 200 | 25 | 625 | 3.1 |
| High (30%) | 75 | 150 | −75 | 5625 | 37.5 |
| Totals | 500 | 100 | | | $\chi^2 = 57.3^*$ |

O, observed frequencies; E, expected frequencies.
* $p \leq .05$

The degrees of freedom would be $3 - 1 = 2$, and the critical value at the .05 level would be 5.99. Since the calculated chi square of 57.3 is greater than the critical value of 5.99, the null hypothesis is rejected, and the researcher concludes that there is a significant difference between what was observed and what was expected. Therefore, the observed data from the health educator's community differ significantly from findings in the government report. It may further be concluded that there was not a good fit between the government and the researcher's data sets. Also, his hypothesis that the town would fare better is supported. Further inspection of the summary shows that the largest difference from what was expected was 75 fewer high readings (that part of $\chi^2 = 37.5$).

## Two-Way Chi Square

The two-way chi square is used to determine whether there is a significant difference between the frequency of observed and expected observations in two or more categories with two or more levels. This arrangement is similar to the two-way factorial ANOVA. The simplest version of a two-way chi square uses a $2 \times 2$ table. The following example is used.

A famous college football coach who is also trained in research thinks his team plays better on grass fields than on artificial turf. He would like to suggest to the booster club to contribute funds to put a new surface in the stadium and would like objective evidence to support his hypothesis. So he performs a two-way chi square analysis on the win-loss record for playing on natural and artificial surfaces for the previous 80 football games.

The two categories and levels are performance (won or lost) and surface type (artificial or natural). The first step in the analysis is to place the observed frequencies of each type of event in a **contingency table** and determine the expected values. As always, the expected and observed frequencies must equal one another, and therefore, the marginal sums of the columns and rows must always equal the total number of frequencies. The $2 \times 2$ table appears in Table 12-5.

The expected values appear in parentheses and are easily determined from the marginal frequency sums for each column and row. The expected frequency for each cell is obtained by multiplying the row total by the column total and dividing by the total N.

**TABLE 12-5. 2 × 2 Table for Two-way Chi Square Analysis**

| | | Natural O | Natural E | Artificial O | Artificial E | Marginal Total |
|---|---|---|---|---|---|---|
| | | *Type of Surface* | | | | |
| Performance | Won | 39 | 33.75 | 21 | 26.25 | 60 |
| | Lost | 6 | 11.25 | 14 | 8.75 | 20 |
| Marginal total | | 45 | | 35 | | Grand Total = 80 |

O, observed frequencies; E, expected frequencies.

| TABLE 12-6. Two-Way Chi Square Analysis of Football Performance | | | |
|---|---|---|---|
| *Category* | *O* | *E* | $(O–E)^{2/E}$ |
| Natural/won | 39 | 33.75 | 0.82 |
| Natural/loss | 6 | 11.25 | 2.45 |
| Artificial/won | 21 | 26.25 | 1.05 |
| Artificial/loss | 14 | 8.75 | 3.15 |
| Totals | 80 | 80 | $\chi^2 = 7.47^*$ |

O, observed frequencies; E, expected frequencies
$^*p \le .05$

The expected values for this problem would be

$$\text{Natural/won} = (60 \times 45)/80 = 33.75$$

$$\text{Natural/loss} = (20 \times 45)/80 = 11.25$$

$$\text{Artificial/won} = (60 \times 35)/80 = 26.25$$

$$\text{Artificial/lost} = (20 \times 35)/80 = 8.75$$

Once the expected frequencies are determined, a two-way chi square is calculated the same as a one-way. The summary appears in Table 12-6.

### Interpreting the Two-way Chi Square

For a two-way chi square hypothesis test, the degrees of freedom are calculated as $(r - 1)(c - 1)$, where $r$ = the number of rows and $c$ = the number of columns in the contingency table. In this problem, there are two rows and two columns, so the degrees of freedom are $(2 - 1)(2 - 1) = 1$. The critical value of chi square at the .05 level is 3.84, which is smaller than the calculated value of 7.47 (see Fig. 12-2). Therefore, the observed performance and surface frequencies differ significantly from what was expected. The coach's hypothesis that the football team performs better on natural turf is supported.

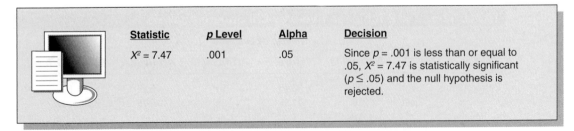

| Statistic | *p* Level | Alpha | Decision |
|---|---|---|---|
| $X^2 = 7.47$ | .001 | .05 | Since $p = .001$ is less than or equal to .05, $X^2 = 7.47$ is statistically significant ($p \le .05$) and the null hypothesis is rejected. |

**Figure 12-2.** A sample computer printout of a two-way chi square analysis.

Further examination of the summary indicates that the greatest contribution to the total chi square comes from more losses on artificial turf than expected (14 versus 8.75 losses, that part of $\chi^2 = 3.15$). So hopefully now he can convince the boosters to put natural turf in the stadium!

Further interpretation of a significant two-way chi square can be done by computing a **Cramer's phi coefficient,** or $\varphi$:

$$\varphi = \sqrt{\frac{\chi^2}{N(k-1)}}$$

where $\chi^2 =$ the calculated chi square, $N =$ the total frequencies, and $k =$ the largest number of categories. For the previous example

$$\text{Cramer's phi} = \sqrt{\frac{7.47}{80(2-1)}} = .30$$

The $\varphi$ statistic may be interpreted like a correlation coefficient. The size of the value is an indicator of the strength of the relationship or difference depicted by the significant chi square. In this example the $\varphi = .30$, suggesting only a weak relationship between surface type and performance. Consequently, the effect of playing surface on winning and losing is real, but it is not strong. Hence, the booster club shouldn't expect a great change in the team's win-loss record because of putting artificial turf on the field.

## Other Two-Way Chi Square Applications

The 2 × 2 is the most basic type of two-way chi square, but it may be used for more than two levels of two categories. One could have a two-way chi square such as a 2 × 3, 3 × 5, 4 × 4, and so on. Here is an example of a 2 × 3 analysis.

An exercise physiologist is interested in determining the aerobic fitness habits of former collegiate athletes to see whether there is a difference in adherence frequencies across different sports. Her hypothesis is that cross-country runners are more compliant than the other athletes. She surveyed 150 former football, cross-country, and tennis athletes and determined whether they conformed to the minimal recommendations for aerobic fitness as established by the American College of Sports Medicine (ACSM). Table 12-7 summarizes the observed and expected frequencies; the analysis is summarized in Table 12-8.

Since there are two rows and three columns, the degrees of freedom would be $(2 - 1)(3 - 1) = 2$, with the critical chi square value at the .05 level being 5.99. The calculated chi square of 43.01 exceeds the critical value of 5.99, so the null hypothesis is rejected. Therefore, the observed ACSM standard/sport type frequencies differ significantly from what was expected. The research hypothesis that the cross-country runners would be more compliant than the others is upheld. Inspection of the summary indicates that the greatest discrepancies were in the frequencies of the cross-country runners, followed by the tennis players, whereas the compliance to ACSM standards of football players were fairly close to what was expected (Fig. 12-3).

| TABLE 12-7. 2 × 3 Two-Way Chi Square Table for Exercise Compliance | | | | | | | |
|---|---|---|---|---|---|---|---|
| | | | | *Sport* | | | |
| | | *Football* $O$ | *Football* $E$ | *X-Country* $O$ | *X-Country* $E$ | *Tennis* $O$ | *Tennis* $E$ | *Marginal Total* |
| ACSM Standard | Yes | 25 | 32 | 45 | 26.7 | 10 | 21.3 | 80 |
| | No | 35 | 28 | 5 | 23.3 | 30 | 18.7 | 70 |
| Marginal total | | 60 | | 50 | | 40 | | Grand Total = 150 |

O, observed frequencies; E, expected frequencies

A Cramer's phi for the significant chi square is

$$\varphi = \sqrt{\frac{43.01}{150\,(3-1)}} = .38$$

This indicates a moderate to weak relationship between type of athlete and compliance with ACSM standards.

## RESTRICTIONS AND ASSUMPTIONS FOR CHI SQUARE

Certain conditions must be met to use chi square analysis. The primary assumptions and restrictions are:

1. Data must be frequency counts.
2. Observations have to be independent of one another.
3. Expected and observed frequencies have to equal one another.

| TABLE 12-8. Two-Way Chi Square for Exercise Compliance | | | |
|---|---|---|---|
| *Category* | $O$ | $E$ | $(O-E)^{2/E}$ |
| Football/yes | 25 | 32.0 | 1.53 |
| Football/no | 35 | 28.0 | 1.75 |
| X-Country/yes | 45 | 26.7 | 12.54 |
| X-Country/no | 5 | 23.3 | 14.37 |
| Tennis/yes | 10 | 21.3 | 5.99 |
| Tennis/no | 30 | 18.7 | 6.83 |
| Totals | 150 | 150.0 | $\chi^2 = 43.01^*$ |

$^* p \leq .05$

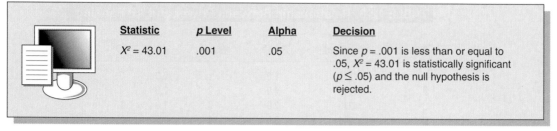

| Statistic | *p* Level | Alpha | Decision |
|-----------|-----------|-------|----------|
| $X^2 = 43.01$ | .001 | .05 | Since $p = .001$ is less than or equal to .05, $X^2 = 43.01$ is statistically significant ($p \leq .05$) and the null hypothesis is rejected. |

**Figure 12-3.** A hypothetical computer printout of a two-way chi square analysis.

**4.** The N size has to be adequate. A one-way chi square with only two categories must have expected frequencies of at least five. When there are more than two categories for one-way or for two-way tables larger than 2 × 2, no more than 20% of the categories or cells may have expected frequencies less than 5, or none of the categories may be less than 1. Also, a two-way chi square using a 2 × 2 table cannot be used for N less than 20.

## SPEARMAN *r*

The Spearman *r* (sometimes referred to as *rho*) is the nonparametric version of the Pearson *r*. It is used when data are ordinal level or for problems with small data sets. Parametric data may be used in this analysis if the observations are first converted to ranks. The equation for the Spearman *r is:*

$$\text{Spearman } r = 1 - \left[ \frac{6(\sum D^2)}{N(N^2 - 1)} \right]$$

where $\sum D^2$ is the sum of the squared differences in rank and N is the number of pairs of observations. Let's look at an example.

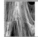 ***The Spearman r is the nonparametric version of the Pearson r.***

A physical educator is interested in examining the relationship between the final season Associated Press (AP) ranking of NCAA Division I football teams and team scores of anaerobic power. Table 12-9 summarizes the Spearman *r* analysis.

Ranks are assigned by giving the highest score a rank of 1, the next highest a rank of 2, and so on. Teams E and H have the same anaerobic power score and therefore share the average rank of the tied positions. These scores were competing for the ranks of 6 and 7, so the average rank would be $(6 + 7)/2 = 6.5$. The ranks of 6 and 7 are now used up, so the next lowest score is ranked 8. Since the AP ratings are already in rank form, no conversion is necessary. The difference between the ranks is obtained, squared, and summed. One virtue of Spearman *r* is the ease of calculation.

| Team | Power (kg/sec) | Power Rank | AP Rank | D | D² |
|------|---------------|------------|---------|-----|------|
| A | 220 | 1.0 | 1 | 0.0 | 0 |
| B | 195 | 4.0 | 2 | 2.0 | 4 |
| C | 210 | 2.0 | 3 | 1.0 | 1 |
| D | 200 | 3.0 | 4 | 1.0 | 1 |
| E | 185 | 6.5 | 5 | 1.5 | 2.25 |
| F | 182 | 8.0 | 6 | 2.0 | 4 |
| G | 190 | 5.0 | 7 | 2.0 | 4 |
| H | 185 | 6.5 | 8 | 1.5 | 2.25 |
| I | 180 | 9.0 | 9 | 0.0 | 0 |
| J | 175 | 10.0 | 10 | 0.0 | 0 |

**TABLE 12-9. Relationship Between Power and AP Ranking**

$$\Sigma D^2 = 18.5$$

Spearman $r = 1 - [6(18.5)/10(100 - 1)] = 1 - (111/990) = 1 - .112 = .89$

## Interpreting the Spearman *r*

The Spearman *r* is interpreted exactly the same way as the Pearson *r*. Therefore, a Spearman $r = .89$ between the final ranking and anaerobic power suggests that the higher the team anaerobic power, the higher the final ranking (Fig. 12-4). In addition, a hypothesis test for $r = 0$ or $r \neq 0$ may be performed. A sampling distribution for Spearman *r* values may be seen in Table A-2, where N is the number of pairs of observations. For this example the critical value of *r* at .05 and .01 would be $r = .648$ and $r = .818$, respectively. Since the calculated $r = .89$ exceeds both of these critical values, $r \neq 0$, and in this sample there is a real relationship between final ranking and team anaerobic power. As with Pearson r, the Spearman r is squared and multiplied by 100 to express the magnitude or strength of the relationship. Consequently, more than 79.2 % of the variance is explained in the example.

One limitation of Spearman *r* is that it cannot be substituted for the Pearson *r* in calculating the standard error of estimate or be used in a regression equation. Also, if

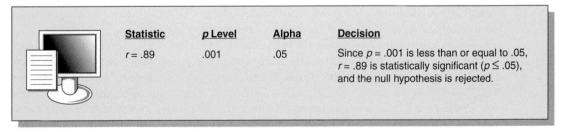

| Statistic | *p* Level | Alpha | Decision |
|-----------|-----------|-------|----------|
| *r* = .89 | .001 | .05 | Since *p* = .001 is less than or equal to .05, *r* = .89 is statistically significant ($p \leq .05$), and the null hypothesis is rejected. |

**Figure 12-4.** A sample computer printout of a Spearman *r* analysis.

there are no tied ranks, the value obtained with the Spearman $r$ will be almost identical to the Pearson $r$. However, if there are several tied ranks, the values will only approximate each other.

# SOME OTHER NONPARAMETRIC TESTS

The following is a brief description of some nonparametric tests that are alternatives to the parametric $t$ tests and ANOVAs. No equations or sample problems are provided for these statistics. These are tests of differences in medians rather than differences in means. The symbol for a population median is H, or eta. Hypotheses for a two-median comparison appear as $H_0$: $H_1 = H_2$ and $H_A$: $H_1 \neq H_2$. The interested student may refer to Bartz (1999) or other statistics texts for more detail.

## Mann-Whitney *U*

The Mann-Whitney $U$ is the nonparametric version of the independent $t$ test. For this statistic, data must be at least ordinal level. Like the independent $t$, this statistic determines whether two independent groups have been sampled from the same population. Its basis is a comparison of the number of scores from each distribution that are larger than the other. If more scores are larger than expected in one group because of sampling error, it is concluded that the groups were not drawn from the same population and are significantly different from one another.

## Wilcoxon Matched Pairs Test

The Wilcoxon matched pairs test, the nonparametric alternative to the correlated $t$, also requires that data be ordinal level. In this analysis the amount and sign of the difference between paired observations are determined. The sizes of the differences are then ranked. The premise is that there should be about the same number of small and large differences that are positive and negative values. This is determined by taking the sum of the ranks of the positive and negative differences and comparing them. If there is too great a disparity in these sums that can be attributed to sampling error, a significant difference exists between the paired observations.

## Kruskal-Wallis One-Way ANOVA

The **Kruskal-Wallis ANOVA,** the nonparametric equivalent to the one-way ANOVA, is the statistic of choice when comparisons of more than two independent groups must be made. Essentially, all of the observations in the analysis are given a rank, and the sum of the ranks for each group is determined. If there is no significant difference among the groups, the sums of the ranks of the groups should be similar. If the difference in the sums is too large to be attributed to sampling error, it is concluded that they were drawn from separate populations and are significantly different.

| TABLE 12-10. Selected Parametric and Nonparametric Tests | | |
|---|---|---|
| **Purpose** | **Parametric** | **Nonparametric** |
| Compare expected vs. observed frequency counts | None | Chi square |
| Compare two independent groups | Independent *t* | Mann-Whitney *U* |
| Compare two related groups | Correlated *t* | Wilcoxon matched pairs |
| Compare more than two independent groups | One-way ANOVA | Kruskal-Wallis ANOVA |
| Compare more than two related groups | One-way ANOVA repeated measures | Friedman's ANOVA |
| Relationship between two variables | Pearson *r* | Spearman *r* |

## Friedman's ANOVA

Friedman's ANOVA is similar in theory to the Kruskal-Wallis test. It is used when more than two repeated measurements have been made on the same subjects. Therefore, Friedman's ANOVA is the nonparametric version of the one-way ANOVA for repeated measures.

## Summary

In this chapter, we have examined a variety of nonparametric statistics that must be used when data are nominal or ordinal level and when the assumptions for parametric analyses can't be met. Overall, nonparametric tests are not as powerful as their parametric counterparts. In addition to the chi square analysis for frequency data, there are nonparametric versions of correlation coefficients (Spearman *r*), *t* tests (Mann-Whitney *U* and Wilcoxon), and ANOVAs (Kruskal-Wallis and Friedman). A summary of these statistics appears in Table 12-10.

## Learning Activities

1. Have you accomplished the objectives stated at the beginning of the chapter? If not, go back and reread the concepts you're uncertain about. Also, ask your professor about these topics.
2. Examine several research articles that used nonparametric statistics and do the following:
   - Identify what statistics were used.
   - Justify the use of the statistics.
   - Identify the type of variables that were used in each analysis and their level of measurement.

**Statistics Exercises**

Perform all tests at p = .05 level.

1. A physical educator is interested in comparing exercise habits, using minimal accepted guidelines, of former varsity athletes (softball players, cross-country runners, and golfers). The following table summarizes the findings. Perform chi square and Cramer's phi analyses and provide a practical conclusion.

| Minimum Standard | Softball | Cross-Country | Golf |
|---|---|---|---|
| Yes | 20 | 45 | 10 |
| No | 30 | 5 | 40 |

2. A recreator studied a group of men and women to determine their approval or disapproval of contact sports. The following table summarizes the results of the survey. Perform a chi square analysis and determine whether men and women differ on their approval of contact sports. Perform a Cramer's phi analysis if the chi square is significant. Provide a practical conclusion.

| Gender | Approve | Disapprove |
|---|---|---|
| Men | 50 | 10 |
| Women | 22 | 38 |

3. An athletic trainer is interested in determining whether there is a relationship between the type of playing surface and injury status. The following table summarizes the results of the research. Perform a chi square analysis and determine whether any relationship exists. Calculate a Cramer's phi if the chi square is significant. Provide a practical conclusion.

| Surface | Injured | Not Injured |
|---|---|---|
| Artificial | 41 | 59 |
| Natural | 27 | 73 |

4. The following data represent team ranking at the beginning and end of the season. Calculate a Spearman *r*, perform a hypothesis test, and provide a conclusion.

| Team | Beginning Rank | End Rank |
|---|---|---|
| A | 5 | 8 |
| B | 1 | 2 |
| C | 2 | 1 |
| D | 4 | 3 |
| E | 6 | 5 |
| F | 7 | 7 |
| G | 3 | 4 |
| H | 8 | 6 |

5. The following data represent the finish time in a 10-km road race and maximal oxygen uptake ($VO_{2max}$) scores for a group of runners. Calculate a Spearman $r$, perform a hypothesis test, and provide a conclusion.

| Runner | Time (min) | $VO_{2max}$ mL/kg/min |
|---|---|---|
| A | 39 | 62 |
| B | 44 | 52 |
| C | 31 | 68 |
| D | 32 | 68 |
| E | 40 | 58 |
| F | 43 | 50 |
| G | 41 | 60 |

# PART IV

# Measurement and Research Design

13. Measurement and Data Collection Concepts

14. Experimental Validity and Control

15. Experimental Research and Designs

16. Nonexperimental or Descriptive Research

17. Qualitative Research Methods

# CHAPTER 13

# Measurement and Data Collection Concepts

## KEY CONCEPTS

- Validity
- Logical validity: face and content
- Statistical validity: criterion-based, concurrent, predictive, construct
- Sensitivity
- Reliability
- Stability
- Equivalence
- Internal consistency
- Spearman-Brown $r$
- Objectivity
- Measurement error
- Standard error of measurement

## AFTER READING THIS CHAPTER YOU SHOULD BE ABLE TO:

- Describe the concepts of validity, reliability, and objectivity.
- Differentiate among the categories and types of validity and reliability.
- Give examples and uses of various types of validity and reliability.
- Describe the concept of measurement error and explain how it may be minimized.
- Discuss how validity and reliability coefficients are interpreted.

A researcher must carefully and logically consider the blueprint, or design, of a study so that it will yield meaningful and accurate results. However, even the most carefully planned study may have faulty results if the investigator doesn't consider the choice of instruments used to collect the data. Usually, a researcher may select from many possible instruments or tests that measure the same variable. Two important qualities to be considered relative to the research tool are its accuracy and its consistency of measurement. Therefore, it is important for an investigator to not only know how to use a measurement device but also to know the quality of the data it generates. The precision and reproducibility of research instruments are discussed in this chapter. Other concerns about measurement procedures are also presented.

## VALIDITY

Upon hearing a political candidate's remark in a debate, you may have challenged a statement by asking, "How valid is that comment?" Essentially you want to know the accuracy of the statement. In research, **validity** is the extent to which a test measures what it is supposed to measure. For example, do pull-ups accurately measure upper body strength? Most of us agree that they do. Do pull-ups measure lower body strength? The answer is obviously no.

Validity is a trait of the test or instrument. That is, once the validity of an instrument is established, it need not be demonstrated again; it more or less goes along with the proper use of the instrument or test. When a new test or procedure is developed through research, the investigators report some measures of validity in a journal article. The instrument should be accurate when used properly and in the conditions for which it was validated. For example, a skinfold test for body fat may be valid for women but not men, or a test for aerobic capacity may be accurate for adults but not children. In this regard, validity is a highly specific trait.

*Validity, from a research point of view, is the extent to which a test measures what it is supposed to measure.*

Several types of validity are used to demonstrate test or instrument accuracy. To understand the nature of validity and make interpretations related to it, one needs to become familiar with the common types of validity used in health, physical education, and recreation (HPER).

### Logical Validity

Varieties of validity in this category are the weakest types, because they are taken either at face value or qualitatively rather than quantitatively determined. In other words, no statistics or numerical values are used to express the degree of accuracy of a test or instrument.

**Face Validity** Face validity is the weakest type of validity because all that can be said about the accuracy of the instrument is that it appears obvious that the test or device is measuring what it is supposed to measure. No statement can be made about the degree of precision of the data generated with its use. A commonly used test to measure balance is standing and balancing on the ball of one foot on a small stick. Its validity is taken at face value, because it is obvious that it measures balance, but one doesn't know exactly how accurately. The 40-yard dash used to assess running speed is an example of another test whose validity is typically taken at face value.

| **TABLE 13-1. Specifications for a 50-Item Test for Measurement and Evaluation in Physical Education** | | | |
|---|---|---|---|
| **Content** | **General Knowledge (50%)** | **Comprehension (25%)** | **Application (25%)** |
| Test administration (15%) n = 8 | 4 | 2 | 2 |
| Test selection (15%) n = 8 | 4 | 2 | 2 |
| Health-fitness tests (45%) n = 22 | 11 | 6 | 5 |
| Motor fitness tests (25%) n = 12 | 6 | 3 | 3 |

**Content Validity** Content validity usually applies to written tests in educational settings, questionnaires, and other written instruments when a comparison to a standard is not possible. The primary concern with this type of validity is the extent to which the items or questions accurately measure the desired information.

One way to approach the development of such an instrument is to construct a table of specifications. Table 13-1 contains specifications for a written knowledge test. Basically, it is a blueprint that allows the researcher to quantify the number, type, and proportion of the questions or items on the instrument. Once the instrument is complete, a number of authorities or jury of experts in that research area may examine it and provide comments and critique on how it may be improved. They may also provide a qualitative judgment on the instrument's validity by describing it as weak, fair, good, or excellent. For instance, someone wanting to conduct a survey may develop a questionnaire and have several experts in survey research critique the instrument to establish its content validity before collecting data.

Again, there is no statistical value related to content validity. This is a bit stronger type of validity than the face type, since it uses both logic and authoritative expertise.

## Statistical Validity

Statistical measures of validity are considered to be stronger than logical types for two reasons. First, there is some type of numerical or statistical index of the accuracy of the instrument, such as a correlation coefficient. This makes statistical validity quantitative. Second, usually some type of comparison is made to a standard that is thought to be a good measure of the variable in question.

**Criterion-Based Validity** Measures of criterion-based validity are established when the results of one test are compared with the results obtained when using an accepted standard or criterion. The criterion or standard usually is the most accurate available measure of the variable in question, and its selection is perhaps the most important point to consider with this type of validity. The most accurate and definitive measure of a variable is sometimes referred to as a **gold standard.** Measurements of some variables in exercise physiology, for example, have gold standards. Underwater weighing to determine body composition and laboratory assessments of maximal oxygen uptake are the methods that all other similar but less accurate tests are compared against. In biomechanics, use of a force platform serves as the gold standard to measure forces while walking or running. In other instances, there is no clear-cut gold standard for a variable.

Suppose a researcher has developed an instrument that is supposed to measure sportsmanship and wishes to determine its accuracy. Sport psychologists may argue at length about what criterion or standard is acceptable for validation of a sportsmanship test, since there is no definitive measure of this trait. Therefore, when judging an index of criterion-based validity, we need to know something about the model test or instrument used in validation. A test that has a high validity index generated from a poor criterion may in fact not be accurate at all. There are two types of criterion-based validity: concurrent and predictive.

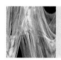 What might be considered the gold standard test for assessing physical activity level? Does the test have limitations?

***Concurrent Validity***  A measure of concurrent validity is made when two measures of the same variable are obtained within a close period (e.g., minutes, hours, a few days). One of the tests that is applied is the criterion, and the other is the test or instrument to be validated. The accuracy of the test is determined by the degree of statistical relationship between the two measures. An example of concurrent validity is correlation on a large group of subjects of the results of underwater weighing determinations of percent body fat and those from a skinfold test. A correlation analysis provides an index of accuracy of the skinfold test as a measure of percent of body fat.

***Predictive Validity***  The purpose of predictive validity is to show the accuracy of estimating the occurrence of some future event through the present use of a test or instrument. In this case, the event to be predicted is considered the criterion measure, and the present test is the one to be validated. Perhaps a health educator is interested in determining whether an inventory that she developed is capable of predicting whether a person is likely to become a regular cigarette smoker. This inventory may contain questions relative to age, gender, education, job type, exercise habits, income, and so on. The responses on the inventory are summed to yield a composite score. She administers the inventory to a representative sample of subjects who vary in terms of their smoking habits. The level of smoking is also quantified by a score and is considered the criterion. Once again, a correlation and prediction analysis is performed to examine the degree of relationship between the two sets of scores. The statistical analysis provides an index of the validity of the health educator's inventory as a predictor of smoking habits. Assuming that a reasonably large representative sample is used and the validity statistics are judged satisfactory, predictions can be made on subjects similar to those used in the validation procedure.

Remember that one of the critical factors in this type of validity is an acceptable criterion measure—in this example, the health educator's definitions of smokers and nonsmokers.

**Construct Validity** Construct validation is used when the variable of interest has no definitive criterion, is difficult to measure, or cannot be directly observed. The variable of interest in this instance is referred to as the construct. For example, we know that sportsmanship exists, but how is it measured? There are many tests of anaerobic power but no acceptable criterion. How do we establish a statistical measure of validity for these constructs?

One approach is to establish two distinct groups: one that is thought to possess a high degree of the construct and the other a low amount. The test in question is applied to each group and the results are analyzed, usually with an independent *t*. If there is a marked difference in the results between the two groups favoring the group that has a high degree of the construct, the test is said to have construct validity. Suppose a recreation professional has developed an instrument to determine whether someone has an inclination to participate in high-risk recreational activities. This particular construct may not be easily observed or may be difficult to measure. After the instrument is developed, it is administered to a group of high-risk recreators (sky divers, bungee cord jumpers, fire eaters) thought to possess this trait and a group of low-risk recreators (bowlers, gardeners, quilt makers) thought not to. If the high-risk group scores are judged significantly higher than the low-risk group, the instrument is considered to have construct validity.

## Sensitivity

Sensitivity of measurement is the degree that small differences can be detected. For example, some skinfold calipers mark each millimeter, whereas others mark every .2 millimeters. The second type thus has greater sensitivity and allows greater precision of measurement. Similarly, if a weight machine permits setting the load in increments of 10 pounds rather than 20 pounds, then the former allows more sensitive measurement of strength than the latter. A study in which strength was assessed with a sensitivity of 20 pounds would be limited because if a person succeeded with 100 pounds but then failed to lift 120 pounds, one does not know exactly how strong the person is as her true strength is somewhere between 100 and 119 pounds. Consequently, more sensitive instruments allow greater precision of measurement and so enhance validity.

## RELIABILITY

When someone is referred to as a reliable worker, we typically imply that this person is dependable and capable of producing at an expected level of consistency. In research, the concept of reliability means much the same thing. Reliability measures the consistency or repeatability of test scores or data. For example, if someone's grip strength is measured every hour over 6 hours, the scores would be expected to be similar to one another but not exactly the same. This would typify a good measure of test score reliability. High levels of reliability are critical in research, because it informs us about the dependability of test results. It is important to point out that a measure of reliability refers to the scores or data and not to the instrument itself. Also, if two people use the same instrument, they may obtain different results, meaning that the test and the tester are different components. Therefore, reliability is not a generalizable trait of a test or instrument and has to be established when it is important to consider or report reliability values.

As with measures of validity, investigators who have developed a new test or procedure will provide measures of reliability to demonstrate the level of consistency of scores they obtained. This doesn't mean that if you were to use the test, you would get the same results, but they should be close if the test was administered in much the same way. Reliability measures should be made whenever a question may be raised about the consistency of test performances. This is particularly true for measurements made with new instruments or administered with a protocol that varies from the norm. For instance, if cholesterol levels are measured using a new analytical procedure, it is important to demonstrate the consistency of these measurements. In journal articles dealing with lipids, lipoproteins, and hormones, the reliability of the results is typi-

 *Reliability is the consistency or repeatability of test scores or data.*

cally quantified by expressing the correlation between two different measures of the same variable. Thus, a study may report that the reliability in measuring serum testosterone was $r = .98$, indicating a very high agreement in results between two blood samples.

As with validity, there are several types of reliability measures. Each measures the repeatability of scores, but they are used under different conditions. The following explains some characteristics of each.

## Stability

A measure of **stability reliability** is determined when the same test is administered on two separate occasions and the results are correlated. The purpose is to determine how closely a test performance can be repeated on second, third, or more occasions. The size of the correlation between the trials is evaluated to determine if an acceptable level of consistency was achieved. This approach is known as the **test–retest method** and probably best defines the concept of reliability. Although applying a test more than one time is relatively easy (but time consuming), several points should be considered about this particular method. Because the same test is administered more than once, recall of items is quite likely on tests of knowledge. Therefore, stability measures should not be used for knowledge or paper-and-pencil tests. It is better suited for variables such as physical fitness and motor performance tests. Also, the time between administrations should not be so long that factors such as growth, learning, or maturation may affect test performance or too short so that fatigue may be a concern.

One time that it would be appropriate to use a stability measure is in a study that includes measuring blood pressure. It is important to demonstrate the repeatability of assessments of this type. Therefore, the test–retest correlation of the researcher's measurements should be high. In some research labs, technicians are not permitted to assist in data collection until they can obtain consistent results in measurements. If a researcher measured the blood pressure of 10 persons on 2 different days and found the correlation to be low, then one would question the accuracy and hence the consistency of measurement.

## Equivalence

A measure of **equivalence reliability** is made when scores from two tests that measure the same variable are correlated. The purpose is to see whether test performance can be repeated using a similar but distinct test or instrument (thus the term *equivalence*). Once again, the size of the correlation between the two sets of scores is evaluated to determine whether an acceptable level of consistency between the two sets of test scores was achieved. This particular approach is known as a **parallel** or **alternate forms method** (e.g., forms A and B). Because different tests that measure the same thing are used, recall of items is not as much of a concern. Therefore, this method is better suited for knowledge-type tests and is used in establishing reliability indices for standardized tests such as the ACT or SAT. As you might imagine, one of the major drawbacks of this method is the difficulty of developing two sound tests that have different items and that measure the same thing.

## Internal Consistency

The two methods of determining reliability just described are based on the administration of a test on two occasions. Measures of internal consistency may be established from one single test administration. This measure of reliability is used to show how consistent the scores of a test are within itself. This approach is commonly used with written tests and performance tests that incorporate many test trials. The most common means of determining this type of reliability is to use the **split-half method.** Essentially, the test is divided in half (usually the odd items are compared with the even items), and the scores from each half of the test are correlated to one another. If the correlation between the halves of the test is judged satisfactory, the test scores are deemed internally consistent. For example, a physical educator is interested in determining the reliability of scores from an archery test consisting of 10 trials of shooting 5 arrows. A score is generated for each of the 5 arrows shot. The composite scores from trials 1, 3, 5, 7, and 9 would be correlated with the scores from trials 2, 4, 6, 8, and 10 for all of the subjects. If there was good internal consistency, one would expect a suitable correlation between the odd and even trials for the group.

In using the split-half method, the reliability of test scores is fairly proportional to the number of items or trials on a test. That is, the more items or trials a test has, the higher its reliability will be. In the split-half approach, a test was divided in half and the halves were correlated to one another. This process reduces the original number of items by 50%, which makes the resulting correlation smaller than it would have been otherwise.

An equation called the **Spearman-Brown r** is used to boost the half-test correlation to what it would be if the test were its original length:

$$Spearman\text{-}Brown\ r = \frac{2 \times r}{1 + r}$$

where $r$ is the half-test reliability coefficient. For example, if a Pearson $r = .60$ was calculated for the odd and even trials on the archery shooting test, the corrected correlation would be

$$Spearman\text{-}Brown\ r = \frac{2 \times .60}{1 + .60} = .75$$

The $r = .75$ indicates good consistency in performance between the odd and even trials of the test.

## Interrater Reliability or Objectivity

Interrater reliability is a special type that is used to determine the consistency of scores obtained by more than one tester. Sometimes this is referred to as a measure of **objectivity.** For example, if two researchers are hand-timing 40-yard dash times as part of a study, it is important to show that they produce measurements that are in very close agreement with one another. The same holds true if two individuals are rating children's playground behavior, because with subjective assessments it is difficult for a single evaluator to be consistent. The statistical correlation between or among the evaluators' scores is used to determine the level of consistency.

This type of reliability is important in studies with large sample sizes in which multiple testers assist in data collection. If blood pressure was being assessed in hundreds of grade school children in a study examining the relationship between body mass index and blood pressure, several persons would probably be needed to do the measurements. To ensure that similar results were being obtained by different testers, interrater reliability or objectivity would need to be determined and reported in the study.

## THE RELATIONSHIP BETWEEN VALIDITY AND RELIABILITY

Validity and reliability are both important aspects of an instrument or test scores but are different traits. However, they are related to each other as shown in the following example (Best, 1981). Imagine an archer shooting 10 arrows at a target. If all 10 hit the bull's-eye, the archer is very accurate, which is an illustration of validity. Since all of the arrows hit the target close together, it can also be said that the archer was consistent, which is the definition of reliability. What if the next 10 arrows were shot at the target and none of them hit the bull's-eye? In fact, assume that all of them missed by 12 inches but were clustered together on the outer edge of the target within a 3-inch circle. Since the

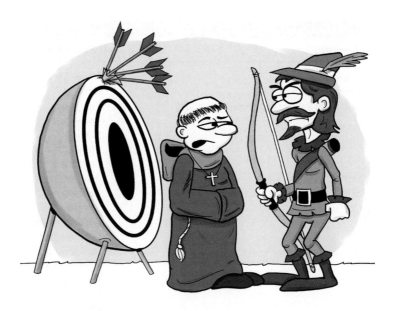

"Well, I'd say your shooting is highly reliable but not valid!"

archer was aiming at the bull's-eye and missed all 10 times, he was not very accurate—an example of poor validity. However, because all of the arrows were grouped closely together, he was consistent, or reliable. So what can be concluded about the relationship between validity and reliability? Quite simply, if a measurement is valid, its scores will be reliable, and scores may be reliable without being valid. Moreover, measurements must be reproducible for a test to be deemed valid. Consequently, these two traits must be evaluated independently.

Consider the measurement of body composition to further illustrate this idea. One method for measuring body composition is called bioelectrical impedance analysis, or BIA. BIA has been researched fairly thoroughly and has been shown to have questionable validity (McArdle, Katch, & Katch, 2001). However, the test–retest reliability of the measurements is almost perfect ($r = .99$). This means that when using this method, one would get the wrong values consistently. If the device was in error by 3% body fat, there is an excellent chance that it would be off by that much every time. So having excellent reliability does not ensure the accuracy of an instrument or test, although if a test has a high degree of validity and is used correctly, the scores should be highly reproducible.

## INTERPRETING VALIDITY AND RELIABILITY COEFFICIENTS

Table 13-2 contains some of the statistics used for assessing validity and reliability. Almost all of them are based on some type of correlation procedure, which was discussed in

| **TABLE 13-2. Commonly Used Statistics for Validity and Reliability** | |
| --- | --- |
| *Measure* | *Statistics* |
| Face validity | None |
| Content validity | None |
| Concurrent validity and predictive validity | Pearson $r$ |
| | Spearman $r$ |
| | Multiple $r$ |
| | Standard error of estimate |
| | Coefficient of determination |
| Construct validity | Independent $t$ |
| Stability and equivalence reliability | Pearson $r$ |
| | Spearman $r$ |
| | Multiple $r$, intraclass |
| | Coefficient of determination |
| Internal consistency | Pearson $r$ (half test) |
| | Spearman-Brown $r$ (whole test correction) |
| Objectivity | Pearson $r$ |
| | Spearman $r$ |
| | Multiple $r$ |
| | Coefficient of determination |

Chapter 10. As with any correlation, the size and the sign of the coefficient allow for a strict interpretation of the value. However, the interpretation, as has been said before, must go beyond that. Here is where knowledge of research in the field is invaluable. For instance, a validity coefficient of $r = .60$ may be quite acceptable for a health–lifestyle inventory predicting longevity but would be very low for a skinfold test to predict percent body fat. There is no question that reading research in your discipline will assist you in interpreting these measurement characteristics.

Safrit and Wood (1995) suggest that in general, validity coefficients of $r = .90$ or higher are desirable but values above $r = .80$ are acceptable. They further advise that for tests used to make predictions, lower validity coefficients ($r = .50$ to $r = .60$) are acceptable if no better prediction method exists. On the issue of reliability, Safrit and Wood indicate that for maximal physical effort tests and precise laboratory tests, reliability coefficients should be $r = .85$ or higher. However, with performance tests that require replication of accuracy (e.g., skills testing, measuring strength with barbells), reliability coefficients will be lower. In any case, they recommend that any reliability coefficient below $r = .70$ is unacceptable.

In addition to a correlation method, other statistics may be used or reported to assist in the assessment of validity and reliability. Statistics that describe error in prediction, such as the standard error of estimate, commonly accompany some type of correlation coefficient. Statistics such as the coefficient of determination ($r^2 \times 100$) and omega squared are also helpful in establishing these measures. (These statistics and their interpretation were discussed previously.) Researchers routinely report several statistics to support validity. The more statistics that are provided, the better the overall ability to judge accuracy. For example, validity statistics for a skinfold body fat test correlated to underwater weighing may appear as: $r = .90$, $r^2 \times 100 = 81.0\%$, and $SEE = 2.0\%$ fat. Each statistic provides interpretive information to help draw a conclusion about that test's validity. These particular statistics indicate that there is a strong positive relationship between the skinfold test and underwater weighing, that 81% of the variance in underwater weighing scores can be explained by the skinfold scores, and that a 68% confidence interval around a predicted score would be ±2.0% fat. Overall, the results indicate that the skinfold test has acceptable validity.

## VALIDITY: IS THERE REALLY SUCH A THING?

Some philosophers argue that the concept of validity cannot be justified logically. The following example may demonstrate why. Assume a scale in a laboratory must be calibrated prior to a study. The researcher uses certified calibration weights that are supposed to be very exact. You may wonder how the accuracy of the calibration weights was determined. Assume it was with weights certified as being accurately measured for mass by the U. S. Bureau of Standards. But how was the accuracy of the bureau's calibration weights established? This line of reasoning is endless. Technically, one could challenge any criterion standard, no matter how precise it may be, and ask how accurate it really is. So can the concept of validity truly be justified if one can dispute the accuracy of any measurement? Obviously, at a certain point one must accept the given level of precision of a test; otherwise, there could be no measurements made or research conducted. Without research our world would be a very dark and cold place!

## MEASUREMENT ERROR

When a measurement is made on a subject, the result is called an **observed score.** The observed score is a combination of what one wants to assess, which is the **true score,** and any error that was made in the process, which is referred to as measurement error. Mathematically, then,

$$\text{Observed score} = \text{true score} \pm \text{measurement error}$$

The true score is one that is free of measurement error. Unfortunately, a true score may never be known; it is more or less a theoretical construct because measurement error always exists to some degree. One of the basic ideas

*Any mistake in data collection is measurement error.*

related to conducting sound research is to minimize measurement error so that you can increase the level of confidence that you are accurately measuring the variables of interest. This also makes the researcher more certain that any observed changes in behavior or an experimental variable are attributed to the treatment and not errors in measurement.

## Sources of Measurement Error

Anything that can contaminate a true score can be regarded as measurement error. Some of the sources of this error may be traced to the **instrument** used in testing, to the **testing procedures,** or to the **performance of the subject.** The instrument that is used should be in proper working order, properly calibrated, and properly used. The testing procedures should be clearly defined and executed in the same manner for all subjects. This means that the researcher should go through several mock trials or pilot tests to work out any possible bugs or inconsistencies and to practice and review testing skills. Attention should be given to how the measurement will be scored and recorded. Data collection forms typically are needed. Finally, the subject should be properly instructed in and familiarized with the testing procedures. The subject's level of motivation, health, fatigue, and previous testing experience all affect the quality of test performance and may contribute to measurement error.

Although it is difficult to control the psychological and behavioral aspects of the subject, the researcher can reduce many sources of measurement error. Research testing should be conducted in a careful, attentive, and professional manner. The end result of collecting research data is usually a mass of numbers, and only the researcher ultimately knows exactly how accurate those numbers are. The phrase "garbage in, garbage out," or GIGO, should come to mind! Succinctly stated, measurement error detracts from the accuracy of the data and hence the quality of the research. Working with or observing an experienced investigator is a good way for the novice to learn to avoid some of the common sources of measurement error that affect particular types of research.

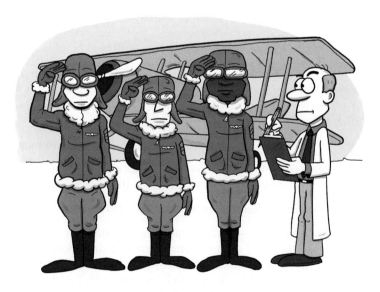

**A pilot study.**

Many measurements made in HPER can be easily tainted by lack of thorough planning for data collection. Something as simple as measuring a skinfold to assess body fatness can pose a number of potential problems. For example, how long should the calipers be applied to the skin? A longer period of measurement tends to reduce the thickness as the pressure from the spring squeezes fluid from underlying tissue. Exactly where on the body is the measurement made? Precise anatomic locations are specified for skinfold assessment, and failure to measure at the exact spot introduces measurement error. Were the calipers calibrated? To ensure accuracy calipers should be calibrated before use in a study. How many times should each site be measured? Should the mean or median of the measures be used for data analysis? These questions should make it obvious that accurate measurement requires special attention to the instrument itself as well as to procedures for using the instrument. Numerous sources of measurement error exist in most situations.

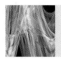

What potential sources of measurement error exist in assessing blood pressure?

## Quantifying Measurement Error

Can measurement error be quantified to some degree? The answer is yes, to a certain extent. A statistic called the **standard error of measurement** (*SEM*) can be calculated and used as an index of the accuracy of an obtained test score. It may also be used to compute confidence intervals for the true test score. The equation for *SEM* is as follows:

$$SEM = SD_{TEST}\sqrt{1 - r_{TEST}}$$

where $SD_{TEST}$ is the *SD* of the test scores and $r_{TEST}$ is the reliability of test scores. Therefore, if $SD_{TEST} = 5$ and $r_{TEST} = .90$,

$$SEM = 5\sqrt{1 - .90} = 1.6$$

Confidence intervals for the true test score may now be calculated, with the obtained test score being the midpoint of the interval:

$$68\% = \text{obtained score} \pm 1.0(SEM)$$

$$95\% = \text{obtained score} \pm 1.96(SEM)$$

$$99\% = \text{obtained score} \pm 2.58(SEM).$$

A 68% confidence interval for an obtained score of 75 is

$$68\% = 75 \pm 1.0(1.6) = 73.4 - 76.6$$

The interpretation of this interval is similar to that for a predicted score (Y′); that is, we are 68% confident that the true test score (one that is free of measurement error) is contained within the interval. Intervals for 95% and 99% may also be computed and used.

A higher test reliability coefficient results in a smaller *SEM;* hence less measurement error. The reliability coefficient is actually a statistical expression of how free the test scores are of measurement error. So having high test score reliability and a small *SEM* is desirable.

Other correlation methods, such as the intraclass correlation, are based on estimates of true score, observed score, and error variance. With this technique, measurement error can be estimated and its influences removed from the observed score. Even though this statistical technique exists and can help buffer the presence of some measurement error, researchers still need to be meticulous in their testing techniques.

## Summary

In this chapter, we focus on concepts related to measurement and data collection. Validity is the accuracy of an instrument or test, which can be determined logically or statistically. Reliability relates to the consistency or reproducibility of test scores, which may be classified as a measure of stability, equivalence, internal consistency, or objectivity. The validity and reliability of any test should be evaluated before its selection or use. Finally, recognize that measurement error always exists, but the researcher can minimize it by detailed planning and practicing skills related to administering a test.

## Learning Activities

1. Have you accomplished the objectives stated at the beginning of the chapter? If not, go back and reread the concepts you're uncertain about. Also, ask your professor questions about these topics.
2. Examine several research articles for information regarding the validity of instruments used and the reliability of test scores.
3. Inspect research articles specifically addressing the development of a new test or procedure. Determine the validation techniques used and their associated statistics. Was test score reliability reported? If so, what methods were used and what were the reliability levels? Did these methods and results seem adequate to you?
4. Select a test in your discipline and identify as many possible sources of measurement error as possible.

# CHAPTER 14

# Experimental Validity and Control

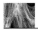

## KEY CONCEPTS

- Internal validity
- Threats to internal validity
- External validity
- Threats to external validity
- Controlling for threats to experimental validity

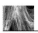

## AFTER READING THIS CHAPTER YOU SHOULD BE ABLE TO:

- Define and give examples of internal and external validity.
- Identify and provide examples of threats to internal and external validity.
- Describe several methods that might improve the internal or external validity of a study.
- Explain when a particular type of validity is important.


Researchers must design experiments in such a way that they have a high degree of confidence in the results. This may be accomplished in part by logically considering things that may possibly go wrong and flaw the experiment. Some contaminating factors are unique to a particular type of study; others are generic to virtually any type of research. Also, some of these conditions are easily controlled for, whereas others are not. Another consideration for investigators is the extent it is possible to apply the results of their research to other subjects, conditions, and situations. In this chapter, these research concepts are addressed.


## INTERNAL VALIDITY

Previously, the concepts of independent and dependent variables were discussed. For quick review: The independent variable is the one that the researcher manipulates. It is the variable that is referred to as the treatment, the one that is tested to determine whether it caused an effect. The dependent variable is the behavior that is affected or that the investigator is observing for change. Internal validity, then, is the extent to which the research condition is controlled so that the independent variable causes an effect or change in the dependent variable. The stronger the controls over an experimental condition, the higher the degree of internal validity. Unfortunately, no statistical value is associated with internal validity, so one must carefully examine how the research was conducted to judge the soundness of a study.

Many factors have been identified as key threats to the internal validity of a study. Campbell and Stanley's report on these factors in their classic 1963 book,

 ***Internal validity is the extent to which the research condition is controlled so that the independent variable causes an effect or change in the dependent variable.***

*Experimental and quasi-experimental designs for research.* has been presented in most research textbooks since then. A discussion and illustration of some of these threats follow. When each of the factors is presented, it will be helpful to understand how each may cause a change in the dependent variable other than the independent variable. In a perfect study, the only factor altering behavior would be the independent variable. However, in the "real world," many variables may and probably do change behavior.

For example, in a study designed to assess the effect of weight training on bone mineral density, numerous factors other than the weight training are likely to have some effect on bone mineral density. Variables such as diet, amount, and intensity of physical activity besides weight training, hormonal status, exposure to sunlight, and medications that affect bone density are all possible extraneous variables. The challenge to the researcher is to minimize the influence of outside variables while maximizing the effect of the independent variable. The most common **threats to internal validity** are summarized in Table 14-1.

## Maturation

Undoubtedly, study subjects change in many ways over time. They may become heavier, more or less anxious, smarter, better coordinated, leaner, and so on. Any time growth,

| **TABLE 14-1. Primary Threats to Internal and External Validity** | |
|---|---|
| ***Internal Validity*** | ***External Validity*** |
| Maturation | Reactive effects of pre-testing |
| History | Subject–treatment interaction |
| Testing | Artificial nature of experimental condition |
| Instrument accuracy | Multiple treatment interference |
| Statistical regression | |
| Experimental mortality | |
| Selection bias | |
| Selection maturation | |
| Placebo effect | |
| Hawthorne effect | |
| Halo effect | |

learning, or maturation occur during the conduct of a study and influence the dependent variable, it raises uncertainty as to the effect of the independent variable. Maturational effects are of high concern when using children for subjects because of their rapid and unpredictable growth rates. Similarly, studies using older subjects must be concerned with the effects of aging. Maturation is a problem, especially in studies that last for several months or even years.

Perhaps the best means of controlling for the effect of maturation is the inclusion of a control group in the design of the study. By comparing the degree of change in the control and experimental group, the effect of maturation can be determined. For example, suppose a group of seniors lift weights twice weekly and their mean gain in knee extension strength over 1 year is 20 pounds. If the mean loss of strength in a control group is 8 pounds, the effect of the independent variable, weight training, was actually 28 pounds rather than 20 pounds. Consequently, interpretation of the study is enhanced when the effect of maturation is known. The change in the control group provides this information.

## History

History relates to all of the things outside of a study that happen to the subject and that may influence the dependent variable. Typically, these factors are recognized as possibilities but can't be controlled. For instance, perhaps a health educator is examining the effects of a smoking cessation program that uses a nicotine gum. Several subjects in the study may work for the same company that instituted a "no smoking policy" in the workplace during the time the research was occurring. This may have created a condition of increased peer pressure to quit smoking. At the end of the study it would be difficult to determine whether the nicotine gum or the peer pressure caused an effect. Of course, there could be many such outside influences besides this one. Controlling the effects of history becomes more difficult as the duration of the study increases.

A means of reducing the potential effect of history is having a reasonably large sample size and randomly assigning subjects to groups. One can better assume that with more subjects, the impact of a no smoking policy on some subjects may be minimized. Furthermore, with randomization to groups, subjects working in companies with such a policy in theory would be randomly distributed to groups, and no one group would be affected more than another.

## Testing

The process of testing provides a subject with some experience about the test that may influence test performance a subsequent time. This is called a *practice* or *learning effect* and is a confounding problem with many physical performance tests that are done more than once, which in pre-post designs is the norm. The effect is particularly strong with novel tests or assessments. For example, a person being tested for the first time on a strength testing instrument such as a Biodex may find that moving a limb while the body is stabilized with straps to be constraining and awkward. Hence, the resulting strength assessment score may be reduced. Upon retesting, the initial experience makes the subject less inhibited and perhaps more comfortable, and thus able to more fully exert to true maximum. The threat to internal validity is that it is unknown how much of the improvement in strength that occurred in a study is due to actual strength increase and how much to the experience gained from testing itself. The testing experience may also provide an increased incentive to improve in some manner that is independent of the experimental treatment. For example, if one knew the initial score on a skills test, the desire to improve on retesting may be an incentive to try harder.

## Instrument Accuracy

As emphasized in the last chapter, it is critical that tests and instruments be valid, reliable, and in good working order. Instruments not properly calibrated limit the accuracy in measuring change in the dependent variable and so limit the internal validity of a study. Strict adherence to a previously determined protocol for testing is also needed to ensure accuracy. In well-conducted studies, practice or pilot testing is done before collecting data on the research subjects to ensure the highest possible accuracy.

## Statistical Regression

Statistical regression occurs when an extreme performance on a test is followed by a less extreme performance. The term regression refers to the tendency for the second score to regress toward the mean or more typical performance on a retest. The phenomenon frequently is observed in sport. If a baseball player's batting average one season is .525 for May and the player is a career .300 hitter, his average will probably regress toward the more typical .300 level as the season goes on. Statistical regression may operate in the same fashion on group performance if the group was formed on the basis of extreme pre-test performance. So for the individual or group with a low pre-test score, it is legitimate to ask whether their post-test or retest score improved because of the independent variable or because of statistical regression. The effect of statistical regression can be minimized by having an adequate sample size. The mathematical effect of a few scores affected by this phenomenon is reduced with more subjects.

## Selection Bias

When groups are formed nonrandomly, the possible effects of selection bias must be considered. This is most likely to occur when volunteers are free to select one group or treatment. The basis of their option may indicate a stronger sense of motivation or predisposition than someone who didn't select that group. This is especially confounding when subjects are asked to volunteer to be in a control group (no treatment) versus an experimental group (treatment). Using intact groups, such as teams or classes, also introduces a form of bias. The major drawback with selection bias is that the researcher does not know whether a pre-post difference between groups was due to original discrepancies or to the independent variable.

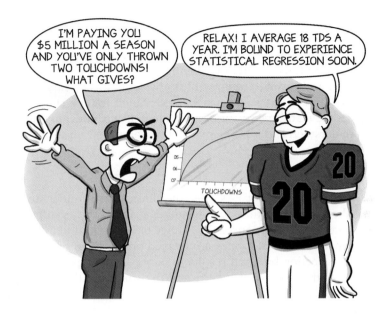

Statistical techniques are available to counter the possible effects of selection bias. Analysis of covariance (ANCOVA) can be used to control for initial differences in groups on a key dependent variable at the outset of a study. For example, suppose physical activity level is assessed in two schools. One school serves as the experimental group being exposed to an intervention to increase physical activity and another school is not exposed to the intervention and serves as the control group. The initial differences in physical activity can be controlled for using ANCOVA. Any differences between the groups at the end of the study can more likely be attributed to the intervention.

## Experimental Mortality

Experimental mortality does not mean that subjects died during a study. Strictly speaking, experimental mortality refers to the **loss or dropout of subjects** in a study. This happens for many obvious reasons, such as disinterest, sickness, inconvenience, injury, and discomfort. What problem in research does experimental mortality cause? Assuming that groups were formed in an unbiased manner at the beginning of a study, it may be concluded that they are reasonably similar to one another. After subject attrition occurs, the remaining subjects may be unique from the standpoint of motivation, health, interest, or some other factor. If most of the attrition occurs in one group, it may alter their characteristics and hence the mean value of the dependent variable. Consequently, groups that were equivalent initially now may be different. This creates essentially the same problem as selection bias. The researcher doesn't know whether differences at the completion of a study arose from the unique attributes of the remaining subjects or were caused by the independent variable.

The best countermeasure for experimental mortality is adequate sample size. The change in a group's mean score due to subject attrition is minimized if the size of the group is relatively large. Researchers typically anticipate some loss of subjects, particularly if the study duration is lengthy. An investigation by one of the authors was longitudinal and involved women lifting weights for 2 years. Some loss of subjects was expected and so extra subjects were recruited for the study. The loss of subjects also reduces the statistical power or ability to detect significant differences. These effects are well understood and it is one reason that sample size is always reported in studies.

## Selection Maturation

Selection maturation occurs when the characteristic under study will improve naturally over the passage of time (e.g., a physical injury); it is difficult to know whether the independent variable caused the change or the condition improved by itself. This threat is compounded when groups are formed on the basis of this characteristic, which is a form of selection bias and results in nonequivalent groups. Since the groups were not similar at the onset of the study and the condition that distinguishes the groups may resolve itself over time, strict comparisons between the groups are difficult to make.

## Other Threats to Internal Validity

The threats to validity just described are the classic ones presented by Campbell and Stanley. However, other threats to external validity exist.

**Placebo Effect** It has long been observed that mere participation in a study may elicit an effect that is separate from the independent variable. In medical studies, control subjects who participate in a drug study are given a placebo, which is simply an inactive substance or procedure. To avoid tipping off the subjects, drugs and placebos are usually administered in what is called a **blind** fashion, which prevents subjects from knowing what treatment they are receiving. Sometimes subjects in the placebo group show an improvement due to **expectation,** which is called the **placebo effect.** The true effectiveness of a drug then is the difference between what is observed in the experimental group and the placebo group. Without a placebo group it would be difficult to know what effect was attributed to the treatment and what amount the placebo was responsible for. A **double-blind** study prevents both subject and experimenter from knowing who receives the placebo and experimental treatment. This technique prevents the researcher from exerting any bias when conducting the study. For example, a researcher might influence a subject in an experimental group by encouraging the person more than a subject known to be in the control group. The bias may even influence measurement procedures.

The placebo effect may exist in many types of research and the effect may be more powerful than previously realized. Eliminating its effect on behavior is difficult in many research situations. Recent studies indicate that the placebo effect is strong enough to require additional steps by the researcher. For example, in a published study of patients with knee arthritis, the effects of surgery were compared with the placebo effect, which

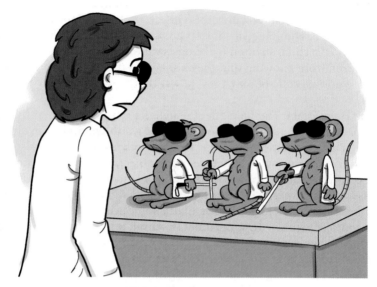

**"This isn't going to be easy."**

"Double-blind studies are really difficult to do!"

consisted of sham surgery. The sham procedure included making an incision at the knee so that patients were unable to detect whether or not they actually had surgery. Interestingly, on follow-up patients having the sham surgery reported significantly less pain and discomfort with the level of improvement rivaling that of the group actually having the surgery. Consequently, the placebo effect can be powerful, and researchers should acknowledge its potential effect. Traditionally, the placebo group has been thought to represent the absence of any effect. Based on these newer findings, it appears reasonable to have an experimental group, placebo group, and also a control group having no exposure to the independent variable in any fashion. This would allow a truer means of determining the effect of the independent variable, real or imagined.

**Hawthorne Effect** A similar phenomenon in behavioral research was highlighted by studies on workers at the Hawthorne plant of the Western Electric Company in Chicago years ago. The investigators were studying the relationship between lighting brightness and work output. It seemed that as the lights were made brighter, work output increased. After a certain point was reached, the investigators reduced the lighting intensity to see whether the relationship continued. To their surprise, as the illumination decreased, the workers' productivity continued to increase. What did they conclude? The increase in work output was probably due to the attention the subjects received under observation by the researchers and/or management. Therefore, because subjects know they are being observed, they work harder.

The placebo effect is one induced by expectation; the **Hawthorne effect is produced by observation.** They are similar in nature in that each may affect the dependent variable and make it difficult to know the true effect of the independent variable. The Hawthorne effect can be eliminated if subjects are unaware of being observed. Studies observing play behavior in children often make observations behind one way windows that prevent the children from knowing that they are being studied. One thus hopes to see children in a more normal state of play.

**The Halo Effect** The halo effect usually is introduced when the **researcher has some expectation about the performance of a subject** and is involved in assessing the person. This expectation may bias the researcher's judgment. Also, it may lead the investigator to exert undue influence on a subject, such as providing encouragement or no encouragement or leading the subject to respond a certain way. The more subjectively assessed the experimental variable is, the greater the halo effect becomes. For example, an exercise physiologist knows that a subject is a distance runner and provides strong encouragement during a maximal treadmill test to exhaustion because of the belief that any distance runner should do well on such a test. However, the same researcher has lower expectations for a nonrunner and so offers only minimal encouragement to that subject. The strong verbal encouragement given the runner encourages the person to work longer and possibly achieve a better score.

Another illustration might be a recreation leader observing playground activity levels of children from two different economic strata. If the researcher expects children from the lower stratum to be more active for whatever reason, she may look for more signs of activity in that group, thus biasing the observations and assessments she is making.

It is important for the researcher to be as objective as possible and avoid affecting the performance status of the subject. Halos of any type may cloud the investigator's impartiality or may lead to coercing the subject in a manner that affects the dependent variable.

One approach to reducing the halo threat to internal validity is to have outsiders who are skilled in the area being studied make the experimental measurements. This, of course, is assuming that they are not familiar with the subjects. Sometimes this is not possible because of the skill needed to make measurements or the limited availability of such personnel. Another approach is to use what is called a **double-blind** method. With the double-blind method, neither the researcher nor the subject knows what group the subject is in or what treatment (if any) the subject is getting. This approach may remove any expectations of researchers about the subject because they are not biased to how the participant should respond.

## EXTERNAL VALIDITY

External validity refers to the generalizability or potential for applying the results of a study to other conditions or settings. For example, if the results of a study showed that walking 1 hour daily lowered cholesterol for men, will it do the same for women? If a method of teaching health education is effective for elementary school children, will it be so for college students? The greater the ability to generalize the results of a study,

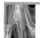 *External validity is the ability to use the results of a study in other conditions or settings.*

the higher the degree of external validity it has. In general, the more similar the subjects in the original study are to the group for whom one is considering generalizing the results to, the more likely it is that similar results might be expected. For example, a health education technique found to be effective in elementary school age children is more likely to be effective in middle school children than in college students.

No statistical tool is available to determine the potential for generalizing. Hence, it is dependent on the reader's judgment. Several factors that threaten the external validity of an investigation are noted by Campbell and Stanley. These **threats to external validity** are summarized in Table 14-1.

## Reactive Effects of Pre-testing

Previously, it was explained that pre-testing a subject may enhance the person's performance on a retest. Another possible consequence of pre-testing subjects is that it may alter their perception of the experimental treatment in such a way that they are motivated to perform better than if they had not been exposed to the pre-test. When this occurs, there is a reactive or interactive effect of the testing experience with the experimental treatment. Why is this a threat to external validity? Essentially, because the treatment may have an effect only if preceded by the pre-test, making the treatment generalizable only under those conditions.

## Subject and Treatment Interaction

Sometimes a unique characteristic of the subjects in a study makes the treatment effective only for them or others possessing that trait. For instance, a sports psychologist interested in examining the effect of a program designed to improve exercise adherence might find different results with a group of college freshmen who are not athletes from those of a group of varsity athletes. If there is group selection bias, the effectiveness of a treatment and generalizability of a study are limited to subjects with that trait. Examples are numerous in medicine. For example, a certain drug may be found to lower LDL cholesterol in those with hypercholesterolemia. However, the same effect may not be observed in those not having elevated cholesterol levels.

## The Artificial Nature of the Experimental Condition

At the heart of this threat to validity is whether a subject will perform in the same manner under experimental conditions as he/she would in the real world. Seldom are the conditions the same in a laboratory or tightly controlled environment as they are in the field. Should one expect subjects to perform or behave differently, particularly when they know they are participating in a study? The Hawthorne effect may also affect this condition. The more artificial and constrained a research setting becomes, the lower the ability to generalize from it. For example, a stress reduction technique may be effective when the technique is used in a quiet laboratory setting and then followed by a series of tests to measure stress such as blood pressure and stress hormone levels. However, outside the laboratory where people are exposed to multiple sources of stress, they may find it more difficult to use a stress reduction technique, and so measures of stress may be more difficult to reduce.

## Multiple Treatment Interference

When a researcher is interested in studying more than one experimental variable or more than one level of one variable on the same subjects, there is a risk of the **treatments interfering with or facilitating one another.** The performance of one task may inhibit or enhance the performance of a different task. Fatigue, learning effects, and other such factors all may interact with test performance in such a way that the ability to generalize study results is reduced. For instance, perhaps performing a test for balance allows someone to do better on a subsequent reaction time test. Hence, improvement may be influenced by performing the first test before the second test. Interference can also occur with multiple tests. For example, fatigue from a treadmill test may interfere with a second test measuring strength. To counteract the possible influence of one test with another, researchers usually randomly assign the sequence of tests.

## CONTROLLING FOR THREATS TO INTERNAL VALIDITY

All studies have limitations and weaknesses. Researchers need to be aware of these factors so they can use methods and designs that minimize their effects. Readers of research need to be attentive to these threats so that informed judgments can be made about the quality of published and presented work. Numerous methods may be used to reduce threats to internal validity. A discussion of some of these follows.

## Making Equivalent Groups: Randomization

One of the key methods for reducing threats to internal validity is to form equivalent groups at the onset of a study. This is most commonly achieved by developing a list of qualifications for the subjects and then to use **randomization,** or chance assignment, when placing them into groups. The premise behind randomization is the presumption that the only initial differences between groups will be those that are produced by chance or sampling error. The statistical estimate of sampling error is called error variance.

How does randomization reduce threats to internal validity? When groups are equivalent at the beginning of a study, it can be assumed that the effects of maturation and history will be similar across groups. It may also be argued that exposure to all of the possible events outside the study during its conduct that may affect its outcome is equally probable in the different groups. However, the researcher must be aware of some of these events and be creative in a way to reduce the subjects' contact with them. Selection bias is removed with randomization, because subjects are not allowed to select their own group. This is also true with selection maturation problems, since the primary factor that causes it is groups that are formed on the basis of a different trait, which is a form of selection bias and results in nonequivalent groups. Rather than forming groups on the basis of extreme scores, randomizing the subjects into groups instead may minimize statistical regression. Randomization is not the only way to make groups equivalent, although it is probably the easiest and most time-honored approach.

## Using Control Groups

Some types of research designs are based on a comparison between the effects of a treatment and no treatment. The group that is used to measure the effects of no treatment is called the **control group.** The control group has characteristics similar to those of the treatment or experimental group, the only difference being that it doesn't receive the independent variable. The best way to develop a sound and representative control group is to randomize the subjects into groups. Theoretically, the subjects in the control group and subjects in the experimental group are equally likely to be exposed to or demonstrate the effects of maturation, history, and testing. So any effects that these factors may exert may be assessed in the control group.

As stated previously, the use of blind and double-blind methods controls for the placebo and halo effects, respectively. To demonstrate the effect of participation without treatment, a placebo group must be used. Therefore, the placebo group is a special type of control group because the subjects actually participate in the study but receive a bogus treatment. A true control group goes through the testing procedures but receives no treatment. The double-blind method is also based on the use of a control group, since by definition neither the subject nor the researcher knows who received the treatment. Control groups may also be used to assess the Hawthorne effect. Control groups are not required all the time but are important when considering means of reducing threats to internal validity.

 *Two effective means of controlling threats to internal validity are making groups equivalent and using a control group.*

## Other Control Methods

Many threats to internal validity are minimized through use of randomization and a control group. Another way of reducing threats to internal validity is ensuring accuracy of the measuring instruments. It is imperative that the instrument be thoughtfully selected, calibrated, if appropriate, and used properly by the investigator, since no research design or other method can minimize measurement error. Experimental mortality is typically beyond the direct control of the researcher. If subjects want to drop out of a study, it is their prerogative to do so at any time without fear of reprisals. Sometimes investigators provide an incentive, such as cash, for the subject to complete the study. If researchers resort to begging or pleading with a subject, they are violating the subject's ethical rights.

## TABLE 14-2. Controlling Threats to Internal Validity

| | |
|---|---|
| Maturation | Randomization, control group |
| History | Randomization, control group |
| Testing | Randomization, control group, no pre-test |
| Instrument accuracy | Researcher |
| Statistical regression | Randomization |
| Selection bias | Randomization |
| Experimental mortality | Researcher hopes subjects stay in study |
| Selection maturation | Randomization |
| Placebo effect | Control group, blind or double-blind design |
| Hawthorne effect | Control group, blind or double-blind design |
| Halo effect | Blind or double-blind design |

Threatening a subject who wants to withdraw from a study is a clear violation of research ethics. Finally, the effects of testing can be assessed with the use of a control group or reduced if it is possible not to pre-test the subject. The primary means of controlling threats to internal validity are summarized in Table 14-2.

## CONTROLLING FOR THREATS TO EXTERNAL VALIDITY

When a high degree of external validity or generalizability is desirable, it is important that the subjects in the study be representative of the population to be generalized to. For example, if an investigator wants to develop a body fat prediction equation for older women, it is important to obtain a large number of subjects through random sampling. This is the best way to ensure that the sample is a good representation of this group, which increases the ability to accurately generalize the study results.

 *For a high degree of external validity, it is important that the subjects be representative of the population.*

The reactive effects of pre-testing can be assessed through the use of a control group or groups. In the ideal case, one group would receive the pre-test only, another would receive the treatment only, and a third would receive both the pre-test and the treatment. A comparison would be made across the groups to measure the influence of each of the conditions. Other research designs are also based on this premise.

The effects of subject–treatment interaction should be appraised by the researcher. The investigator must analyze the nature of the subjects and contemplate whether the treatment in question may work only on them. Also, it is necessary to decide on the desired extent of external validity. If a researcher would like to be able to generalize the results of a study to college students in general, a large representative sample obtained through random sampling in various regions of the country is needed. The use of intact groups or classes as a study sample would be inappropriate.

| **TABLE 14-3. Controlling Threats to External Validity** | |
| --- | --- |
| Reactive effects of pre-testing | Control group or design |
| Subject–treatment interaction | Researcher appraisal |
| Artificial nature of experimental condition | Researcher, if possible |
| Multiple treatment interference | Randomization of treatments, design, or researcher appraisal |
| Overall | Have a representative sample |

The artificial nature of the testing condition is another consideration of the researcher because there is no technique to control for it. Moreover, some measurements can be made only under controlled laboratory conditions, so not much can be done in this regard. In other instances, the investigator may think of creative ways to make the testing condition more closely resemble the real world, but this is effective only if the subject performs in a real world manner. Minimizing the effects of multiple treatment interference is also under the control of the researcher. Attention must be given to whether the treatments may affect one another or not. If they may, the investigator may have to consider perhaps arranging treatments in a unique manner, randomizing the treatment order, or having several experimental groups, with each group receiving only one treatment.

Sometimes a researcher is interested in how treatments may interact with one another. This is the basis for factorial ANOVAs (analyses of variance), with which the researchers study not only the main effect of each independent variable but also any possible interaction between the variables. The basic ways to control for threats to external validity are presented in Table 14-3.

## INTERNAL VERSUS EXTERNAL VALIDITY: WHICH SHOULD BE THE FOCUS AND WHICH IS MORE IMPORTANT?

External validity may not be a major focus with some types of research. For example, a medication tested for efficacy in reducing blood pressure would not be applicable for the general nonhypertensive population. The generalizability then is limited only to those who are hypertensive. Even more limited concern for external validity might be demonstrated in physics research, in which subatomic particles are accelerated to incredibly high velocity and then allowed to collide with each other. Here, the purpose is to observe what happens, and the importance of generalizing is secondary. This research may enhance the development of theories to better understand the composition of matter and ultimately this knowledge may be useful or applicable to a variety of conditions. However, the focus of the initial research is on internal validity.

Both types of validity are important, but it is difficult to have a high degree of each within the same study. The relationship between internal and external validity is inverse.

That is, the more of one means less of the other. The best way to control for most threats to internal validity is to conduct research under very sterile, tightly controlled conditions. When research is done in this manner, a higher degree of internal validity can be reached. However, research that is carried out this way is not at all like the real world, so generalizability of the results is reduced. This is typical of **pure** or **basic** research. On the other hand, if research is conducted in the real world or in the field, some element of control over the experimental condition is lost. So, in the process of making the study more externally valid, the researcher may weaken internal validity. This is characteristic of **applied** research. Although it is not possible to have a high degree of both, it is conceivable to have a reasonable amount of each. When both of these experimental validities are desirable, research can still be done, but not without some loss of the known effect of the independent variable or the ability to generalize the study results.

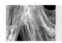 Internal and external validity are inversely related.

Which type of validity is more important depends largely on the type and purpose of the research. If an investigator is conducting basic research that is predicated on theory development and requires a high degree of control, internal validity is critical and external validity is not. When it is desirable to generalize research results, as it is with much of the research done in HPER, external validity is more important. This does not mean that the applied researcher is not interested in internal validity, because every investigator must be. An investigator has to be at least reasonably confident that the independent variable in the study was responsible for the effect on the dependent variable. Without this assurance, no viable research can be done. With applied research, some element of internal validity is lost in favor of external validity. For applied research, striking an acceptable balance between the two is key.

 ## Summary

In this chapter, we examine the issues of experimental validity and methods that can be used to minimize their effect. Internal validity is the extent to which the research condition is controlled so that the independent variable causes an effect or change in the dependent variable. External validity refers to the ability to use the results of a study in other conditions or settings. The producer and consumer of research subjectively determine the degree of both of these types of validity. Methods that may be used to minimize their effects include the use of control groups, the use of randomization, and the researcher's knowledge and logic in designing the study. Some degree of internal validity is important to every type of research. However, strong internal validity is more important in basic research, whereas in applied research good external validity is desirable. Most researchers in HPER should seek a reasonable balance between the two types of validity.

## Learning Activities

1. Have you accomplished the objectives stated at the beginning of the chapter? If not, go back and reread the concepts you're uncertain about. Also, ask your professor about these topics.
2. Examine several research articles and determine whether there are significant threats to internal and/or external validity. Identify practices that were used to reduce these or other threats. Provide an overall rating of the quality of the studies' internal and external validity.

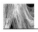

# CHAPTER 15

# Experimental Research and Designs

## KEY CONCEPTS

- Cause-and-effect relationship
- Experimental control
- Experimental research designs: true, quasi, and pre-experimental
- Error and treatment variance

## AFTER READING THIS CHAPTER YOU SHOULD BE ABLE TO:

- Explain the concept of cause and effect, especially as it relates to experimental research.
- Report why experimental research offers the greatest degree of experimental control.
- Describe the characteristics of true, quasi-, and pre-experimental designs.
- Explain the concepts of treatment and error variance.
- Distinguish among the various experimental designs in terms of their ability to demonstrate a cause-and-effect relationship.

Think for a moment about what most people's impressions might be if you said you were going to conduct an experiment. It would probably conjure up visions of seeing you in a white coat, in a laboratory with test tubes, beakers, and expensive electronic devices while mixing chemicals and performing elaborate calculations. You know by now that much research, particularly the type often done in health, physical education, and recreation (HPER), doesn't fit that stereotype at all. However, many studies conducted in our disciplines are of the experimental variety. Therefore, this chapter provides an overview of experimental research and related concepts.

## EXPERIMENTATION AND CAUSE-AND-EFFECT RELATIONSHIPS

The primary purpose for conducting research is to develop new knowledge. The best-organized, best-controlled, and most powerful means of generating new facts is through the use of experimentation. Research that is performed with experimental methods is typified by a careful and systematic approach to minimizing threats to validity and other factors that may contaminate the study. Needless to say, the researcher must be aware of these conditions if attempts to reduce their influence are to be successful. Along with a high degree of control comes introduction and manipulation of an independent variable. The experimental condition is set up to provide a high degree of confidence that the independent variable produced an effect on the dependent variable while simultaneously minimizing the effect of extraneous variables.

When it is logically determined that one factor demonstrates a predictable influence on another, a **cause-and-effect relationship** is said to exist. Experimental research is the most robust way to demonstrate whether this association exists. If there is a true cause-and-effect relationship between two (or more) variables, then one of the more important purposes of research may be met. That aim is to be able to generalize the relationship to other conditions and situations outside the experiment. In this manner, sound experimental research not only determines what happens in the present but also allows for the prediction of future events (i.e., given condition A, one is confident that B will occur). In this regard, experimental research seeks to answer this basic question: What will be?

Experimental research also best embodies the scientific method of problem solving. It allows an investigator to propose a hypothesis, to design and conduct a study in such a way that the hypothesis may be tested, and to draw a logical conclusion from the results. Although the scientific method may be used with other types of research, experimental methods remain the most important tool for discovering new information.

It should be apparent now that because experimental research is typified by much control, it is probably better suited for laboratory or other well-controlled conditions. This is true to a certain extent. However, a considerable amount of good experimental research in HPER is performed outside the laboratory. Regardless of the setting, conducting experimental research involves recognizing the main factors that may weaken the study, controlling for them in the best way possible, and introducing and manipulating the independent variable.

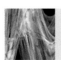

Experimental research is the most robust means of determining cause and effect.

## EXPERIMENTAL CONTROL REVISITED

As previously discussed, a high degree of control is characteristic of experimental research methods. In the previous chapter, we described several approaches to reducing threats to validity, thus increasing **experimental control**. If you recall, the most common methods used were randomization, control groups, having an adequate sample size, and the researcher's ability to logically trouble-shoot the situation. It is important to emphasize that although randomization and control groups are good procedures for establishing an experimental condition, they must accompany other means of diminishing the effects of variables that are extraneous to the study. The use of blind and double-blind techniques minimizes the influence of variables such as the placebo and halo effects. Other contaminants or **extraneous variables** to a study may be controlled for by limiting their influence. Sex, age, fitness level, health status, and race are examples of some factors whose impact may be lessened by using that element as a control variable. This may be accomplished by thoughtfully preparing a list of qualifying characteristics (delimitations) that may affect the dependent variable. For instance, if it is perceived that cigarette smoking in some subjects may produce a differential effect on the dependent variable, the research design could require all subjects to be nonsmokers. Or, if aging has a specific effect on the dependent variable, all subjects could be within a given age range. To be successful at understanding whether variables may have undesirable effects on one another or the dependent variable, researchers must be experienced in their field, knowledgeable about the related literature, and open-minded.

Sometimes the elimination of an extraneous variable raises ethical questions. For example, the issue of gender differences as a confounding variable in biomedical research has been a long-standing problem. The wide fluctuations in female hormonal and biologic cycles and their possible interactions with medications have been the focal point for using gender as a control variable. Women have also been restricted from participating in some types of research for the protection of their childbearing potential. Bernadine Healy, former director of the National Institutes for Health (NIH), brought to national attention the chronic effect of systematically eliminating women from biomedical research as an extraneous variable. She reported that women's health concerns have been seriously neglected and understudied. Because of this issue, the NIH has developed policy statements regarding the inclusion of women in biomedical research to help develop important knowledge in this area.

## EXPERIMENTAL RESEARCH DESIGNS

A research design is the overall plan or blueprint for a study. It gives the study structure and direction, and it dictates the appropriate statistical analysis to test the researcher's hypothesis. Like an architect, researchers must put down ideas on paper and sketch a draft of what is to be accomplished and how it will be done. This, of course, must be done before the actual conduct of the study. Sketching out the design before the study is done provides the researcher with an opportunity to consider many of the elements of the project as well as a time for needed brainstorming. The goal of the study design is to allow the researcher to conduct the study and test the hypothesis with a minimum of contamination from extraneous variables. This allows the investigator to make sound judgments about the relationship between the independent and dependent variables.

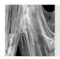

The design of a study is the overall plan or blueprint as to how the study is to be conducted.

Experimental research designs are classified by their sophistication and the degree of control they provide. The categories of these designs are called **true, quasi-,** and **pre-experimental.** One thing all experimental designs have in common is manipulation of an independent variable.

 *In all experimental designs an independent variable is manipulated.*

There are many possible research designs to choose from. The selection of the design is based on factors such as the type of research problem, the number and variety of experimental variables, how groups will be formed, and the threats to validity the researcher wants to control. The following sections describe a few of the basic and common experimental designs used in HPER research. Those desiring more detail on this topic are referred to Kirk's (1968) authoritative text on experimental designs.

## Error and Treatment Variance

Before examining various experimental designs, it is worthwhile to review a few concepts that were discussed previously. Recall that the basis for the use of randomization for group equivalence is the premise that the only differences between experimental and control groups are those produced by chance or sampling error. The statistical estimate of sampling error is called **error variance.** A proper study design should optimize the effect of the independent variable on the dependent variable while reducing threats to experimental validity. The effect of the independent variable on the dependent variable will result in differences known as **experimental** or **treatment variance.** At the heart of any experiment is the desire to enhance the effect of the treatment while reducing sampling error. Thomas and Nelson (2001) refer to this notion as the **minimax principle,** which emphasizes minimizing sampling error variance while maximizing treatment variance. The most effective way of achieving this is through the use of randomization, having an adequate sample size, and the thoughtful selection and use of a sound design.

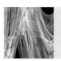

The ideal design of a study maximizes experimental variance while minimizing error variance.

Upon completion of a study an inspection and analysis of treatment and error variance is necessary. If there is considerably more treatment variance than error variance, the difference is judged to be the influence of the independent variable. The basis of statistics such as $t$ and $F$ is the ratio of treatment to error variance. Thus, when obtaining a statistically significant result, treatment variance exceeds error variance by a specified margin.

## Symbols and a Helpful Hint

For the research designs and blueprints in the following sections the following symbols or words will be used:

- Random: groups were formed by randomization
- Nonrandom: groups were formed in a nonrandom manner
- IV: introduction of the independent variable; the treatment
- Test or re-test: measurement of the dependent variable

At this point it may helpful to review the threats to validity and ways to control them (see Chapter 14). This may enhance your understanding as to how and why some designs are stronger than others.

## TRUE EXPERIMENTAL DESIGNS

True designs are the strongest tools for experimental research. They offer a considerable degree of control and minimize threats to validity to the greatest extent possible. These designs incorporate the two key elements of experimental control: randomization of subjects into groups for equivalence, and a control group. Randomization and control groups reduce many threats to experimental validity.

 *True experimental designs incorporate an independent variable, randomization of subjects into groups for equivalence, and a control group.*

## Post-test Only Design

Post-test only design is based on randomizing subjects into either an experimental or control group for equivalence, introducing the independent variable into the experimental group, testing for the effects of treatment and no treatment, and finally determining whether any difference between the two groups is significant. If the groups were equivalent at the onset of the study, any difference between the two groups at the conclusion of the research is presumed to be due primarily to the independent variable. This particular design is the one of choice when there are significant concerns related to controlling the effects of testing. This design may be expanded to two or more experimental groups if there is more than one level of the independent variable to be examined in the study. The appropriate statistical analysis would be an independent $t$ for two groups and a one-way ANOVA for more than two groups. A blueprint of the post-test only design follows:

| | |
|---|---|
| Experimental: Random | IV | Test |
| Control: Random | No IV | Test |

Perhaps a health educator is interested in determining the effectiveness of a particular school-based drug education program. The researcher thinks that exposing the subjects to a pre-test on knowledge of drug use may adversely affect the experiment, so she elects to use the post-test only design. Subjects are placed into groups by randomization (ideally subjects were randomly sampled from a population, then randomized into groups), the drug education program is given to the experimental group only, the drug use knowledge test is given to both groups at the end of the study, and finally the test performances between the two groups are compared. This example can be extended to comparing two or more different programs with the logic of the design remaining the same.

## Pre- and Post-Test Design

Pre- and post-design differs from the post-test only by the addition of a pre-test. This approach may be used when the effects of testing are negligible or when pre-test data are needed to initiate subject selection or group formation. The pre- and post-test design allows the researcher to determine the amount of **change** in the dependent variable that was due to the independent variable. In other words, observing which group changes more is the basis of this design. The pre- and post-design, like the post-test only, may be augmented to two or more experimental groups if there is more than one level of the independent variable. Appropriate statistical analyses include ANCOVA using the pre-test as the covariate and an independent $t$ or one-way ANOVA on **change scores.** A change score is simply the difference between the pre- and post-test performances. Although each of these approaches has advantages and disadvantages, they and other techniques are commonly seen in HPER literature. Below are blueprints of pre- and post-test designs based on one experimental group:

| | | | |
|---|---|---|---|
| Experimental: Random | Test | IV | Retest |
| Control: Random | Test | No IV | Retest |

And two experimental groups:

| | | | |
|---|---|---|---|
| Experimental: Random 1 | Test | IV, level 1 | Retest |
| Experimental: Random 2 | Test | IV, level 2 | Retest |
| Control: Random | Test | No IV | Retest |

Maybe an exercise physiologist is interested in studying the effect of a 10-week aerobic exercise program on high blood cholesterol levels. The investigator wants only subjects with cholesterol levels higher than 250 mg/dL. Initially, the researcher assesses the cholesterol levels of each subject by giving a pre-test. The pre-test data are used for two purposes in this case: one is to provide a baseline for change and the other is used for a subject selection criterion. After the pre-test, the subjects are randomly assigned into groups. The experimental group now participates in the exercise program, whereas the control group does not. The control group is also instructed not to begin an exercise program during the study. The study concludes with post-assessments of cholesterol levels and the appropriate statistical comparisons.

## Other True Designs

Technically, any time a study is designed with the use of randomization of subjects, a control group, and the introduction of an independent variable, it is a true experimental design. Many other permutations of experimental and control groups are possible, such as the **two-way factorial ANOVA,** discussed previously. This statistical analysis may be applied to some of the more elaborate experimental designs. Return to Chapter 11 for a review of factorial research problems.

## QUASI-EXPERIMENTAL DESIGNS

The term *quasi* means to some degree or seemingly, so quasi-experimental designs are like true experimental ones to some degree. One of the major differences is that randomization of subjects into groups is not used. The lack of randomization of subjects raises doubts about the equivalence of groups. Obviously, that raises some problems. Some quasi-experimental designs are based on observing a group of subjects over time, making repeated measurements on them. The subjects serving as their own control group usually characterize these types of designs. Some quasi-experimental research designs and methods are intended for studies conducted in natural settings, such as classrooms or other intact groups. The premise is to study the subject in a real-world setting, introduce the independent variable, and measure its effect. Overall, these designs are typified by good external validity but less internal validity because of the absence of randomization. Discussion of a few of the more common quasi-experimental designs follows.

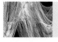 Quasi-experimental designs do not include randomizing subjects to groups.

## Pre- and Post-Nonrandom Design

This design is identical in form with the pre- and post-true experimental design except for randomization of subjects into groups. It is used when the researcher does not have the ability to randomize subjects, desires to use groups that are intact for convenience, or wants to conduct a study in a real world setting. The major drawback to this approach is the matter of the equivalence of groups. As a check for group equivalence, an investigator may perform an independent *t* test, or one-way ANOVA if there are more than two groups, on the pre-test results. If no significant difference is observed between or among the groups, a judgment of equivalence is made. This deduction may be faulty for two reasons. First, a test of significance does not provide reliable information about the magnitude of a difference. It is possible to have a large difference that is not statistically significant. This is a particular problem if the sample size of the groups is small, which reduces the likelihood of detecting significance. The second reason is that although there may be no significant difference between or among groups on the dependent variable, the subjects may be different on another or other factors that may influence the experiment. For example, the subjects in one group may tend to be more adherent to an intervention than another group. Therefore, perhaps the most appropriate statistical analysis for this design is the ANCOVA using the pretest scores as the covariate. This procedure statistically adjusts for differences in pretest scores. A blueprint of this design is as follows:

| Experimental: Nonrandom | Test | IV | Retest |
|---|---|---|---|
| Control: Nonrandom | Test | No IV | Retest |

To illustrate this design, assume that a recreation director is interested in examining the effect of elders' participation in bingo games on social interaction. Both for convenience and to study the subjects in a real-world environment, the researcher decides to use two retirement homes in her community. At one retirement home, games of bingo (with cash prizes) will be added to the recreation program; the residents of this home will form the experimental group. Residents of the other retirement home, which has a similar recreation program without bingo, will be used as a control. Before and at the conclusion of the study, a socialization inventory is administered to both groups. The ANCOVA can be used to adjust for the initial socialization scores and the appropriate conclusions drawn. Obviously, the biggest problem with this study is not knowing what differences may have existed between the subjects of the two retirement homes. For instance, one retirement home may have had a disproportionate number of well-to-do, widowed, or handicapped residents compared with the other group. These factors and others like them may have influenced the study's outcome. This is an example of why the interpretation of results of studies using this design has to be done carefully.

## Repeated-Measures Designs

The repeated-measures approach is commonly used in HPER. In this design, there is only an experimental group that is exposed to more than one level of the independent variable. Usually, the effect of each level is measured on one dependent variable. Because the subjects have repeated measurements made on them, they technically serve as their own control group, making this actually a fairly sound design. This design works best when there is little interaction among the levels of the independent variable and not much time is required between the measurement sessions. To minimize any interaction or testing effect, the order of test administrations should be randomized for each subject. The appropriate statistical analysis for this design is a correlated *t* test to compare two levels of an independent variable or a one-way ANOVA for more than two levels. A blueprint of the repeated-measures design if subjects were measured on three levels of an independent variable would appear as follows:

| Experimental: Nonrandom | IV, level 1 | Test | IV, level 2 | Test | IV, level 3 | Test |
|---|---|---|---|---|---|---|

Suppose a physical educator would like to compare the effect of three seat heights on leg cycle power output. After careful consideration the investigator thinks that there may be some testing or interactive effects, so he decides that the best approach is to randomize the treatment order for each subject. Also, to minimize the effects of fatigue, he tests the subjects on three separate days. Each subject reports to the testing facility three times to be assessed on a randomly selected seat height. The results are compared with a one-way ANOVA for repeated measures and the appropriate conclusions are made.

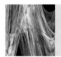

Repeated measures design uses multiple measurements on the same subjects and hence the term "repeated."

A desirable aspect of this method is that fewer subjects are needed than if three separate groups were used for each test. This would not be the correct approach if the levels of the independent variable were some type of long-term treatment, such as an educational program or a method of physical training that may take weeks or months to administer. The most obvious concerns in this case are the length of time it would take to expose the subjects to all the treatment variables and the carryover effect of each treatment on the subsequent one. For long-term treatments, it becomes necessary to use one of the other designs previously described.

Many possible repeated-measures designs exist. For example, when repeated measures are made on the same subjects with more than one independent variable and more than one level of each, a factorial ANOVA for repeated measures is used.

## Time Series Design

An approach fairly similar to repeated measures is the time series design. A single experimental group that serves as its own control is assessed on a dependent variable several times over a specified period. This establishes a constant baseline for the variable. This design is valuable in studying measures that by their very nature fluctuate considerably.

This may characterize variables such as stress, some hormone levels, and anxiety. The independent variable is then introduced, after which several more assessments of the dependent variable are made. Any departure from the baseline is thought to be attributed to the independent variable. However, a major weakness in this design is that without a control group it is difficult to know if the effects of history may have actually been responsible for the change. The blueprint for the time series design is:

| Experimental: Nonrandom | Test | Test | Test | IV | Test | Test | Test |
|---|---|---|---|---|---|---|---|

Suppose a health educator is interested in examining the effect of a smoking cessation program. A group of smokers is identified, and the researcher has decided to use blood levels of carbon monoxide as an index of smoking quantity. These measurements are performed once per week for 3 weeks to establish a baseline. The researcher then introduces the smoking cessation program and repeats the carbon monoxide tests in the same fashion as before. Any reduction in group carbon monoxide level is thought to be attributed to the smoking cessation program. It is entirely possible, however, that an extraneous variable that presented itself simultaneously to the independent variable caused the change. For instance, what if a major news story reported that smoking significantly reduces sex drive! If many of the research subjects were exposed to this type of news, this may have provided a strong stimulus to change regardless of the influence of the smoking cessation program. On the other hand, if there is no marked departure from the baseline, the program was probably ineffective.

## PRE-EXPERIMENTAL DESIGNS

Pre-experimental designs have the weakest degree of experimental control and are characterized by no randomization, sometimes no control group, and no assurance of equivalence between groups if a control group was used. They are classified as experimental designs only because there is a manipulation of an independent variable. These designs offer such poor control that it is difficult to draw any meaningful conclusion about a cause-and-effect relationship. They are illustrated here only as techniques **not** to use. They are seen often in advertising. Any graduate student or faculty using a pre-experimental design should be summarily turned over to the experimental design division of the research police!

 *Pre-experimental designs have the weakest degree of control of all experimental plans.*

### One-Group Pre- and Post-Design

This approach is probably the best of all of the pre-experimental types, which makes it the best of the worst! One experimental group is given a pre-test, treated with the independent

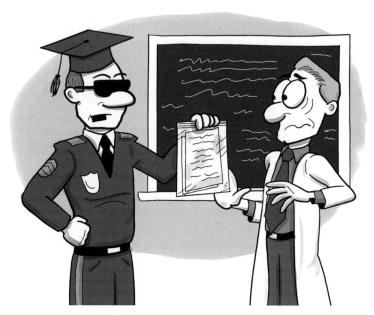

**"Research police, sir.  Citation for poor research design and methods."**

variable, and given a post-test. A major flaw in this design is the lack of a control group. The change between the pre- and post-scores is attributed to the treatment. Of course, too many threats to internal validity are uncontrolled, so one is not at all confident about why the change took place. The blueprint appears thus:

Experimental: Nonrandom

| Test | IV | Retest |
|------|----|--------|

## Static Group Comparison Design

The inadequate design called static group comparison is based on no randomization of subjects into groups. This, in fact, is the main factor that makes it different from the post-test only experimental design. An intact experimental group receives the independent variable and is compared with an intact nonequivalent control group on the dependent variable. Since the groups were probably not comparable prior to the treatment, it is difficult to conclude that any post-test differences between groups are due to the independent variable. Simply, the groups could have been different prior to the treatment. The design looks like this:

Experimental: Nonrandom

Control: Nonrandom

| IV | Test |
|-------|------|
| No IV | Test |

## One-Shot Design

The one-shot design is the least acceptable of all experimental plans. With this technique, an intact experimental group receives a treatment and is tested on its effect on the dependent variable. The results of the treatment are compared against what the researcher *expected to occur if the treatment was not given.* This expectation can be based on previous observation of subjects or supposition on the part of the researcher. There is no pre-test, no randomization, and no control group. Consequently, there is no way to test for any possible effect that the independent variable might have had. Also, there is no control for threats to experimental validity. Any conclusions on the part of a researcher are pure speculations that cannot be supported logically or objectively. The one-shot design can be summarized as:

Experimental: Nonrandom

| IV | Test |
|----|------|

Imagine a sports psychologist who is interested in studying the effect of mental imagery on basketball free-throw shooting accuracy. He has the team use imagery for 10 minutes before each practice for a week before a game. After the game, he examines the team's free-throw percentage and finds that it is higher than what he expected from previous performances. He claims that this improvement was due to the mental imagery practice. There is no control group, no randomization, no control for day to day variation, etc. It should be obvious that numerous flaws exist with this very limited design and method of discovery.

 **Summary**

Experimental designs are the best tools for establishing cause-and-effect relationships and discovering new knowledge. All of the designs are based on causing something to occur by manipulating an independent variable. These designs vary in terms of their ability to minimize threats to experimental validity. True designs are the foremost variety and are characterized by the use of control groups and randomization. Quasi-experimental designs are more real-world oriented and are typified by no randomization of subjects or equivalence of groups. This design generally provides good external validity. Pre-experimental methods are by far the weakest designs because of lack of randomization and equivalence of groups. In some cases, a control group is also lacking. Professionals

| **TABLE 15-1. Typical Experimental Designs Used in HPER** | | |
|---|---|---|
| *True (Best)* | *Quasi (Adequate)* | *Pre (Weak)* |
| Post-test only | Same as True except nonrandom grouping of subjects | One group pre- and post-test |
| Pre-test and post-test | Repeated measures | Static group |
| Factorial | Time series | One shot |

in HPER need to consider the type of design and its ability to reduce threats to validity when producing and reading research. A summary of experimental designs appears in Table 15–1.

 **Learning Activities**

1. Have you accomplished the objectives stated at the beginning of the chapter? If not, go back and reread the concepts you're uncertain about. Also, ask your professor about these topics.
2. Read several research articles and focus on the methods section to determine the following:
   ■ Was an experimental design used? If so, what type?
   ■ Was randomization of subjects used? If so, how was it done?
   ■ Was a control group used? If not, was a rationale provided?
   ■ What was the independent variable? Was there more than one level of it?
   ■ What type of statistical analysis was used? Did it seem appropriate for the design?
   ■ How well did the study design appear to control some extraneous variables?
   ■ What threats to internal validity existed?

# CHAPTER 16

# Nonexperimental or Descriptive Research

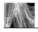

## KEY CONCEPTS

- Nonexperimental research and cause-and-effect relationships
- Survey research
- Correlation research
- Developmental research
- Epidemiological research
- Observational research
- Ex post facto
- Meta-analysis

## AFTER READING THIS CHAPTER YOU SHOULD BE ABLE TO:

- Explain the relationship between nonexperimental research and cause and effect.
- Describe the basic steps in conducting a survey.
- Describe the characteristics of the various types of nonexperimental research commonly used in health, physical education, and recreation.

Nonexperimental research methods are used when the manipulation of an independent variable is not practical, possible, or ethical. This technique of scientific inquiry is also known as **descriptive research,** which asks the basic question: What is? Nonexperimental research is typified by observations or descriptions of the status of a condition or situation. Investigators using this method do not manipulate variables or make things happen. They measure and record events that would have occurred had they not been there anyway.

Much behavioral research is nonexperimental because it would be impossible to replicate some elements of human conduct in a laboratory setting. For example, studying seatbelt usage or sportsmanship may not be feasible in a laboratory environment. It would be unethical to conduct experimental research on some aspects of human behavior. Even if a researcher lacked a certain moral conviction, approval by a human subjects institutional review board (IRB) (see Chapter 18) would be difficult if not impossible for a study based on the orchestration of something that was harmful or dangerous. For instance, a researcher could not deliberately inject athletes with megadoses of anabolic steroids to study their effects on strength or deliberately cause athletic injuries to investigate the healing properties associated with a new type of therapy. Experimental studies causing cancer, car accidents, and other such things would be inhumane. However, these types of behaviors and conditions do exist, and it is important to examine them. Therefore, sometimes the only way to study certain situations or actions is through **descriptive** or **nonexperimental** methods.

Most nonexperimental studies are conducted using the basic elements of the scientific method; that is, a hypothesis is stated and tested, and conclusions are drawn. In fact, the only distinction from experimental research in this respect is that the hypothesis is tested using nonexperimental procedures, and these methods characteristically do not have good control over the experimental condition. Therefore, nonexperimental research is not as robust as experimentation in establishing cause-and-effect relationships. Even though it is not as strong a tool in this regard, it should not be thought of as second-rate research. In this chapter, we examine the nature of several varieties of nonexperimental research that are frequently used in HPER.

## NONEXPERIMENTAL RESEARCH AND CAUSE-AND-EFFECT RELATIONSHIPS

Nonexperimental research is not a rigorous means of verifying traditional cause-and-effect relationships for several reasons. The primary reason is that the researcher does not introduce an independent variable and measure its effect. The investigator only records the presence of a certain variable as it occurs or after the fact. For example, a woman arrives on the scene of an auto accident and sees three cars with extensive damage.

 *Cause-and-effect relationships may not be established when an independent variable is not introduced.*

The only logical deduction she can make is that an accident has occurred. She can't make any valid conclusions about the cause of the crash, because she did not observe it directly, and even if she had, she wouldn't necessarily know for sure what caused it.

In nonexperimental research, no independent variable is introduced and no extraneous variables may be controlled, making it difficult to conclude that variable A caused B to occur. The most logical conclusion that may be drawn with this type of research is that variable A is present, but how this happened is difficult to say.

Another factor that reduces the ability to conclude cause and effect is that subjects are typically not randomized into groups. Subjects are usually identified by some predetermined criterion and are grouped in that fashion. However, this does not mean that subjects are not or cannot be randomly selected from a population. This is an important procedure in any kind of research when it's desirable to make generalizations about a particular population of subjects, and it is commonly done with descriptive research. Lack of randomization raises many threats to internal validity. Because the possible effects of extraneous variables haven't been controlled for and the researcher didn't make something happen, serious questions may be raised about assuming cause and effect.

Nonexperimental research is based on logical deductions about the connections between variables. This type of association is referred to as a **causal relationship.** Essentially, this means that variables are often observed with one another, but the true nature of the relationship may not be known or explained. Nevertheless, an association does not mean causation. This point was emphasized when interpreting correlation coefficients. These statistics depict mathematical relationships between variables, but only the reader or researcher may conclude a cause-and-effect relationship from them.

Most large-scale epidemiologic (research on disease) studies are nonexperimental. For instance, obesity is routinely identified as a risk factor for heart disease. Does this mean that the more body fat one has, the more likely having heart disease becomes? Maybe. Since variables are only observed and not manipulated in this type of study, a careful interpretation might be that in large-scale studies, high body fat levels were more typical in persons who had heart disease than in those who did not. However, some obese people live long lives and don't die of heart disease. Most people would agree that it would be prudent to reduce body fat for this and other health reasons. However, such a decision is not based on a systematic cause-and-effect relationship.

Producers and consumers of research need to use sound logic when making interpretations and speculations relative to nonexperimental research. Nonexperimental research attempts to discover functional relationships between variables and depends on logic and knowledge to rationalize the association. However, adequate logic and scientific substantiation may justify a conclusion that there is a **causal relationship.** Many possible explanations for the existence of variables and their causes must be entertained. A seemingly obvious relationship may be erroneously taken at face value, producing false conclusions. One can see why researchers are reluctant to use the term *cause and effect* when discussing relationships observed in nonexperimental research.

Nonexperimental research is often conducted on topics that have not previously been studied in depth. The initial purpose of the research in this area then is exploratory; relationships are examined and logic used to judge whether or not the relationships *might* be causal. If additional research confirms the existence of the relationship, then experimental research can be conducted to determine whether the relationship is cause and effect. For example, suppose a study reports a significant negative relationship between level of physical activity (measured by the number of steps taken daily using pedometers) and the incidence of type 2 diabetes; that is, more physical activity is associated with reduced incidence. One might think that the reason for the relationship is that greater level of physical activity improves insulin sensitivity and reduces visceral obesity, both of which might logically reduce incidence of type 2 diabetes. The stronger the logical link between the two variables, the more likely it is that a cause-and-effect relationship exists. However, regardless of the logic, experimental research is needed to confirm cause and effect. Thus, if experimental research is conducted and increased physical activity is actually found to reduce the incidence of type 2 diabetes to a level lower than that of a less physically active control group, then stronger evidence for cause and effect is provided.

Nonexperimental research often explores relationships on topics with limited previous research. However, the possible cause-and-effect link between the variables needs to be confirmed with experimental research.

# SURVEY RESEARCH

Survey results are commonly cited in the media today and surveys are frequently used in HPER. A survey is a broad-based information gathering procedure that is designed to measure practices, opinions, or other such variables. Typically, rather than a researcher observing a particular behavior, the subject reports it. With certain variables or behaviors, this may be a significant limitation. However, it's a necessary drawback, because usually no other means exists in obtaining such data. Routine assumptions or limitations to self-reporting of information include whether the subject is capable of making a valid assessment of the variable in question and/or whether the subject is responding truthfully. Survey research should not be considered mere bean counting, because it requires much skill to orchestrate, conduct, and draw conclusions. Many steps and procedures must be attended to in a successful survey. Since a most common type of survey is performed with a mailed questionnaire, discussion is limited here to that variety.

## Steps in Conducting a Survey by Mail

Before survey research can be done, the investigator must develop a detailed plan of action. This plan should present all of the required steps in a logical chronological order. Since so many things have to occur for the study to be successful, it is necessary to write them down. Even a veteran survey researcher can forget an essential item or two. Poor planning such as leaving out an essential step or detail may have ruinous effects.

**Step 1: Decide What You Want to Accomplish** As with any research project, the investigator must have a clear and defined purpose for the study and be able to state a testable hypothesis. The study must then be designed in such a way that the hypothesis can be tested. It is such an obvious characteristic of sound research that often it is not considered as seriously as it should be. In the case of surveys, numerous details, such as the type and number of questions, the variables to be assessed, how to generate a representative sample, allocation of resources, preparation of the questionnaire, and scoring and analysis of data, must be determined before the fact.

**Step 2: Select the Sample** One of the primary purposes of conducting a survey is to be able to make generalizations from a sample to a population. To successfully accomplish this, at least two key factors have to be considered. The researcher must first decide on clear delimitations for subject inclusion and then have a systematic and unbiased means of establishing a representative sample.

In some cases establishing subject delimitations is very easy. For example, in a broad-based public opinion poll, nearly everyone can be in the study. In other cases, subject selection criteria must be more precise. If a health researcher were interested in studying differences in health behaviors between adults who exercise and those who don't, many attributes require distinct operational definitions. What is the criterion for an adult? That may be easy to define, perhaps anyone older than age 21. Is there an upper age limit? How are exerciser and nonexerciser defined? There are many possible definitions here.

The point is that researchers must carefully identify the characteristics of the type of subject they want to study before they recruit them. A standard consideration, however, regardless of any other criteria, is whether the subject in question can accurately provide the investigator with the desired information.

After deciding on the traits of the subjects, investigators need to determine how many subjects they will require and how they will be identified. The number of subjects to include is dictated by several factors. From a statistical standpoint, the sample must be large enough to be considered representative and to make reasonable generalizations. This is largely dependent on the potential size of the population in question. For example, if someone wanted to make generalizations to a population of 200 recreation leaders in a community park district, she would need a large percent (maybe 25% to 50% or so) of the 200 possible subjects in the sample. On the other hand, accurate generalizations and predictions are made in U.S. presidential elections based on polling of less than 1% of the voting population.

The last point to consider relative to sample size is cost. Envelopes, paper, copying, stamps, and so on, all cost money, and these costs have an insidious way of escalating quickly. Students or researchers on restricted budgets may have to make compromises in sample size and statistical power. In some cases, the restriction in sample size may be so great that it is not feasible to carry out the study at all.

The method of subject identification and the sampling procedure are important. Various random sampling procedures were previously discussed, such as the use of random numbers and developing a stratified random sample. Any one of these may be appropriate, depending on the nature and diversity of the population and the size of the sample. It may be helpful to review these procedures to determine which one is best for your situation. To simplify the sampling process, researchers sometimes use mailing lists from organizations. This is often desirable when the group has members who typify the subjects the researcher would like to study. For example, if someone is interested in studying the exercise habits of professionals in HPER, a quick way to generate a sample of subjects may be to get a mailing list from an organization like the American Alliance of Health, Physical Education, Recreation, and Dance. However, it would be an incorrect approach if the researcher used this list as a sample of average Americans.

**Step 3: Develop the Instrument** With surveys conducted by mail, the questionnaire is the instrument used to measure the experimental variables. The development of a valid questionnaire requires considerable time and skill. Many a survey has failed to yield any meaningful information because of a sloppy or badly prepared instrument. The type and number of questions, their format and wording, how they will be evaluated, and so on must be considered in the planning process.

Before preparing any questions or items, researchers should develop a list of the variables to be measured in the survey. There should be a clear understanding of exactly what is to be known or learned. When these have been itemized, a table should be prepared. This table should include the areas or variables that the researcher would like to assess and the number and type of items to be used. These procedures reduce the likelihood of using a disorganized shotgun approach to constructing the instrument.

The type of questions or items to be used has a large influence on the success of the survey. A concise, easy-to-answer survey instrument is much more likely to be completed and returned than one that takes considerable time or effort. Generally, questions or items may be classified as **open-ended** or **closed-ended.** Open-ended items allow the respondent an opportunity for free expression. An item such as "Describe your attitude toward sex education in the public schools" is an example. Although they allow for free expression, these items have some undesirable aspects. One is that they are highly subjective to interpretation, making them difficult to analyze and quantify. Another factor is that they take longer to complete and perhaps require the respondent to think too much about the answer. If faced with any or too many of these types of items, the return rate of the surveys may be reduced. Obviously, an open-ended item can provide only some kinds of information. Information such as an annual income or the number of years lived in a city are open-ended items but are completely objective. If subjective items are used, they should be kept to a minimum, with attention given to how they will be scored or analyzed.

Closed-ended items are objective, making them easier to analyze and quantify. One type of closed-ended item is a simple **ranking** process. For instance, from a list of 10 recreational activities, the subject is asked to rank them according to preference with their highest choice receiving a 1 and least favorite getting a 10. Another traditional approach is to use **scaled responses. A Likert scale** is one that assigns point values to statements that indicate the extent of agreement or disagreement. Different words or terms may be applied to the scale, depending on the nature of the question. Here are two examples of Likert scale items:

During soccer practices, do you get mad at your teammates?

|  1  |  2  |  3  |  4  |  5  |
|-------|--------|-----------|-------|--------|
| Never | Rarely | Sometimes | Often | Always |

High school students should be required to take a drug education class.

|  1  |  2  |  3  |  4  |  5  |
|----------------|----------|----------|-------|-------------------|
| Strongly agree | Disagree | Not sure | Agree | Strongly disagree |

Likert scale responses should usually be constructed with an odd number of choices (e.g., five or seven), typically with the middle choice being one of neutrality bound by choices of ascending or descending degrees of association. Incidentally, Likert scale responses are actually ordinal level measurements, which suggest the use of nonparametric statistical analyses.

Some types of information can be provided easily with a **categorical** response. These include responses such as yes/no, true/false, high/medium/low, female/male, and Catholic/Lutheran/Jewish/Hindu. Although these responses are easy to quantify, they lack the ability to show the degree of association to an item. Therefore, categorical questions should be reserved for more outright questions or opinions that can be clearly classified. Examples include "Do you have a university degree? (yes/no)" and "Do you believe that cigarette smoking is the number one preventable public health risk? (true/false)."

There is no clear-cut number of items that should appear on a questionnaire, but a simple rule of thumb is that fewer is better. Items should be pertinent so as to minimize the length of the instrument, which increases the probability of a high rate of return. If an item can't provide the researcher with relevant information, it should be discarded. Borg and Gall (1983) report that longer questionnaires result in a reduced rate of return.

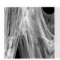 Carefully scrutinize and limit the amount of information sought because longer questionnaires tend to suffer lower return rates.

Regardless of the type of item selected, all should have certain qualities. The items should be concisely and unambiguously stated and convey only one question or idea. "Do you enjoy hiking and camping?" is a poor question because it is asking two things. A yes answer means that one enjoys *both* hiking and camping. A no response may mean that the subject doesn't like either activity or likes one and not the other. Verbiage that leads the subject to respond one way or another should be avoided. Finally, the items should be written in such a manner that they are not too technical but are stimulating and respectful of the knowledge level of the subject.

The quality of the layout and appearance of the questionnaire are also vital for a successful survey. The questions or items should follow a logical sequence and not skip around to different topics. The first several items should be easily answered and be motivators, so that the subject is prone to complete the entire questionnaire and not be immediately discouraged. Finally, the questionnaire should look neat and orderly, using easy-to-read type or lettering and quality paper. Erasures, fingerprints, blotch marks, cheap or torn paper, and other such things convey an unprofessional message. A summary of the steps in the development of the instrument may be seen in Table 16-1.

**Step 4: Write the Cover Letter**  A well-developed questionnaire is very limited without an effective cover letter. As with the questionnaire, the cover letter should be concise, attractive, and professionally written. The letter should appear on the official letterhead

**TABLE 16-1. Factors in the Development of a Survey Instrument**

Variables to be studied
Types of questions to be asked, e.g., open vs closed-ended
Number of questions
Order of questions
Scoring of responses
Layout and appearance of instrument
Exact instructions for completion of instrument
Instrument's content validity

stationery of the organization affiliated with the research. Perhaps the first thing that will catch the eye of potential subjects is their name and how they are addressed. If someone's name is misspelled or doesn't address him or her correctly, the survey may quickly become part of the recycling effort. In any type of professional correspondence, particularly when you do not know someone personally, you should address the person with his or her honorific (e.g., Mr., Ms., Dr.) and last name.

The first few sentences should contain some information about the study, such as its purpose, and should provide some brief background about the researchers and their affiliation. It helps to promote the study's credibility if a noted professional organization or individual is supporting it. A letter of support or endorsement from a prominent officer in an association that encourages the participation of its members would be invaluable in some cases.

Within the letter, let the potential subjects know that they are part of a select group and that you value their participation. Some people participate in a study only if there is something of value in it for them. Therefore, you need to tell them how they benefit (e.g., money, rewards, or feedback about the results of the study). One can always let subjects know that only *they* can provide this information and that it is needed for the advancement of knowledge. This may make subjects feel good about contributing for a societal or professional benefit and may encourage them to take part. One of the authors has received several surveys with a packet of M&Ms included. After indulging in the treat, it is hard not to complete the questionnaire.

Exact instructions for completing the instrument should appear either in the letter or directly on the questionnaire. If the instructions are on the instrument, it is a good idea to mention that fact in the letter. Also, it's helpful to provide an approximate amount of time that it will take to complete the questionnaire. A date of return should be indicated. Trying to determine an appropriate time for completing and returning the survey is a guessing game. If you give subjects too much time, they may forget about it or think it's not important. On the other hand, if you ask for a return date within a short period, subjects may feel their time is not being respected, and they may not complete it.

 *A well-developed questionnaire is functionally useless without an effective cover letter.*

The amount of time required should be based on the length of the instrument and the types of variables being measured. Generally, 7 to 10 days for a short survey and 2 to 3 weeks for a longer one are good ballpark figures. Finally, don't forget to include a stamped, self-addressed envelope that can easily hold the questionnaire.

Research subjects have the right to anonymity and confidentiality, and an assurance of those rights should be included in the letter. Of course, complete anonymity makes following up potential subjects more costly or time consuming. A summary of the major considerations for writing a cover letter appears in Table 16-2.

**Step 5: Check It Out and Make a Trial Run**   After developing the questionnaire and writing the cover letter, an assessment of their quality should be performed. Enlisting the help of a few individuals with experience in this type and area of research effectively accomplishes this. They should examine both documents for clarity, format, grammar,

| **TABLE 16-2. Factors in Writing a Cover Letter** |
| --- |
| Use official letterhead stationery. |
| Address subject properly, e.g., Mr., Ms., Dr. |
| Check for spelling and other grammatical errors. |
| Include letters of endorsement if applicable. |
| Encourage the subject to participate. |
| Indicate any possible benefits to the subject or society. |
| Include directions for completing the survey. |
| Indicate the amount of time to complete the survey. |
| Specify the return date. |
| Include a self-addressed stamped envelope. |
| Include a consent form if applicable. |
| Ensure confidentiality. |

and appearance. The instrument and its items should be evaluated for **content validity,** which was discussed in Chapter 13. Any revisions in the letter or the instrument should be made. A pilot study of the survey to a few select individuals may provide further feedback on the letter or the questionnaire and may give the investigator a good idea of the time actually needed to complete the instrument. The trial run may also furnish an opportunity to identify and correct any oversights before the actual study takes place.

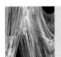 Pilot test the questionnaire and letter before mailing them. This provides one last chance to make revisions.

**Step 6: Send It** To increase the return rate, consider when to mail the survey and where to send it. If it is an occupation-related survey, the preferred place to mail it is to the subject's place of work. The season of the year may have some bearing on return rate. For instance, school-based surveys should not be distributed during the weeks that schools are starting and finishing or over vacation times. A survey dealing with summer recreation choices might yield better results in July than in January. Mailing a survey just before or during holidays is likely to reduce the return rate because respondents will probably not respond at that time anyway and they may misplace the instrument so that even if they had intended to respond, they may not be able to.

**Step 7: Follow Up** A prime goal of any survey researcher is to obtain as high a rate of return as possible. Several strategies that may increase the likelihood of subject participation have already been discussed. However, incorporating these methods into a study doesn't necessarily translate into a high return rate. Even well-meaning subjects may require some subtle persuasion to get involved. Sometimes people forget, get too busy, or just need a little extra encouragement to take part; that is why follow-up tactics are needed.

Follow-up techniques differ slightly depending on whether a study was conducted so that the respondents remained anonymous. If subjects are anonymous, one approach is to send a new questionnaire to *all* of the participants about a week after the return date. This should be done under the guise that perhaps the survey didn't arrive or was lost. Regardless, it is hoped that the subject will take part if given a second opportunity. However, this is an expensive approach but it is the price to pay for anonymity. If the respondents are known, sending a new survey to *just* the nonparticipants is all that is necessary. Another method is to send a postcard to the subjects, either reminding them to complete and return the survey, or if they have done so, thanking them. Of course if the nonrespondents are known, a reminder postcard to them is all that is needed. This may be done once or twice after the return date. After two reminders, it is fairly unlikely that the potential subject is going to take part. Some surveys are done with a few select subjects in mind, and the inclusion of almost all of them is vital to the success of the study. If the respondents are known, placing a follow-up phone call or two may be the right personal touch to get the stragglers involved.

What rate of return is needed for a valid study? That depends on the number of prospective participants and the size of the population that is to be generalized to. Generally, the smaller the sample, the higher the rate of return, where with a larger sample a smaller return rate can be tolerated. Overall, the higher the return rate, the more representative the sample is. Statistical inferences can be accurately made from representative random samples with relatively low N sizes. The key word here is *representative*. With a low rate of return, one must question how representative the sample is. The respondents may tend to be more humane or professionally minded than nonrespondents. A limited return rate introduces a form of selection bias and reduces the experimental validity of the study in many respects. This is why a proper random sampling procedure and a respectable return rate are crucial to valid survey research.

**Step 8: Summarize the Results and Thank the Participants**  One right of a research subject is to be informed of the results of a study. Therefore, the final step in the survey is to provide the participants with a summary of the major findings of the investigation and to thank them for taking part. This is a common courtesy of the investigator. Also, it may increase the likelihood that the subject will participate in future studies. A summary of the major steps in conducting a mailed survey is presented in Table 16-3.

## OTHER SURVEY METHODS

The survey techniques discussed thus far have been related to surveys that are mailed. However, in recent years much survey research is conducted via the World Wide Web. Typically, this is done using a **listserve** of an organization or interest group to distribute the questionnaire. In addition, on-line surveys may be conducted through local applications, such as Blackboard or other websites. Surveys may also be conducted using personal interviews. Interviews may be done by telephone or face to face. These are usually more time consuming and labor intensive than mail surveys, but they may be preferred when depth of information is sought. The basic tenets of carrying out a survey

| **TABLE 16-3. Major Steps in Conducting a Survey** |
| --- |
| Determine the research objectives for the study. |
| Determine the sample, e.g., size, sampling procedure, subjects' characteristics. |
| Develop the instrument. |
| Develop the cover letter. |
| Establish the quality of the instrument and cover letter. |
| Get endorsements for the study if applicable. |
| Conduct pilot survey if applicable. |
| Conduct actual survey. |
| Use established follow-up procedures to get highest return rate possible. |
| Send results and thank you letters. |

are similar no matter what the technique, particularly when it comes to developing the instrument. Typically, only the method of disseminating questionnaires or securing data is different. All survey procedures have distinct advantages and drawbacks. Factors such as time, cost, number, location, and availability of subjects, coding of responses, training and number of interviewers, sensitivity of questions and sampling procedures have to be appraised for selection of the appropriate survey approach.

## INFORMED CONSENT AND SURVEYS

One of the rights of a research subject is informed consent, and this right is not waived in survey research. How does a researcher get informed consent with a survey? One approach is the traditional way, with the subject reading and signing a written document. Informed consent documents may be included in a mailed survey and returned with the instrument or administered before a face-to-face interview or a survey that is completed by a subject in the presence of an investigator. Informed consent may be *implied* in the case of a mailed survey if the subject returns it. If the subject doesn't want to participate in the study, he or she simply need not send it back. If this approach is used, however, the subject should be provided with appropriate background information in the cover letter. Finally, informed consent may be obtained verbally, which is the most appropriate for telephone interviews. No matter what type of survey is used, subjects should have a clear understanding of the nature of the research and their role so they may

 *The right of informed consent is not waived in survey research.*

make a knowledgeable decision about whether to participate. Failure to provide informed consent is a violation of the subject's rights and is unprofessional conduct on the part of the investigator.

## OTHER NONEXPERIMENTAL METHODS

Although survey research is a commonly used and important technique, there are many other nonexperimental procedures. Some of these are quite complicated and difficult to conduct and usually require much skill and expertise. In fact, the core of entire texts, courses, and disciplines may be based on any one of these methods. Because of this, elaborate descriptions are beyond the scope of this text. The following sections present brief overviews of some other types of nonexperimental research.

## Correlation Research

The purpose of correlation research is to examine the relationships between or among variables. By using a variety of correlation statistics, the researcher may answer questions that pertain to the type and strength of relationships, prediction, or the accuracy of the prediction. Perhaps the most common approaches are the simple and multiple correlation techniques that examine relationships between two variables or more than two variables, respectively. Any or all of these procedures have applications in solving correlation research problems. Refer to Chapter 10 for a review of correlation analyses and relevant examples.

One of the most common errors in correlation research is assumption of a cause-and-effect relationship. Correlation statistics depict only mathematical relationships between or among variables. Cause-and-effect relationships depend on logic, knowledge, and reason. However, to *conclude* cause and effect, experimental research should be conducted. Since no independent variable is introduced or manipulated, interpretations of correlation research are bound by the same limitations as other types of nonexperimental research.

Correlation research, though rigorous to conduct, may be viewed as efficient in that subjects routinely are assessed for variables of interest only once or twice. For instance, in a study examining the relationship between blood cholesterol and body fat, subjects could report to a laboratory and have both measurements made in the same testing session. That may conclude their involvement in the study. Many subjects may view this type of commitment as more desirable than participating in a 12-week experimental study.

## Case Studies

The case study is a widely used approach in fields such as medicine, psychology, and the social sciences. Even in our disciplines, cases studies of unique situations appear in the literature. A case study is an in-depth analysis of a unique condition or situation. The subject in the case study may be one person or an intact class, institution, or entire community. The purpose of a study like this is to examine as many aspects of the subject in question as possible and to note how the case is unique or different from what is normal or expected. Usually, the event or situation in question is not well known, not well understood, or rare, making experimental research on it impractical or impossible. For example, a case study of the coping strategies of a blind wrestler may be informative particularly if little or no previous research was available on the topic. Unusual sports injuries and novel rehabilitation strategies are common topics for case studies in athletic training.

Obviously, drawing any broad generalizations from a case study is not warranted. However, when many case studies have been performed on the same topic and similar results are reported, the basis of formulating a hypothesis or theory is made. Therefore, case study research may be the only way to provide a foundation of knowledge when examining exceptional circumstances or conditions. Also, in some instances, case studies may use experimental methods and designs.

## Developmental Research

The purpose of developmental research is to explain changes in factors such as behavior, growth, or knowledge throughout the life cycle or a specified time period. Longitudinal research is study of the same subjects over time. Although this is a preferred method, any long-term study of variables in humans is burdensome to carry out for many reasons. The time needed to conduct the study, subject attrition and mortality, subject familiarity with testing procedures, and the Hawthorne effects are all factors that may negatively influence longitudinal research results. Because of these concerns, sometimes developmental studies are performed using a **cross-sectional** approach. This involves generating a representative sample of subjects across several age group strata. For instance, if a motor learning researcher wants to study the effect of aging on coordination, a stratified sample may consist of 25 subjects in each stratum for every decade of life. Although the cross-sectional methods reduce some of the possible limitations associated with longitudinal research, it has drawbacks. One question is how representative of the developmental process are the subjects in each stratum at that age. Another drawback is that the subjects are not the same in each stratum, so any differences across age groups may be due to the individual variation in subjects and not necessarily due to changes in maturation. Despite these concerns, the cross-sectional method is a common and popular form of developmental research.

## Epidemiologic Research

Epidemiology is the study of diseases. Research in this area may be experimental (both basic and applied) and nonexperimental. Nonexperimental investigations are usually large-scale descriptive studies that use longitudinal or cross-sectional methods. The intent of such studies is to examine subjects in a free-living environment and assess them on a periodic basis. For example, more than 5000 residents of Framingham, Massachusetts, have participated in an ongoing heart disease study since 1948, and the study is ongoing. The Framingham Study is a very famous epidemiological investigation that has provided extensive information about heart disease and cardiovascular risk factors.

The incidence rates of the disease in question are recorded along with the variables associated with the affliction being observed. Causal relationships but not necessarily cause and effect may then be established between the disorder and variables that appear the most frequently with it. Even though cause-and-effect relationships are not confirmed with this type of research, it doesn't mean the results are not useful. For instance, suppose research has shown that of 100,000 confirmed cases of heart disease, 89% of the subjects had cholesterol levels above 240 mg/dL. This would be a very powerful finding, and it would be foolish to ignore it just because it may not demonstrate a cause-and-effect relationship. However, experimental research would still be needed to substantiate the relationship as being cause and effect.

It is considered unethical to introduce diseases to human subjects, so at times animal subjects are used instead. However, there are limitations to the ability to generalize the results of animal research to humans. So in many instances the only means to conduct human epidemiological research is in a nonexperimental manner.

## Observational Research

In observational research, the investigator obtains data by examining or observing a behavior or trait and recording it rather than having the subject report it. This type of research is used when there are serious questions about the subject's ability to provide accurate and honest information. Can you imagine the validity of the data if athletes were asked how many acts of good or bad sportsmanship they displayed in a certain game? The athletes may be unaware of these actions at the time, may not be able to recall all such acts, or may not tell the truth.

Many observations of behavior can be contaminated or altered by the presence of an investigator or if performed in an artificial environment. Therefore, it is important sometimes to observe behaviors or practices in an inconspicuous manner so that the subjects function normally. Observations may be made from a distance, through a one-way mirror, or with other such covert means. Also, since it is difficult to replicate most human behaviors in a laboratory, much observational research is performed in real world settings. Observations can also be made with the assistance of a video camera. This enables the researcher to replay the video allowing for a more accurate analysis. For this approach to be effective, the camera must be positioned in an unobtrusive manner.

Observational studies require special attention to certain details. Before data collection can begin, the observational researcher should specifically and functionally define the behaviors and the delimitations for the subjects to be studied. Careful consideration must be given to studying the subjects in the most natural setting and means possible. The investigator also needs to develop a means of measuring and quantifying the behavior in the most accurate and feasible way. Detailed recording forms are usually developed to permit data entry into specific categories for later analysis. For example, one of our recent graduate students videotaped a basketball game and in later analysis quantified the percentage of playing time each player spent running, jumping, shuffling, walking, and standing. In replaying the video in 3-second intervals, the major activity for each interval was coded into one of the categories. By summing the 3-second values for each activity, the percentage of each activity was calculated for the entire game.

Sometimes ethical questions may be raised relative to the type of the behaviors studied and how the observations of them are made. For example, perhaps a health researcher is interested in conducting an observational study to examine the use of illegal drugs by college students. To provide a setting for observation, the researcher attends a party for students. During the party, the investigator is covertly observing or videotaping and recording the incidence of drug use without the participants knowing. Would this be ethical? How would you feel if some aspect of your behavior, particularly if it were very personal, was being observed and chronicled without your knowledge or consent? There are no easy answers to these questions. The ethics of this type of research center on the sensitivity of the behavior and the amount of deception or concealment that is used to assess it. The example of the party is similar to a study examined by the IRB at the university where the authors teach. After a rousing discussion by the board members, the study was disapproved.

## Descriptive Research

This specific type of research attempts to describe selected meaningful characteristics of a distinct group. The purpose may be to compare these traits with those of other groups, to develop normative information, or simply to profile the group for the sake of knowledge. Numerous studies have examined common physical fitness variables of athletes from different sports. Athletes from many sports, including football, soccer, rugby, karate, track, and cycling, have been studied in this regard. These studies did not involve the manipulation of an independent variable, making them nonexperimental or descriptive.

## Ex Post Facto and Meta-analysis Research

This type of research falls between the cracks because it may be based on past data generated in an experimental or nonexperimental fashion. **Ex post facto** (after the fact) or archival research uses past data to answer present questions or to test new hypotheses. For instance, a health researcher may examine public health records to investigate factors that are related to a particular illness or disorder. A recreator may inspect data on park usage from previous years to estimate current or future participation patterns. Using past data that are appropriate eliminates the need for present information gathering and expedites the research process. Moreover, this method may be the primary means by which some topics (e.g., deaths due to auto accidents or factors related to deaths from a disease) are studied.

Data do not necessarily have to come from records or files. Results in published research may be used as a form of data to be analyzed and to test new hypotheses. This process is referred to as a **meta-analysis.** Essentially, studies examining the same variable may be inspected and relevant data extracted to calculate a statistic known as an *effect size*. The effect size for each study may then be calculated and used as a form of raw data for further analysis and hypothesis testing. The meta-analysis is technically a form of ex post facto research. More details on meta-analysis are presented in Chapter 19.

 **Summary**

In this chapter, the nature of nonexperimental research was examined. Nonexperimental research is typified by making observations or descriptions about the status of a condition or situation. A primary feature of this type of research is that no independent variable is

**TABLE 16-4. Selected Types of Nonexperimental Research in HPER**

Surveys: mailed, Internet, in person, telephone
Correlation
Case studies
Developmental
Epidemiological
Observational
Descriptive
Ex post facto
Meta-analysis

introduced or manipulated. Because of this limitation nonexperimental research is not as robust as experimental research in establishing cause-and-effect relationships. Even though it is not as strong a tool in this regard, it should not be thought of as a lesser form of research. Nonexperimental research may be conducted through the use of surveys and numerous other techniques. A summary of the major types of nonexperimental research appears in Table 16-4.

 ## Learning Activities

1. Have you accomplished the objectives stated at the beginning of the chapter? If not, go back and reread the concepts you're uncertain about. Also, ask your professor about these topics.
2. Read selected nonexperimental research articles and become familiar with the subject selection process, methods, data analysis, approach toward writing the discussion section, and any other unique characteristics of that type of research.
3. Read a study reporting the results of a survey.
   a. What steps were taken to increase the return rate?
   b. What was the return rate? Does this rate influence your opinion as to whether the sample was biased?
4. Read a case study. What made the study unique?
5. Read an observational study. How was the observation made unobtrusive?

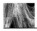

# CHAPTER 17

# Qualitative Research Methods

## Manoj Sharma, MBBS, CHES, PhD*

### KEY CONCEPTS

- Case study
- Focus groups
- Nominal groups
- Content analysis
- Purposeful sampling
- Open coding
- Audit trail
- Axial coding
- Trustworthiness
- Credibility
- Coherence
- Transferability
- Dependability
- Confirmability

### AFTER READING THIS CHAPTER YOU SHOULD BE ABLE TO:

- Describe the assumptions in qualitative research.
- Compare and contrast qualitative and quantitative research.
- Identify the characteristics of common qualitative research methods.
- Discuss the advantages and disadvantages of common qualitative methods.
- Define and use basic terms common to qualitative research.

Qualitative research owes its origin to the disciplines of anthropology and sociology. Many terms have been used to denote the qualitative line of inquiry, such as cultural studies, constructivist paradigm, naturalistic inquiry, phenomenological inquiry, postmodernism, postpositivism approach, and poststructuralism (Schwandt, 2001). Similar to quantitative research, qualitative research is rigorous, disciplined, and systematic, and it often provides a viable alternative approach to quantitative research techniques. In this chapter, four commonly used methods in health, physical education, and recreation (HPER) are briefly discussed.

*Associate Professor, Health Promotion and Education, University of Cincinnati

## QUANTITATIVE VS. QUALITATIVE RESEARCH

In quantitative research, the design and variables are set or defined before data are collected. In qualitative research, however, the design and variables measured are flexible and somewhat dependent on the context of data collection. For example, a health science researcher doing a quantitative study and interested in measuring physical activity levels makes a priori (prior) decisions about measures of exercise intensity, frequency of exercise, and duration of each session. On the other hand, a health science researcher doing a qualitative study and examining physical activity levels is more interested in the meaning of physical activity in the participant's life, that is, why the activity is being done, the participants' feelings during the activity, with whom the activity is done, and so on.

 *In qualitative research, the design and variables measured are flexible and somewhat dependent on the context.*

Quantitative research requires the researcher to carefully define variables that may be quantified with numbers. This method has often been viewed as **reductionism;** that is, the reality is reduced to a number. In contrast, the qualitative researcher is interested in the complete or **holistic perspective,** which includes underlying values and the context as a part of the phenomena (Morse, Swanson, & Kuezel, 2001). For example, a quantitative health education researcher wanting to study healthy dietary behavior will reduce measurements to numbers. He or she may be interested in observing or relying on self-reported data about how many servings of vegetables and fruits are eaten per day by individuals in the sample and then comparing these data against United States Department of Agriculture (USDA) guidelines. The quantitative researcher may not be particularly interested in what fruit or vegetable, personal liking, with whom, where, when, how it was consumed, and other contextual details, which may be the main interest of the qualitative researcher. If the quantitative researcher becomes interested in recording some of those aspects, they will also be reduced to numbers, and the number of variables studied would be limited. In quantitative research, parsimony or brevity is encouraged, whereas in qualitative methods details of the context are emphasized.

 A unique strength of qualitative research lies in its inclusion of many variables in studying behavior. Hence, it is more holistic than is quantitative research.

The quantitative paradigm assumes that variables can be measured objectively. The study of cause-and-effect relationships between or among variables is often of interest in this approach. In contrast, qualitative methods assume that only partially objective accounts of the world can be produced and hence can be interpreted in a variety of ways. For example, a researcher in health science who is examining the relationship between smoking and lung cancer finds the risk of lung cancer in those exposed to smoking 22 times the incidence among those not exposed to smoking. Then the researcher would

| TABLE 17-1. Comparison of Quantitative and Qualitative Research Methods | |
| --- | --- |
| **Quantitative** | **Qualitative** |
| Researcher defines the reality | Reality is defined by the participants |
| Researcher independent | Researcher as an interactive observer |
| Concepts reduced to numbers | Holistic perspective |
| Purpose is hypothesis confirmation | Purpose is hypothesis generation |
| Deductive reasoning (general to specific) | Inductive reasoning (specific to general) |
| Fixed research design | Dynamic research design |
| Statistical manipulation required | Statistical testing not required |

be interested in looking at evidence from other similar studies (consistency), examining the time sequence, dose–response relationship, and possible biological mechanism, and only then might he or she conclude that smoking is likely to cause lung cancer. On the other hand, the qualitative researcher may be interested in looking at different facets of the life of victims of lung cancer or at different facets of the life of the smokers. The latter researcher may be less interested in establishing any causal relationships but only in describing the observations.

Quantitative research is based in part on deductive reasoning, in which the logic proceeds from general to specific. For example, if a study found estrogen replacement therapy to increase bone density of postmenopausal women, the results might be applicable for one's 60-year-old aunt. In the qualitative research paradigm, the logic is reversed or is inductive: It proceeds from specific to general. For example, a qualitative study of elderly American women done by a cross-cultural researcher from Nepal may find them taking some "hormone pills" and being able to jog. She may recommend study of the role of hormone pills in Nepalese elderly women to improve functioning in later years of life.

Finally, quantitative inquiry entails measurement instruments and data analysis that is expressed in statistics. On the other hand, qualitative research allows a more open-ended and flexible approach to assessment. The differences between quantitative and qualitative paradigms are summarized in Table 17-1.

 *Qualitative research allows an open-ended and flexible approach to assessment.*

## CASE STUDIES

Case study has been defined by Yin (1994) as an empirical inquiry that investigates a contemporary phenomenon within its real life context. It is much like quantitative research in that it includes stating a research question, determining an appropriate design, establishing data collection and analysis methods, and making an assertion or generalization about the results.

The case study may be **simple,** dealing with only one decision, or **complex,** dealing with many intricate and interrelated decisions. For example, a recreation therapy researcher may illustrate a simple case study dealing with a community reentry decision of a traumatic brain injury (TBI) patient (simple case study). The same researcher may present the readers with an account of all of the dilemmas, cultural adaptations, and modifications made during rehabilitation of a recent immigrant TBI patient (complex case study). An example of a case study in HPER research is a study by Sharma and Deepak (2002) describing a community-based rehabilitation program in Mongolia that examined the various dimensions of the program, several governmental decisions, and explored alternatives to some decisions.

The chief advantage of the case study method is its rich documentation of the context. The case study method also provides an opportunity for critical reflection on different alternatives. It is a method for bringing to the reader an account of a reality that may not be easily perceptible. Furthermore, evidence from different case studies on the same topic helps to identify patterns. One disadvantage of the case study method is inability to tell the entire story. One also needs to remember that the case study method, like most qualitative methods, cannot demonstrate causality.

*The chief advantage of the case study method is its detailed documentation of the context.*

## FOCUS GROUPS

The field of marketing is well known for using and popularizing the technique of focus groups. Marketing researchers primarily use this method for testing the negative and positive perceptions of a target audience regarding various new products or potential ideas. Focus groups are gaining importance in HPER as researchers and practitioners use them to assess needs and to gain early impressions for program planning. For example, Yoon and Byles (2002) used focus groups to document perceptions of stroke among the members of general public and patients. Focus groups are indispensable for gathering early impressions. As an illustration, Smith, Blake, Olson, and Tessaro (2002) used focus groups to begin work on diabetes in rural settings in West Virginia. Focus groups are especially important in determining which populations to target. An example in HPER is a study by Frohlich, Potvin, Chabot, and Corin (2002) that identified the context of neighborhoods in smoking behavior among youth. Focus groups are also used in developing and modifying psychometric instruments. For instance, a study

*Focus groups are indispensable for gathering early impressions.*

by Ford et al. (2002) modified a breast cancer risk factor survey for African-American women using focus groups.

The focus group method entails developing a detailed protocol. In developing the protocol the researcher first decides the research topic. The time planned for conducting a focus group session is usually between 1 and 2 hours. The guidelines start with directions for recruitment of the focus group members (8 to 12 persons with a minimum of

4 groups for each topic). It is important to keep the recruitment instructions simple and brief and give participants some incentive or reward for participation. The first decision in recruitment is whether to select one gender or to combine them. If the possibility of any threat to openness is perceived because of gender influence, the focus group must be restricted to only one gender. Similarly, where appropriate, efforts must be made to have similarity with regard to race, age, socioeconomic status, ethnicity, national origin, and spoken language. Finally, to ensure that discussion is honest, it is important that participants not know each other.

The focus group protocol includes direction for conducting the discussion. Each discussion starts with introductory comments from the moderator thanking the participants, explaining the process, and making clear that everyone's input is important. Rules such as one person to speak at one time and people should speak frankly about what they think and not what someone else wants to hear are presented. It is very important to instruct the participants that there are no correct or incorrect responses but that the purpose is mainly to elicit opinions. An opportunity must be given for the participants to introduce themselves. The questions that follow must be open-ended with an aim to stimulate the discussion and not tally responses. The protocol must have examples of questions that prevent a yes/no response.

In conducting the focus group, one must choose a convenient location and try to create as relaxed and familiar an atmosphere for participants as possible. Name tags with first name only (to allow confidentiality) must be provided. It is also advantageous to have an observer who should note interactions and body language and record content exchanges. Having an experienced and competent moderator is an important prerequisite. The roles and competencies of a moderator are summarized in Table 17-2.

The focus group discussion may be tape-recorded after consent from the participants to ensure accuracy and completeness. It is also helpful if the moderator can use visual

---

**TABLE 17-2. Roles and Competencies of a Moderator in Conducting Focus Groups**

Adequate training and sufficient experience
Well informed about the project
Able to express thoughts and feelings clearly
Able to draw reticent members into the group and keep the vocal ones from dominating
Encouraging and motivating disposition
Receptive and flexible
Attuned to important information
Intuitive, able to probe for further information to clarify a participant's meaning
Culturally sensitive
Empathetic, conveys genuine interest
Kind but firm
Able to pose sensitive questions to the whole group rather than to one person
Must note interactions, body language, and record content exchanges

aids to document the data and seek clarity from participants. In analyzing the data, the analyst must first listen to the whole tape recording and read its transcript to get an overall impression, then tabulate and organize discussion group findings and pertinent quotations. Emphasis must be made to evaluate differences among the thoughts, beliefs, and emotions of different people. The analyst must pay special attention to participants' hesitations, silences, and emphases, as well as actual words used.

An important advantage of focus group discussion is that these are inexpensive and relatively quick means of collecting data. One disadvantage is that the group members may not be representative of the target audience. Often when the moderator is not experienced, the moderator and dominant participants influence the responses. On sensitive topics, group members may be inhibited from discussing private topics in public. A major disadvantage is that the nature of the data precludes drawing firm conclusions. Finally, focus group findings are easily subject to misuse through absence of the required moderating skills and through misinterpretation of the data.

## NOMINAL GROUPS

Nominal group process is a qualitative technique commonly used for needs assessment from a target population. Its chief advantage is that it allows for ranking of the problems (Gilmore & Campbell, 1996). The nominal group does not aim to find solutions to a problem but is used only to prioritize problems elaborated by target audience members. In health education conducted in community settings, it is a very potent tool for an applied researcher to determine community-driven priorities. In an example of this methodology in HPER, Ginsburg et al. (2002), while working with inner city youth, used the nominal group process to prioritize information about what solutions would

 *The nominal group method does not aim to find solutions to a problem but is used only to prioritize problems elaborated by target audience members.*

most influence the likelihood of inner city youth in achieving a positive future. In another study, Reed, Pearson, Douglas, Swinburne, and Wilding (2002) used the nominal group method to prioritize motivations among older adults in being discharged from hospitals and going home.

The first step in conducting nominal group process is to articulate the problem in a single question. For example, a question in physical education might be, "What is the most popular moderate-intensity leisure time physical activity in middle-aged African-American women in Alabama?" In the second step, 8 to 12 participants (found to be an optimum number) directly affected by that problem or directly involved in the situation are recruited. In dealing with this issue, 8 to 12 middle-aged African-American women in Alabama will be recruited. In the third step, the participants are provided an opportunity to reflect on the question or the problem. No discussion is allowed, and an index card may be provided to organize thoughts. In the fourth step, all of the responses are collected and documented on a flip chart or a blackboard. No discussion is allowed until all responses have been recorded. In the fifth step, discussion seeking clarification and exploring logic behind the choice is done, with the moderator ensuring that no lobbying or argumentation on any point is happening. In the sixth step, participants rank the choices or select five top items, with 5 being the most important and 1 the least important. Sometimes this may be done by a secret ballot. Finally, a summation of the voting results is done and a priority list established.

Nominal group process is a tool to assist arriving at a priority from the perspective of the target audience. A research study cannot be based solely on this method, but this qualitative method can be a useful adjunct in any study. For a graduate student writing a thesis, this method is useful in establishing the significance of any study of practical importance.

## CONTENT ANALYSIS

Content analysis is the process of organizing and integrating narrative qualitative information according to themes and concepts. It is a procedure for analyzing written or verbal communications in a systematic and objective fashion (Polit & Hungler, 1999). This method can be applied to analysis of diaries, letters, speeches, books, articles, newspaper stories, and other linguistic materials (Wiederman & Whiteley, 2002) A study by Malone, Wenger, and Bero (2002) conducted a content analysis of tobacco articles in high school newspapers. In the analysis, the authors found that the most common framing was around "kids" (46%), followed by "killer" (31%), "nonsmokers' rights" (10%) and "choice" (5%). In another study, Marx and Chavez (2002) used content analysis in examining outdoor recreation magazines to ascertain whether textual information in magazines is created and sustained by value differences between different recreation groups.

 *Content analysis is a procedure for analyzing written or verbal communication in a systematic and objective fashion.*

The common units of analyses in content analysis are the **size of the article, individual words,** and **themes** (namely, phrase, sentence, or paragraph). Sometimes a unit of analysis may include an **item,** such as an entire e-mail, editorial, diary entry, conference presentation, article, or special journal issue. Finally, unit of analysis may also include a **space and time measure,** such as number of pages, number of words, or number of speakers (Polit & Hungler, 1999).

The chief advantage of content analysis is its ability to combine a qualitative method with quantitative methodology. Content analysis also helps the researcher in HPER to plan and evaluate programs. It is a useful technique in identifying themes and patterns and is the only method for some research problems. A disadvantage of this method is the risk of subjectivity.

## QUALITATIVE DESIGN, SAMPLING, DATA COLLECTION, ANALYSIS, AND INTERPRETATION

As mentioned earlier, the design in qualitative research is not fixed but dynamic. The forces in the environment and participant input shape the design. Nonetheless, it is

---

**TABLE 17-3. Considerations in Planning a Qualitative Design**

Plan for flexibility but begin with some boundaries, including inclusion/exclusion criteria that may and can be altered.

Decide on what, where, and from whom to collect data.

Decide on specific qualitative methods to be used matching it with the research need.

Seek to understand and describe; do not attempt prediction.

Seek to look at the complete picture.

The researcher must aim to become the research instrument.

Plan for ongoing data processing that will help decide when to complete inquiry.

Plan logistics for data collection including scheduling and budgeting.

Plan techniques for ascertaining trustworthiness of the data.

---

important to keep some guidelines in mind. Some guidelines that may be helpful for a qualitative researcher in planning qualitative design are presented in Table 17-3 (Denzin & Lincoln, 2000; Polit & Hungler, 1999).

Sampling in qualitative research is termed **purposeful sampling.** The common types of purposeful samples used in HPER qualitative research are as follows (Patton, 2002):

1. **Convenience samples** that entail use of conveniently available people as study participants
2. **Snowball** or **network** or **chain samples** that entail asking early members of the sample to make referrals
3. Politically important case samples that entail seeking information from leaders or participants identified by leaders

Despite the flexibility accorded by purposeful sampling, the reader must be cognizant of three common kinds of errors identified by Patton (2002) in the sampling process:

1. Insufficient breadth in sampling (e.g., collecting information from only an urban site of a project and neglecting data from rural sites)
2. Distortions due to data collection spread over a long period (e.g., a study in which data collection lasted for a couple of years or a stress-related study that collected data before and after the September 11, 2001 event)
3. Distortion due to inadequate depth at each site (for example, the researcher at the beginning collects data intensively and then toward the end collects perfunctory data because of fatigue, shrinking resources, and other factors).

For qualitative research, **interviews** and **observation** remain the predominant means for collecting data. Qualitative interviewing generally entails open-ended questions. They could be informal conversational interviews, semistructured interviews, or standard open-ended interviews (Patton, 2002). In an informal conversational interview, the researcher does not plan a priori and is merely guided by his or her inquisitive self. This allows for rich exploration but makes summarization difficult, especially with multiple subjects. In a semistructured interview, a script, interview guide, or schedule is prepared, but the interviewer is free to probe, skip questions, and add questions. This provides some flexibility while making it easier to summarize data. Finally, standard open-ended interviews have a set of questions that have been pretested, and the interviewer asks only these questions. These are most useful when multiple sites have to be covered and time is of the essence. Most qualitative researchers generally advocate use of tape-recording and transcribing when conducting interviews, which is helpful in accurate data collection. However, some researchers recommend against their use because of intrusiveness, lack of feasibility in remote locations, and technical failures.

The other data collection method of observation for qualitative research is a little more time consuming and necessitates that the researcher become the true instrument for research. Depending on the research topic, opportunity, feasibility, and institutional review board (IRB) approval, the observer may choose to be a (1) hidden observer; (2) passive, unobtrusive observer, (3) limited-interaction observer, or (4) completely participatory observer. The chief advantage of observation over interview is its ability to capture the context. The chief disadvantage of observation is higher degree of skill on the part of the observer, who must be adept at noticing verbal content and nonverbal cues, must have command over local language and dialect, and must be versatile with field-based note taking.

The data analysis in qualitative research is an ongoing exercise in which the researcher is processing data and analyzing his or her strategy on a daily or weekly basis during data collection, at least on a preliminary basis. It must be easy for the reader to imagine by now that in qualitative research the amount of data collected is usually quite copious. Therefore, this ongoing data analysis is helpful. This also provides the researcher with an input to decide when to stop collecting data. Ongoing data analysis also provides insight for identifying concepts for open coding.

The first step in summative data analysis of qualitative research is what is called **open coding,** in which the researcher decides on tentative conceptual categories into which the data will be coded. Words, phrases, items, events, timings, and so on may be chosen for this purpose. The second step is the **audit trail,** for which the researcher must have a means of linking the data identified in open coding with the source and context. This can be simply done in a tabular format in a notebook or word processor or through the use of some qualitative software. It is also important to keep actual quotations from the sources. The third step in data analysis is called **axial coding.** In this step the researcher begins to put together the complete picture, in which events pertaining to the research topic, related topics, implications from research, and description of a proposed conceptual model are tied together and presented. Finally, the researcher addresses concerns of data interpretation, namely, trustworthiness, credibility, coherence, transferability, dependability, and confirmability.

The issue of **trustworthiness** pertains to how much the researcher has adhered to procedures specific to the chosen method, has exercised rigor in inquiry, and is open about describing the procedures. The concept of **credibility** is similar to the concept of internal validity of quantitative research. To establish credibility, Patton (2002) recommends using **triangulation.** Triangulation is the use of multiple methods to aid in decision making. Triangulation can be of methods or of the data or through use of multiple analysts or theory (Patton, 2002). The issue of **coherence** is essentially about the extent to which the final research write-up makes sense, the degree to which conclusions are supported by data, and use of triangulation (Eisner, 1991). The issue of **transferability** is similar to the concept of external validity. In qualitative research, the researcher cannot specify the generalization but can give some idea about similarity of the research situation studied with other similar settings. Patton (2002) recommends use of the term **extrapolation** for depicting this concept. **Dependability** is a concept similar to reliability. Denzin and Lincoln (2002) note that this concept has not been adequately considered by many qualitative researchers and is essentially a function of detailed description of the method by one researcher being consistently used by another. **Confirmability** is the extent to which neutrality of research interpretations can be established. It is difficult to achieve in qualitative research because it depends on values and is subjective.

Several computer programs are available to aid the qualitative researcher. Although discussions on merits, demerits, and usage guidelines are beyond the scope of this discussion, a brief description of some commonly used software developed by Scolari (www.scolari.com) may be useful.

 ## Summary

In qualitative research, the meaning of any situation is perceived from the participant's viewpoint, and the researcher is a mere observer. Qualitative research is also holistic in its orientation, and the reality is multiply constructed and interpreted. Qualitative design is dynamic and is based on inductive reasoning. Commonly used qualitative methods in HPER are case studies, focus groups, nominal groups, and content analysis. Case studies entail empirical inquiries about investigation of contemporary phenomena within their real-life contexts. Focus groups are thematic interviews with a group of 8 to 12 individuals assembled to answer questions on a given theme. Nominal groups are a qualitative ranking method for identifying needs, problems, and/or possible solutions through voting. Content analysis is a process of organizing and integrating narrative qualitative information from diaries, letters, speeches, books, articles, newspaper stories, and other linguistic materials.

The sampling in qualitative research is purposeful sampling. For qualitative research, interviews and observation remain the predominant means for collecting data. Data analysis is ongoing and also summative. Summative data analysis entails open coding, audit trail, axial coding, weaving the complete picture, and polishing the narrative account. In data interpretation, the researcher must pay attention to trustworthiness (adherence to procedures and rigor), credibility (consensus or triangulation or using multiple methods), coherence (extent to which the final research write-up makes sense), transferability (idea about similarity of the research situation studied with other similar settings), dependability (similarity with work of other researchers), and confirmability (extent to which neutrality of research interpretations can be established).

**Learning Activities**

1. Have you accomplished the objectives stated at the beginning of the chapter? If not, go back and reread the concepts you're uncertain about. Also, ask your professor about these topics.
2. Locate several qualitative research articles and classify them by method. Explain why the information obtained could be achieved only through qualitative techniques.

## REFERENCES

Denzin, N. K., & Lincoln, Y. S. (Eds.). (2000). *Handbook of qualitative research*. (2nd ed.). Thousand Oaks, CA: Sage.

Eisner, E. W. (1991). *The enlightened eye: Qualitative enquiry and the enhancement of educational practice*. New York: Macmillan.

Ford, M. E., Hill, D. D., Blount, A., Morrison, J., Worsham, M., Havstad, S. L., et al. (2002). Modifying a breast cancer risk factor survey for African American women. *Oncology Nursing Forum, 29*, 827–834.

Frohlich, K. L., Potvin, L., Chabot, P., & Corin, E. (2002). A theoretical and empirical analysis of context: Neighborhoods, smoking and youth. *Social Science and Medicine, 54*, 1401–1417.

Gilmore, G. D., & Campbell, M. D. (1996). *Needs assessment strategies for health education and health promotion*. Madison, WI: Brown & Benchmark.

Ginsburg, K. R., Alexander, P. M., Hunt, J., Sullivan, M., Zhao, H., & Cnaan, A. (2002). Enhancing their likelihood for a positive future: The perspective of inner-city youth. *Pediatrics, 109*, 1136–1142.

Malone, R. E., Wenger, L. D., & Bero, L. A. (2002). High school journalists' perspectives on tobacco. *Journal of Health Communication, 7*, 139–156.

Marx, M., & Chavez, D. J. (2002). Conflict and coalitions: An examination of outdoor recreation magazines. *Environmental Management, 29*, 207–216.

Morse, J. M., Swanson, J., & Kuzel, A. J. (2001). *The nature of qualitative evidence*. Thousand Oaks, CA: Sage.

Patton, M. Q. (2002). *Qualitative research and evaluation methods*. (3rd ed.). Thousand Oaks, CA: Sage.

Polit, D. F., & Hungler, B. P. (1999). *Nursing research. Principles and methods*. Philadelphia: Lippincott.

Reed, J., Pearson, P., Douglas, B., Swinburne, S., & Wilding, H. (2002). Going home from hospital: An appreciative inquiry study. *Health & Social Care in the Community, 10*, 36–45.

Schwandt, T. A. (2001). *Dictionary of qualitative inquiry*. Thousand Oaks, CA: Sage.

Sharma, M., & Deepak, S. (2002). A brief case study of community-based rehabilitation program in Mongolia. *Asia Pacific Disability Rehabilitation Journal, 13*, 11–18.

Smith, S. L., Blake, K., Olson, C. R., & Tessaro, I. (2002). Community entry in conducting rural focus groups: Process, legitimacy, and lessons learned. *Journal of Rural Health, 18*, 118–123.

Wiederman, M. W., & Whiteley, B. E. (Eds.). (2002). *Handbook for conducting research on human sexuality*. Mahwah, NJ: Lawrence Erlbaum.

Yin, R. K. (1994). *Case study research, design, and methods*. Thousand Oaks, CA: Sage.

Yoon, S. S., & Byles, J. (2002). Perceptions of stroke in the general public and patients with stroke: A qualitative study. *British Medical Journal, 324*, 1065–1068.

# PART V

# Quality Control and Application of Research

18. Quality Control in Research

19. Assessment and Application of Research

# CHAPTER 18

# Quality Control in Research

### KEY CONCEPTS

- Internal quality control
- Peer review
- Student colloquia and defenses
- Institutional review board
- External quality control
- Blinded review
- Publish or perish research quality
- Research quality versus quantity
- Research dishonesty

### AFTER READING THIS CHAPTER YOU SHOULD BE ABLE TO:

- Distinguish between internal and external quality control measures.
- Describe the role of the institutional review board in regard to quality control.
- Discuss the journal review process, especially as it pertains to blinded and unblinded review of manuscripts.
- Understand the nature of publication demands and the potential impact on research quality and quantity.

N ow that the foundations of the research process have been covered in this text, you may wonder what individuals watch over research to make sure that it is done correctly, safely, and honestly. This is not an easy question because no single process ensures or protects the quality of these factors. The individual researcher ultimately exerts the greatest influence over the quality of most facets of research. Consequently, the training, integrity, and work habits of the investigator are of vital importance. In this chapter, some of the factors that affect research quality control are discussed.

## INTERNAL QUALITY CONTROL

Internal quality control in research may be regarded as any individual or unit within an institution that either approves research projects or protects the rights of subjects. This measure affects research quality up to the point where the researcher attempts to publish or present the results of the study. Because much research in health, physical education, and recreation (HPER) is conducted in universities, the internal quality control mechanisms in higher education are highlighted. Most departments have some type of peer review of research proposals for faculty members as well as colloquia and defenses for student theses and projects.

 *Internal quality control includes peer review, student defenses, and institutional review boards.*

Also, virtually every university has some type of institutional review board (IRB) that approves research projects prior to their initiation. Each of these is now discussed.

## Peer Review

Most departments have a person or committee that is responsible for reviewing research proposals before their submission to the IRB or before the research is conducted. Much of what is accomplished with the peer review process is editing the proposal for content and methods and evaluating its scientific merit. One of the major problems with this procedure is related to one faculty member's ability to evaluate the work of another. For example, if a recreation researcher is reviewing a proposal for a biomechanics study, it is difficult for the recreator to pass reasonable judgment on the methods used or the scientific worthiness of the project. So the best outcome of the review may be only editorial suggestions or ethical questions related to the safety of subjects. Therefore, peer review works best when someone with a similar level of expertise in the same area of study critiques the proposal. In small academic departments, this may not be possible. In such circumstances, a faculty member may contact a colleague with the necessary expertise at another institution to request a review.

Often peer review takes place at an informal level. That is, faculty members approach colleagues and ask them to read a proposal and give frank and sincere feedback. When faculty members respect each other's opinions and welcome constructive criticism, this approach works well. In this regard, successful researchers need to be open-minded and willing to accept and provide critique.

## Student Colloquia and Defenses

Students who elect to write a thesis or dissertation have their work reviewed numerous times by their committee members. Perhaps the two most important reviews are the formal presentation of the research proposal and the final thesis. The forum for presenting the proposal or final thesis is known as a colloquium, or oral defense. Typically, these are public presentations that all faculty and students are invited to attend. Contrary to popular belief, the purpose of these presentations is not to humble the student but to provide helpful critique and suggestions in the attempt to have the best study possible. It is important to understand that this process is a learning experience for the student. Students are asked questions that allow them to consider a problem and are guided toward a logical conclusion. Although this may seem intimidating, one should approach it with a positive frame of mind.

At our institution students must successfully present their proposal and obtain the approval of their committee before they may submit the plan to the IRB. These steps and IRB approval must be completed before any data collection can take place. Needless to say, the student must also successfully defend the final thesis for the degree to be awarded. Approval of the final thesis must be obtained from the committee and then usually the graduate dean for research. Some institutions have a thesis editor who gives final endorsement of the thesis. The thesis editor is concerned only for checking format, style, and grammar, and not the content or merit of the study.

By its nature, the thesis is a very structured and guided experience with many quality control measures. Ultimately, the goal of any research project is to publish or present the results and make a scholarly contribution to the discipline. This should also be the projected outcome of a thesis or dissertation. Publication or presentation of research is another benchmark of research quality and a type of control measure to be discussed later.

## Institutional Review Boards

We have mentioned the IRB several times in this and other chapters. For many reasons the IRB is one of the most important internal quality control mechanisms. What exactly is an IRB, and what quality control functions does it serve?

The IRB exists primarily to assist researchers in the protection of research subjects. When scientifically sound and ethical studies are conducted, not only are the research subjects' rights upheld but also indirectly the reputation of the institution and researcher are safeguarded to some extent. Research subjects may be categorized as human or animal, and usually a specific IRB serves the needs of each. Since animal subjects are used only in a small number of highly specialized areas in HPER, our discussion here will be limited to the human subject IRB.

U.S. government regulations (e.g., Code of Federal Regulations [45 CFR 46], 1983, updated 1991) specify that any institution that is receiving federal money to support research must have a committee competent to review research proposals involving human subjects. Technically, any institution that is not receiving federal dollars is not legally required to have an IRB. However, it would seem logical that any institution that

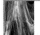 *The IRB is one of the most important internal quality control mechanisms.*

allows human subject research has a moral and ethical charge to ensure subjects' welfare and therefore should have an IRB.

The IRB consists of members who represent a wide variety of academic specialties in which human subject research is likely to be done. Depending on the size and needs of the institution, the IRB membership may be quite large and diverse. Representatives often include physicians, psychologists, educators, lawyers, philosophers, sociologists, and nonscientist community members. Faculty in HPER often serve as well. The research conducted by biomechanists, athletic trainers, and exercise physiologists, for example, is somewhat unique in the university setting, and inclusion of such expertise is often needed on an IRB. This assorted membership is important so that experts from various areas may assist the IRB in competent review of research.

The material that an investigator submits to the IRB is usually some form of a detailed written proposal and an informed consent document. The proposal contains many of the components of a research paper previously discussed, in addition to some others. The informed consent document (see Chapter 2) is examined for its clarity, simplicity, and completeness.

Not all research studies involving human subjects have the same element of risk. So it is not necessary for an entire IRB to deliberate over studies that are routine and pose little or no risk to the participant. There are various levels of IRB review for proposals, depending on the risk to the subject. Federal guidelines classify the review of proposals three ways: exempt, expedited, and full board. Exempt research studies typically have little or no risk associated with them and involve the collection of data from routine practices or procedures. Most educational research (e.g., research involving normal educational practices) is classified as exempt. The chairman of the IRB approves this type of proposal on behalf of the board. Expedited review is done on studies that involve no more than minimal risk to the subject. Examples of studies that qualify for this level of review include the use of moderate exercise, noninvasive electronic monitoring of the subject, examination of preexisting records, and obtaining small amounts of blood. Usually one or two expert board members are selected to review and approve the proposal for the IRB. The full board must review any study that does not qualify for exempt or expedited status. These studies usually expose the subject to greater than minimal risk. An example of a study requiring full board approval is one with subjects over age 40 performing treadmill exercise to exhaustion.

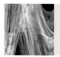

Research proposals are classified for IRB review into three levels: exempt, expedited, or full board.

At the heart of every review a basic question is asked: What is the risk to the subject in relation to the possible benefit? This risk/benefit analysis must always favor benefit; otherwise, the proposal is not approvable. There has to be direct benefit to the subject or to society but not necessarily to both. Since the risk/benefit ratio is subjectively determined, IRB members may have lengthy debates about whether some studies are approvable. The decisions of the IRB basically influence what human subject research can or cannot be done at that institution. A thumbs-up or thumbs-down ruling on a controversial study may have lasting impact on, among other things, the research agenda of an investigator (which may alter a career) or the growth of a scientific discipline. For example, the IRB at the University of Utah debated at great length before allowing human research on the artificial heart. After the 1982 experiment headed by Dr. William deVries, further human studies in this area were disapproved at that university.

Every proposal that involves the use of human subjects has to be approved by the IRB before it is initiated. The study then must be conducted in the manner in which it was approved and under full IRB guidelines. The IRB doesn't have a police force to ensure that investigators are in compliance with these guidelines. It is accepted in good faith that investigators will conduct research within this framework. So it is the researcher who has the primary responsibility for complying with all guidelines and regulations. Violations of this obligation could result in serious penalties for the institution as well

*The researcher has primary responsibility for complying with all IRB guidelines and regulations.*

as the investigator. Ask your professor for details regarding the IRB at your university.

Recent federal regulations governing IRB regulated research now require that all persons involved in the conduct of research at a university undergo periodic training. The procedure involves completing a web-based certification program. All students and faculty involved in a research project must be currently certified. IRB approval for a study requires evidence of this certification. The process ensures that all researchers are fully aware of the ethics and principles underlying research. Consequently, this process is a component of internal quality control.

## EXTERNAL QUALITY CONTROL

External quality control is any process or procedure outside of an institution that regulates the publication or presentation of research results. After a research project has been completed and the results are determined, the investigator has the challenging task of presenting and/or publishing the study. Of these two media for transmitting re-

*Publication in a well-respected journal is a high benchmark of research quality.*

search information, publication in a well-respected journal is considered a higher benchmark of research quality.

### Publication of a Research Article

After completing the data collection phase of the study and performing the appropriate statistical analyses, the researcher must determine whether the study is worthy of being shared with the professional community, including students and practitioners. In other words, will the work contribute to a discipline's body of knowledge? Everyone who does research would like to think that his or her work is meaningful, but frankly, it varies. The same study may have been done elsewhere previously (although it is important to replicate studies), or it may have been conducted with unacceptable methods or a faulty research design, all of which reduce the value of the outcome. Sometimes even a well-conducted study yields little value because of incomplete interpretations or lack of clarity in writing. Obviously, there are many things to consider and evaluate about a study to deem it worthy of publication. Who makes these decisions, and what is the process?

The investigator must decide on which journal to submit the study to and then write the manuscript according to that journal's style. The researcher then sends the article to the journal editor to initiate the review process. The editor selects two or three expert reviewers, sometimes called *referees* because of their impartiality, who volunteer their services to the journal to provide a critique of the manuscript. In most instances, these reviews are done in a blinded fashion. A **blinded review** means that there are no names or identifiers on the paper, so reviewers do not know the names of the authors or their institutional affiliation. Similarly, the authors do not know the names or institutions of the reviewers. The blinded review process provides for an objective review, since it limits a halo effect (both positive and negative) that may be associated with the study. Many but not all journals in HPER use the blinded review method.

The reviewers submit their critiques to the journal editor, who ultimately makes a decision to accept or reject the manuscript for publication. There are usually three fates for an article on its initial submission: accepted (a rare event for a first time submission), resubmission with revisions needed for further consideration, and rejection. When a verdict of resubmit is reached, the author(s) revise the paper in accordance with the feedback provided by the reviewers and then resubmit the manuscript for a second review. The revised paper is then reviewed again, and the reviewers vote to recommend acceptance or rejection of the paper. The final decision is made by the editor. Each review takes about 2 to 4 months and depending on the time needed by the author to revise and resubmit the paper, the total process typically takes at least a year or more. The original submission and acceptance dates are often printed with the article. It also takes about another 6 months for it to appear in print after being accepted. When an article is rejected by one journal, the investigator usually makes some revisions and sends it to another journal. Then the entire process starts all over. It should be obvious that perseverance and having "thick skin" are essential traits of those who publish regularly. It is unethical to submit the same article to two separate journals simultaneously (in case you're wondering).

## Limitations with the Review Process and Publication

This procedure sounds as if it should provide effective external quality control, and for the most part it does. However, think for a moment about the importance of the judgments of the reviewers and the editor. They are not only making a determination about what will be published in a journal but also about what will be part of a discipline's body of knowledge. This decision has far-reaching effects. It influences what teachers teach, what students learn, what is printed in textbooks, and what professionals in a discipline practice. Needless to say, these are very important decisions. Assume that the reviewers and editors are well qualified to make these decisions. What, then, may limit the process?

Perhaps the biggest limitation to this procedure is the inconsistency of the critiques of the reviewers. Morrow, Bray, Fulton, and Thomas (1992) reported on the interrater reliability of blind reviews done by independent evaluators on 363 manuscripts submitted to the *Research Quarterly for Exercise and Sport* (RQES). RQES is a respected HPER journal. Several reliability analyses were performed on the data, with not very impressive results. Overall, only 40% of the reviewers' ratings were in perfect agreement, and with an intraclass reliability coefficient (consistency indicator) of $r = .37$. Although these results are similar to those reported in other disciplines, it indicates that the review process is far from perfect. The authors concluded by suggesting that reviewers need more orientation and experience and better review guidelines to improve the procedure. Most experienced researchers have experienced exactly what Morrow and colleagues found.

Another interesting study on this topic was done by Peters and Ceci (1982). They obtained 12 studies from different authors in highly respected psychology departments around the United States. These studies had been published 18 to 32 months before and were resubmitted to the same journal in which they were published. The editorial staffs detected 3 of the 12 resubmissions and prevented a second review. Of the remaining 9 studies reviewed, 8 were rejected.

Because of the subjectivity of the review process, it is now and always will be less than perfect. Studies such as that of Morrow and colleagues stress the continued need to improve the soundness and dependability of the process. In spite of the limitations surrounding it, the review process remains one of the most important and time-honored quality control measures of research.

Finally, it should be understood that not all published studies are of high quality. Furthermore, in all disciplines some studies are published but when read or reviewed by others, flaws may be apparent. The review and revise process then is not perfect, but it undoubtedly enhances the overall quality of most published research. Students and readers of research should be aware that occasionally an inferior study may receive favorable evaluations from reviewers and be accepted for publication by an editor. Therefore, the readers of research must take an active role in assessing the quality of any study, whether it is published or presented, because they are the ultimate judges of its value.

## PUBLISH-OR-PERISH AND RESEARCH QUALITY

Most universities have a research mission to some degree. Because of this mission, faculty are expected to conduct research and are evaluated accordingly. Let us digress for a moment regarding the tenure process for a faculty member, since it is intimately related to publish or perish. Typically, new faculty members with a doctorate initiate their employment at the rank of assistant professor and strive to become tenured and to be promoted to associate and eventually full professor. Many universities use a 7-year tenure model: at the end of a 6-year period, a tenure decision is made. If tenure is granted, for all practical purposes, the professor has a job at that university for the rest of his or her career. As you might imagine, receiving tenure is the ultimate in job security for a faculty member, making it a very desirable goal.

If the university requires a high evaluation in the area of research for tenure, the faculty member may be placed in a publish-or-perish situation. Because considerable time is needed to conduct and publish research, young faculty experience some anxiety to produce a given volume of research in this short period. This is particularly true at many universities where much time is devoted to teaching and service. When the pressure to publish is considerable, there is an increased potential for research quality to be adversely affected and hence, the publish-or-perish phenomenon rears its head.

## Research Quality versus Quantity

The mindset of research as a numbers game is at the root of this problem. One may hear professors talking about the number of studies they have published or how long their resumés or curriculum vitae are. University administrators often use the number of articles their faculty have published as a benchmark for research productivity. It is far easier to count the number of published papers of a faculty member than to judge their quality. Hence, the tenure decision is often affected strongly by the number of publications. This proclivity for research numbers can be a principal source of the dilution of research quality.

Since the conduct of research is a mission of a university, there is an obligation to uphold its quality. In an attempt to address the quality-versus-quantity issue, some universities are attempting interesting changes. One approach is to lengthen the time to a tenure decision from 6 or 7 years up to 10. That allows a faculty member to develop a quality research agenda with less pressure of limited time. Another strategy is to allow a faculty member to submit only a specified number of publications for a tenure decision. For instance, an institution indicates that only four publications can be submitted for tenure review. It wouldn't matter if the professor had 20 articles, since only the best 4 are presented. Therefore, the emphasis is placed on quality. Universities need to continue to address this dilemma.

Institutions vary considerably on research and productivity standards for faculty. The publish-or-perish syndrome occurs at universities with unreasonable expectations of faculty or when there is a poor match between the professor's work output and the institution's demand. For example, some professors simply don't enjoy doing research and may think having to publish a requisite number of articles for tenure or promotion is too demanding. It may be tempting in such situations for a faculty member to pursue rather simple topics for their research in hopes that the minimal number of publications may be met. However, this greatly limits the quality of the work and defies to some extent the purpose of doing research.

## RESEARCH DISHONESTY

No one knows the incidence rate of research dishonesty, but on occasion it has been reported with dire consequences for the researcher. Recently, in 2005, a South Korean university professor had to resign his position after his stem cell lines were found to be fraudulent. Another example in 2006 was the discovery of a pioneering oral cancer researcher in Norway who was discovered to have fabricated much of his data. Logically, when it does occur, it affects the quality of published and presented research, and endangers the reputation of researchers in general. Since there is no easy way to detect fraudulent work, we must put our trust in those who conduct and publish research.

 **Summary**

In this chapter, several aspects of research quality control have been discussed. Internal quality control relates to institutional guidelines on what type of research may be done

| **TABLE 18-1. Summary of Quality Control in Research** |
|---|
| Internal quality control |
|     Peer review |
|     Student colloquia and defenses |
|     Institutional review boards |
| External quality control |
|     Blinded review of journal articles |
|     Unblinded review of journal articles |
| An important judge of research quality is the consumer of research! |

and the protection of research subjects. This is accomplished by departmental peer review, colloquia and defenses of student research, and the IRB. External quality control relates to the publication or presentation of research results. The blinded review process best enforces this. Table 18-1 provides a summary of the primary sources of research quality control.

Research quality control has many components, but the sources of control can be traced to two key individuals. One source is the producer of research. This person must be knowledgeable, diligent, and honest to support a major part of research quality. The other source is the consumer of research. Consumers must also possess knowledge of the research process and of their field. Even if one never takes part in the production end of research, that person has an obligation as a professional to be active at the consumer level. Because the consumers of research ultimately decide whether or not to use research information, they are important judges of research quality.

 **Learning Activities**

1. Have you accomplished the objectives stated at the beginning of the chapter? If not, go back and reread the concepts you're uncertain about. Also, ask your professor about these topics.
2. Attend a student defense of a proposal or thesis. Describe the format. Also identify several features you consider to be quality control mechanisms.
3. Discuss the issue of faculty publish-or-perish syndrome in class with your professor, sharing his or her perspective on the topic.
4. Discuss the journal article review process in class with your professor. See if he or she has any special insights or experiences with this procedure.

# CHAPTER 19

# Assessment and Application of Research

## KEY CONCEPTS

- Assessing the quality of research
- Internal validity
- Sample size
- Level of significance
- Statistical power
- Post hoc error
- Treatment effect
- Interpreting and summarizing the results of research
- Meta-analysis
- Application of research

## AFTER READING THIS CHAPTER YOU SHOULD BE ABLE TO:

- Assess the quality of research based on internal validity, limitations, and treatment effect.
- Discuss the importance of sample size and power in research.
- Describe factors affecting power.
- Discuss the merits of using significance levels lower and higher than .05.
- Distinguish between significance and treatment effect.
- Describe several ways of quantifying treatment effect.
- Explain why the reputation of people and publications should not be used to assess the quality of research.
- Describe post hoc error.
- Discuss several means of collating and interpreting the findings on a topic across numerous studies.
- Discuss several criteria to use in applying research.

This chapter focuses on improving your ability to interpret research, integrate the findings on a given topic, and determine what information can be applied to the real world setting of your professional life. These skills are necessary for professionals with graduate training in health, physical education, and recreation (HPER). Your own professional development as well as progression within our disciplines depends heavily on the quality of work routinely performed by individual professionals. Unless we stay informed by reading professional literature and use updated information on the job, the quality of work carried on by professionals in our disciplines is limited. Therefore, this chapter highlights some strategies to use in interpreting research and making decisions about using research findings in your professional work.

## ASSESSING THE QUALITY OF RESEARCH

Blind acceptance of the written word may be more common than it should. The authors frequently note this based on comments our own students frequently make. Today, information can be electronically searched. The number of sources available on the Internet as well as in print is staggering; this perhaps explains why it is easy to feel confident that what one reads must be accurate. Obviously, this is not necessarily the case. A major goal of graduate study should be providing the knowledge and insight for soundly assessing the quality of published work, including research and the professional literature. Several assessment criteria are discussed here.

### Evaluate All Research for Adequate Sample Size

Every study must be judged on its academic merits, including its overall soundness or **internal validity** (e.g., adequate treatment, design, methods, and statistics) and limitations. A primary criterion for internal validity is adequacy of **sample size**. A number of times, particularly in the statistics section of this text, we have emphasized that a large sample size facilitates achieving **statistical significance**. The capacity for a statistic to detect significance when the null hypothesis is false is termed **power**. Thus, sample size and power are directly related. A large sample aids achieving significance because it reduces the error term or denominator of a statistic. Recall that

$$t \text{ or } F = \frac{\text{treatment variance}}{\text{sampling error variance}}$$

The error term shrinks with a large N because sampling error is reduced; that is, a large N better represents a population than does a small N. A larger $t$ or $F$ ratio increases the probability of statistical significance being achieved. The limited power of any statistic used with a small N tends to make acceptance of the null hypothesis and the probability of a type II decision error more likely. Unfortunately, this may lead to the conclusion that no real difference or relationship exists when a larger sample might have shown a significant difference. Consequently, it behooves researchers to use an adequate N so as to draw sound conclu-

*The capacity for a statistic to determine significance when the null hypothesis is false is called power.*

sions. One can understand why inadequate sample size might be a reason for rejecting a paper for publication because of the relative loss of statistical power.

Formulas exist to assist estimating appropriate sample size. No single threshold for N exists because significance and power depend on several factors, each of which vary from study to study. When comparing the means of two groups, the following formula provides an estimate of the sample size needed to achieve significance at a specific level (Borg & Gall, 1979).

$$N = \frac{2\ SD(t^2)}{D^2}$$

where

        $SD = SD$ in other similar studies
        $t = t$ ratio that is significant at .05 level in similar studies
        $D$ = Difference in the two variables that is of practical significance

For example, we will estimate the number of subjects needed in a study in which the SD reported in other similar studies on the subject is 2, the $t$ ratio is 5, and the practical difference for the variable is 3. The number of subjects needed in this instance is 11 ($N = 4(5)^2/3^2 = 100/9 = 11$). Selecting appropriate values for each component of the equation is based on previously published work on the topic and an educated feel for practical difference. The formula provides only an estimate rather than a definitive value. Cohen (1988) is an excellent reference that is widely used by researchers. It includes tables that facilitate estimation of sample size.

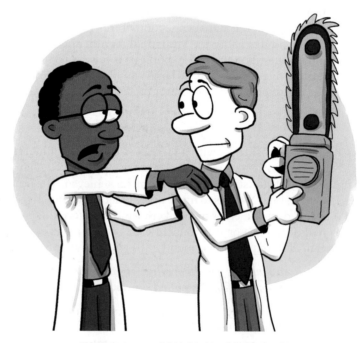

"I know you need 141.6 test subjects, but how about we just round up the number to 142?"

Estimating sample size is well worth the effort if for no other reason than the study is far more likely to be accepted for publication. But even more important, the purpose of research is to carefully examine a condition and test whether an occurrence of something is real or due to chance. Therefore, principles of good research demand that an adequate sample size be used to provide a fair test of the hypothesis.

Some years ago the power for studies appearing in one volume of a major research journal was analyzed. Studies were categorized into small, medium, and large effects, referring to the magnitude of change in the dependent variable. In studies with small and large effects, the chances of detecting significance were only 20% and 40%, respectively. Thus, the average study was going against the odds of finding significance given the sample size used. It was concluded that studies reporting no relationship or no significant effect be cautiously interpreted. When such a finding is reported, one should certainly judge to what extent the lack of significance may be explained by a small sample size. The reporting of **statistical power** or a rationale for the sample size used is now required by many journals in our disciplines.

Certain types of studies require a larger sample than others. Studies conducted outside the laboratory often require a larger sample size because of the possible influence of numerous extraneous variables. For example, suppose a researcher wishes to compare the effectiveness of various teaching techniques in the public schools. Many variables operate in the school and home environment to influence learning. The teachers vary in personality, inherent teaching ability, and so on; each classroom environment varies. Thus, student learning is affected by all of these forces, and the problem is to determine whether one teaching technique—the independent variable— differs from another technique enough to overcome the effects of the contaminating variables. In such cases, a larger sample is needed to reduce the variance in the subjects such that initial differences in subjects is minimized or statistical adjustment such as use of ANCOVA (analysis of covariance) is needed to make the groups more equivalent. One can see why studies in the real world, where so many variables are operating to influence behavior, require a large sample size. This would include studies of worksite wellness programs and studies in recreational settings and health agencies. Such studies have inherently high external validity but at the same time are limited in internal validity. One partial solution to the latter problem is using a reasonably large sample.

When the expected difference in the outcome measure is small, a larger sample size should be used. Suppose a researcher wished to determine whether two types of stretching techniques for the hamstring muscles in professional football players have a differing effect on hamstring pulls over a season of play. Most likely all of the players regularly stretch anyway, so any gain in flexibility is likely to be small, regardless of the stretching technique used. Also, hamstring pulls may be caused by factors other than hamstring flexibility, such as strength imbalance, fatigue, and contact. Thus, a large sample is needed to elicit a significant effect when the expected outcome measure is anticipated to be small. In designing the study, the researcher might conduct the study using several different teams to obtain enough subjects. In comparison, a study assessing whether or not flexibility of the hamstrings can be improved in the general middle-aged population would probably require fewer subjects to obtain a significant effect simply because most such people probably do not stretch regularly and so are likely to experience improvement.

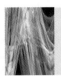 A large sample size is needed in studies where numerous extraneous variables may affect the dependent variable and when anticipating a small effect in the dependent variable.

## Critique the Measurements

Accuracy of measurement is critical in research, which is why journal articles describe the measurements in the Methods section in such detail. Typically, several paragraphs are required to provide the necessary detail. Some of this material may seem unnecessary, but it is important for the careful reader who realizes that the calibration and operation of instruments, use of multiple trials, amount of warm-up, etc., all may affect the data obtained. Failure to provide these details leaves much to the imagination of the reader. The detail allows the reader to judge the degree that accuracy was likely attained.

## Examine the Variance of the Subjects

The variance of subjects affects statistical power. As *SD* increases within a group, note the effect on the formula to estimate sample size when comparing two groups. A large *SD* increases the numerator, thereby increasing the number of subjects needed. Put another way, a large *SD* increases the error variance for *t* and *F* ratios, thus denoting a reduction in *t* and *F*. Therefore, researchers should strive to select subjects with limited variance on the dependent variable to optimize internal validity. For example, if investigating the effects of walking on aerobic fitness, the investigator may select subjects with similar levels of fitness and physical activity. This reduces sampling error. However, researchers often wish to use subjects with considerable dissimilarity because the results of the study can be more broadly applied to a larger segment of the population. In such cases, concern for external validity compromises the degree of internal validity and tends to reduce power. Knowledgeable researchers understand this trade-off. Insightful readers of research might examine subject variance when wondering why a given statistic was not significant. As pointed out in previous chapters, the mean difference in groups may be substantial, yet statistical significance may not occur simply because of the large amount of variance. In reading research, a simple way of doing this is to examine the *SD*s reported in tables. When they are large in relation to the means, one may have uncovered much of the reason for a statistic not being significant. The same mean difference may have been significant in subjects who did not vary as much on the given measure.

## Critique the Significance Levels Used and Reported

An interesting argument made by Franks and Huck (1986) contends that although increasing sample size to boost statistical power is sound, it is impractical for many researchers because of time and financial constraints. As an alternative they suggest changing the significance level from the commonly used .05 level to a higher level such as .10. The probability of making a type I error is increased, but they contend that such an error in one study does not seriously undermine previous work because most researchers and readers understand the hazard of making decisions based on a single study. Furthermore, they explain that using an alpha of .05 is not without problems. For example, failure to find significant results using the typical standard of .05 may tend to steer other investigators away from a potentially meaningful area of study. This may be true in particular in studies with numerous extraneous variables and in studies in which the degree of change is expected to be small. Research on the training of elite athletes is sparse perhaps because of the small gains that can be made in performance and limited control over diet, injury, psychology, etc. Consequently, researchers seemingly avoid studying the elite athlete. More research might be generated if investigators had a better probability of achieving significant results by using an alpha of .10 instead of .05.

Franks and Huck also recommend reporting significance levels for all variables studied, which allows the reader to judge the potential for type I error. Only indicating whether or not a finding is significant omits important information. An alpha level of .051 may be very differently interpreted from a level of .60, yet neither falls into the significant category if alpha = .05. The former narrowly misses meeting the common criterion for significance, whereas the latter is wide of the mark. This information should be available to the reader. However, more often than not, alpha levels are reported only for findings that are significant. One might argue that all *p* levels should be given, but particularly when close to the .05 level.

Feinstein (1983) reminds us that the .05 significance level was never meant by its originator, Sir Ronald Fisher, to be used in all research. Rather, it was intended to serve as a guideline. The .05 level was suggested largely because of its mathematical advantages, including the fact that all but about 5% of scores will be within about 2 *SDs* of the mean. Through the years, however, the .05 level has become rigidly used. Manuscripts failing to achieve significance at the .05 level are sometimes rejected, regardless of the size of the treatment effect. Imagine a researcher finding that a new drug is 50% more effective than any other traditional treatment, yet having the manuscript rejected because the difference with a small sample size fails to meet the .05 standard. One wonders how many sound ideas and findings died because of lack of statistical significance.

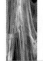
*It is recommended that significance levels be reported for all variables studied, which allows the reader to judge the potential for type I error. Only indicating whether or not a finding is significant omits important information.*

## Determine How Large the Treatment Effect Is

As indicated, statistical significance and treatment effect are distinctly different characteristics of a study. Significance relates to the probability that a difference or relationship is real, whereas **treatment effect** refers to the magnitude of the differences between groups. Nearly all studies report significance, but many do not quantify the treatment effect or variance explained. This is unfortunate, because significant differences are not necessarily large or meaningful. Such a paradox may occur because of the effect of N size in determining sig-

*Statistical significance and treatment effect are distinctly different characteristics of a study. Significance relates to the probability that a difference is real, whereas treatment effect refers to the magnitude of the differences between groups.*

nificance. With sample sizes exceeding 100, small differences or relationships of little practical consequence can be significant. Quick examination of a statistics table in Appendix A clearly reveals this.

Obviously, treatment effect should be quantified wherever possible. There are several ways to do this. The simplest is reporting the percent difference between groups. Calculation and interpretation are easy. A second method of determining treatment effect is the calculation of omega squared or coefficient of determination ($r^2$). Recall that omega squared indicates the percent variance attributed to the experimental variable, which is a different way of quantifying the treatment effect. The third method is to calculate what is termed the **effect size.** The equation appears as

$$\text{Effect size} = \frac{M_e - M_c}{SD}$$

where

$M_e$ = mean of experimental group
$M_c$ = mean of control group
$SD$ = standard deviation of control group

The calculation is simple and often is the most useful and interesting result of a study. How different are various treatments? Cohen (1969) proposed that in the behavioral sciences an effect size of 0.2 indicates a small difference; 0.5, a moderate difference, and 0.8, a large difference. It may be helpful here to interpret how much change a given effect size represents. For example, an effect size of 1.0 is large using Cohen's standard, but how else might this be quantified to help us interpret the amount of change? If an aerobics exercise class improved their maximum aerobic capacity after 10 weeks by 1 full *SD*, this is equivalent to an effect size of 1.0. This means that their score improved from a percentile rank of 50 to 84! Recall that the area under the curve for a score 1 *SD* above the mean represents about 34%. This amount of change most certainly is large! Even an effect size of .50 represents improvement from the mean of 50 percentile rank to a percentile rank of 69. This also probably represents good improvement or what Cohen describes as moderate.

Direct comparison with other studies can be made if effect size is expressed directly or even indirectly, the latter by providing the *M* and *SD* of variables. It may be more meaningful to analyze effect size than significance, because the latter is so strongly affected by sample size and variance. This may aid the interpretation of new studies and hence the development of new knowledge. Thomas, former editor of the *Research Quarterly for Exercise and Sport* (*RQES*), for years strongly advocated the reporting of either omega squared or effect size. However, little or no change at that time was noted in published articles in the *RQES* (Thomas, Salazar, & Landers, 1991). Obviously, both faculty and students should be encouraged to familiarize themselves with the merits of reporting magnitude of the treatment effect.

## Realize That Well-Known Names and Prestigious Journals Do Not Guarantee Sound Research

Dr. Linus Pauling received a Nobel prize in science years ago. Shortly thereafter, articles appeared in magazines and newspapers about his extolling the virtues of vitamin C in preventing and treating the common cold. His opinion was initially based on observations on himself and his wife. Although no research data were available to support his conclusion and recommendation, the American public assumed that the advice of an esteemed scientist must be sound. Thus was born the selling of vitamin C in every drugstore and grocery store. We are familiar with several examples of misguided information from reputable scientists in other disciplines as well.

Although the standards for publishing in most professional journals are high, not everything printed is actually sound, and none of it is perfect. All manuscripts submitted to juried publications are peer-reviewed by experts. However, this does not guarantee that every study appearing in a given volume used the best design, methods, or even statistical approach. All studies have their limitations, and readers should appreciate this.

In the disciplines of HPER, we must be especially aware of the commercial approach to people's problems. Weight loss, health food, running shoes, and exercise clothing are multibillion-dollar businesses. The approaches used to market products include star athletes and Hollywood personalities. They lend excitement to products and techniques that honestly is not found in research (except perhaps for the authors of this text!). A widely used strategy is the "super claim," that is, a benefit that is far larger than actually occurs. Some years ago 10 minutes of rope jumping was touted by one company as being equivalent to 30 minutes of jogging. New weight loss diets promise impossible results. Books such as *The 120 Year Diet and Nutrition Plan* tempt people because of their staggering implications. Pearson and Shaw, authors of *Life Extension: A Practical Scientific Approach,* claimed to be research scientists, but in fact neither had graduate degrees, and neither had ever published a paper in a reputable research publication. Their book is filled with case histories that cannot be verified. The point is that the expertise and claims of any author should be carefully examined, particularly if the claims seem extravagant. The cliché "If it seems too good to be true, it probably is…" seems valid from a common sense point of view.

## Understand That Not All Changes During and After an Experimental Period Should Be Attributed to the Independent Variable

The tendency to violate the above principle is called **post hoc error.** If a woman started a running program and 6 months later was divorced, is it valid to conclude that running caused the divorce? If a person starts taking vitamin supplements and 3 weeks later has a cholesterol reading lower than ever previously, is it logical to assume that the vitamins caused the low reading? Common sense makes these examples illogical, but when put in a more professional context, logic can easily be swayed.

Suppose a company begins a wellness program and hires a health educator or exercise science professional to administer it. To justify the merits of the program and its continuation, the administrator compares the job absenteeism of those who regularly attend various activities of the wellness program, such as exercise, blood pressure screening, and health fair, with absenteeism of those who never participate in these activities. The absenteeism rate is found to be significantly higher in those who never attend the wellness program, much to the delight of the administrator, who proclaims that the program reduced absenteeism. Is this a valid conclusion? To demonstrate cause and effect, an experimental research design is needed. Groups would have to be randomly assigned to participant and nonparticipant groups and then compared. At the beginning of the study, the participants may have been different in terms of job absenteeism as well as a variety of health habits. Unless these differences are controlled experimentally or statistically, no sound conclusion can be drawn. Some of the early studies assessing the influence of health and wellness programs in the workplace made conclusions based on post hoc error. The more one wishes to see good things happen, the more good things will be found. Being

*Not every beneficial change in behavior during and after an experimental period can be attributed to the independent variable.*

enthusiastic about a program or treatment is fine, but be aware of the possibility of post hoc error.

Figure 19-1 is a checklist to be used in evaluating research. It includes design, methods, threats to internal and external validity, and so on. It may be useful in assessing the many aspects of a study.

## INTERPRETING AND SUMMARIZING THE RESULTS OF RESEARCH

A difficult task for most people is summarizing the findings on a topic across many studies. Typically, most research questions studied are somewhat controversial by nature, which results in a variety of findings and conclusions. Furthermore, across the studies subject characteristics differ, as do the details of measurement, treatment, research design, and statistics. Therefore, it is hardly surprising that results differ across studies. How can one collate the findings from this mass of information? Several approaches are presented here.

### Read Current Reviews of the Literature

Most research journals periodically include review articles. In addition, some professional associations annually sponsor a review publication. For instance, the American College of Sports Medicine publishes *Exercise and Sport Science Reviews*, which consists entirely of review articles written by experts on a given topic. Reviews typically include

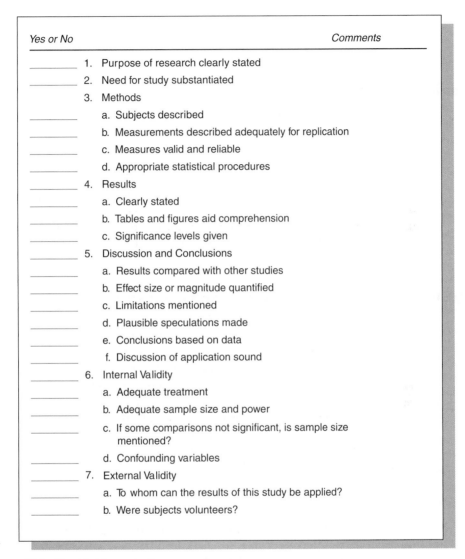

*Yes or No*                                                                      *Comments*

_____  1. Purpose of research clearly stated

_____  2. Need for study substantiated

          3. Methods

_____      a. Subjects described

_____      b. Measurements described adequately for replication

_____      c. Measures valid and reliable

_____      d. Appropriate statistical procedures

_____  4. Results

_____      a. Clearly stated

_____      b. Tables and figures aid comprehension

_____      c. Significance levels given

_____  5. Discussion and Conclusions

_____      a. Results compared with other studies

_____      b. Effect size or magnitude quantified

_____      c. Limitations mentioned

_____      d. Plausible speculations made

_____      e. Conclusions based on data

_____      f. Discussion of application sound

_____  6. Internal Validity

_____      a. Adequate treatment

_____      b. Adequate sample size and power

_____      c. If some comparisons not significant, is sample size
                 mentioned?

_____      d. Confounding variables

_____  7. External Validity

_____      a. To whom can the results of this study be applied?

_____      b. Were subjects volunteers?

**Figure 19-1.** Checklist for evaluating research.

a discussion of the points of disagreement, possible causes of the disagreement, and recommendations for research on the subject.

How do these experts actually synthesize and weigh the literature? Probably their involvement as active researchers and readers over many years develops a level of familiarity that few could achieve without spending equivalent time and undergoing similar training. Thus, they know the subject matter so well that every published study that adds something new to the knowledge is fitted in at a logical conceptual point in their frame of reference. So take advantage of their expertise. Read review articles to assist in interpreting what the current state of knowledge is.

## Construct a Summary Table of Studies

This suggestion was made in Chapter 4 dealing with the review of literature. A table with column headings of authors, date, subject characteristics, results, and comments is helpful in tallying the characteristics and results of a number of studies. Several pages of such tables can be used to summarize and even categorize the major findings. For example, one table might summarize studies having the same finding (e.g., that technique A is superior to other techniques) whereas a second table may summarize studies with a different finding (e.g., technique B is superior). Then, one can look for common factors among studies reporting the same result; for example, technique A is superior mostly or only in children 6 to 12 years old. This process can facilitate making generalizations across many different studies.

## Tally Studies Showing Significant and Nonsignificant Results

This method is sometimes used in review articles but is limited because studies not finding significance may have methodological and statistical flaws. For example, measurement error and small sample size may have prevented a finding of statistical significance, although the treatment effect was strong. Furthermore, a mere count does not include factors such as subjects' characteristics, magnitude of the treatment, and sample size. Also, this technique treats all the studies as being of equal value. That is, the results of a well-conducted study are treated the same as those of a lesser-quality study. The same is true of studies with a large number of subjects and those of a small number of subjects. Consequently, the tally technique is only a quantitative measure and is limited qualitatively.

## Use Meta-analysis

Meta-analysis statistically treats the result of each study as one data point. The value used from each study is the **effect size,** which is the difference in the mean of the experimental group(s) and the control group divided by the standard deviation of the control group.

Effect size is expressed in units of *SD* and is therefore fairly easy to interpret. For example, an effect size of 0.73 means the experimental mean was .73 standard deviations greater than the mean of the control group. The effect size of each study is calculated and used to determine the *M* and *SD* of all the effect sizes. Thus, the mean effect of an independent variable across a number of studies can be quantified. The significance of the difference in effect size can be determined by using the *M* and *SD* of categories compared in an independent *t* test, if there are two means to compare, or by using an analysis of variance (ANOVA) if there are more than two means. Examples of meta-analysis in HPER include comparison of maximum oxygen uptake in males and females

(Sparling, 1980), effect of exercise on blood lipids and lipoproteins (Tran, Weltman, Glass, & Mood, 1983), gender differences in motor performance (Thomas & French, 1985), long-term weight loss maintenance (Anderson, Konz, Frederick, & Wood, 2001), trainability of senior citizens (Lemura, von Duvillard, & Mookerjee, 2000), and effects of exercise on bone mineral density in men (Kelley, Kelley, & Tran, 2000). The technique offers great potential for quantitatively comparing the results of many studies, which in turn facilitates making sound conclusions about the literature. Meta-analysis pools the results from many studies, and by incorporating effect size into its analysis it allows making conclusions based on statistical power and magnitude. Hence, it is an effective means of interpreting the overall results across many studies in a way more powerful than the typical review article. The advantages are too strong to ignore, and the technique will undoubtedly be used far more commonly in the future.

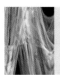

Meta-analysis quantifies the effect size across many studies and allows drawing firm conclusions from the literature. It's what we all wish we could do in our heads after reading several articles!

## TIPS FOR INTERPRETATION OF RESEARCH

Several tips are provided here to enhance your ability to make sound interpretations when reading research.

### Tip 1: Realize That Statistics Can Be Abused

Statistics and numbers seem to be much respected in this country; perhaps overly so. Everyone seems to use numbers to justify something. But in some cases, the logic behind the statistics is faulty. For example, statistics and results of studies can be presented to exaggerate the findings. It all depends on the context. For example, one often hears statistics about a medical problem that seems to be getting worse. At this writing, obesity and overweight are rapidly increasing. If data that depicted the accelerated rate of persons becoming obese from 1990 to 2000 were extrapolated over the next 50 years, it might appear that nearly all Americans would be obese in the year 2050. Let's hope not! Obviously, we hope that the rate of increased obesity will decelerate in the coming years with continued educational and medical efforts. The point is that one should not assume that a rate of change over one decade will remain constant over future decades.

Another example of predicting beyond the data is the notion that female athletes may eventually surpass males in running the marathon, because their progress has strongly exceeded that of males in the last several decades. One major reason for much of the rapid progress for women may be that many more female athletes have trained for and competed in the marathon in the past 20 years or so in comparison with earlier years. Women didn't compete in the marathon in the Olympics until 1984. In the years following such a change, women had more room for progress than men. Will the initial rapid rate of improvement continue for women? Examination of world records across all running distances from the 100 meters to the marathon in both men and women suggests an ever-descending rate of improvement as the years pass. The limits to training, nutrition, equipment, and other factors have progressed to the point where future changes in performance in most sports will most likely be smaller and smaller. Furthermore, if extrapolation beyond the data were a sound method of prediction, women marathoners would be predicted eventually to run the distance in several minutes rather than well over 2 hours, which is absurd. Consequently, when reading studies that involve prediction, realize that the estimate was made on past data and as time marches on, the slope of the prediction line or the rate of change may not stay constant. The longer one attempts to predict into the future, the more unsure the accuracy. Simply said, don't predict very far beyond the data.

Be cautious in interpreting percent change. Although percent is a common and effective means of conveying the degree of change, it can exaggerate the interpretation. For example, suppose two people both improve their one repetition maximum in a specific lift by 10 pounds: subject A from 10 to 20 pounds, a 100% increase, and subject B from 400 to 410 pounds, a 2.5% increase. How different the progress seems when expressed as a percent. Obviously, a small absolute change can be large or small when expressed as a percentage, depending on the initial value. Another example may emphasize the point. A child learning to shoot free throws in basketball might initially make only 1 out of 10. Several days later after additional practice, an improvement to 2 successful shots out of 10 represents a 100% increase! That value certainly sounds better to our young player than saying "Your score improved by one." Percentage is used so widely by the media as well as in research because it is relatively easy to understand, but it also can exaggerate the actual amount of change. Next time you are reading your quarterly stock statement, think about these implications! Therefore, when using percent to judge the amount of change in a variable, express change as an absolute value as well as a percentage to improve the interpretation.

## Tip 2: When a Finding Is Found to Be Nonsignificant, Check Sample Size

As previously stated, statistical significance is strongly influenced by sample size. Consequently, make it a practice to focus on sample size whenever reading a study in which significance was not found. If the N was quite small, you know that the probability of making a type II decision error is increased. Interpret the findings of such a study cautiously. Do not assume that the independent variable had no effect or is not worthy of additional study. With a larger sample, perhaps the same degree of difference might well be statistically significant.

## Tip 3: Be Cautious of Biased Sampling

Interpretation of results from studies should include consideration of the sample to determine whether it is biased. For example, public school officials wish to report student data on standardized tests that reflect well on their school districts or school. However, comparison of student achievement across schools and districts may be unfair because of differences in socioeconomic level, proportion of students with special needs, and so on. Similarly, comparing performance on college entrance tests in different states may be unfair. In some regions of the country, the ACT may be the more common test for students to take while the SAT is more common in other areas. If one state has only 7% of students taking the ACT and those who do so have mostly excellent grades and hope to be accepted into prestigious universities in a certain region of the country, they are a biased sample. If the scores from that state are compared with scores in a state where 64% of students take the ACT, the comparison is also biased. The latter state may have an equivalent percentage of excellent students, but the mean score for the state would be driven down by the mass of students taking the exam who are closer to the mean.

## Tip 4: Examine Figures Closely: They Can Distort Meaning

Sometimes this is done purposely to impress readers with the findings of a study. By using different size increments for the variable representing the Y or vertical axis, differences and trends can be magnified or diminished. For example, Figures 19-2 and 19-3 contain mock data for depicting the improvement in vertical jump performance before and after a 10-week training program. Both figures attempt to convey the same information. Note how much more impressive the improvement in jumping ability appears to be in Figure 19-2, where values on the Y-axis begin at 21 inches. In comparison, the improvement looks much smaller in Figure 19-3, where values for the Y-axis begin at 12 inches. The key here is to examine the increment used in presenting the data and to judge accordingly. Don't fall into the trap of interpreting data from a figure solely by the slope of the line (line graphs) or the absolute differences (in bar graphs). Check the increment used for the Y-axis and the lowest value plotted on the Y-axis, and then make an interpretation. Your interpretation will be much sounder.

It is best to portray data in a figure without trying to manipulate an interpretation. Don't use figures trying to convince readers of how impressive the results were. That

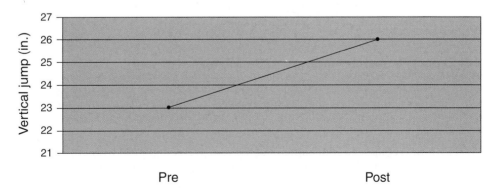

**Figure 19-2.** Vertical jump performance pre- and post-training: magnifying the difference.

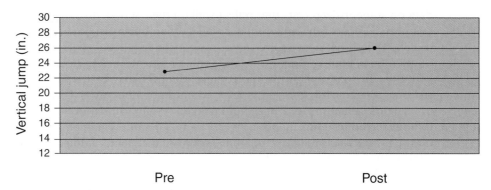

**Figure 19-3.** Vertical jump performance pre- and post-training: minimizing the difference.

may be the goal in selling products, but it isn't when reporting the results of research. Facilitate the reader's interpretation by letting the data speak for themselves.

## Tip 5: Correlation and Statistics Based on Them Do Not Mean Cause and Effect

For example, people wear more and heavier clothes in cold weather, and the relationship is probably quite strong. One might conclude that wearing of heavier clothing makes the weather cold! Recall that experimental research with control group, random assignment, and manipulation of an independent variable is the strongest research design to assess cause and effect. However, it is very easy to make the jump in logic, particularly when logic may suggest a mechanism as to why A might cause B to occur.

Suppose a researcher finds a strong correlation between vegetable intake and longevity. There may well be mechanisms quite logically suggesting that people will live longer by eating more vegetables such as greater intake of fiber, antioxidants, vitamins and minerals, and so on. However, by itself the correlation does not mean that A causes B to happen. It remains for other studies using a more experimental approach to document that vegetables affect longevity. The tendency to forget this principle is particularly likely when examining your own data.

## Tip 6: Expect Research Findings to Be Mixed

Studies addressing the same research question use different subjects, different techniques in measurement, different pieces of equipment, and different people to administer the tests. Is it any wonder that their results vary? It's almost a wonder perhaps that similar results can be obtained in different studies. One researcher may find that vitamin D enhances bone mineral content in premenopausal women, whereas another study may report no such effect. A third study reports that vitamin D enhanced bone mineral content in women over age 60 but not in younger women. This variety of findings is typical in research on most topics. Here's why. Think of the number of variables that need sorting out in such research. The effect of vitamin D needs to examined in relation to age, dosage, interaction with other nutrients, type of vitamin D (D2 or D3), length of study, and so on. Obviously, many of these variables differ across studies, which explain the mixed results. Numerous studies are usually needed before strong, consistent trends can be detected. Meta-analysis helps a great deal in drawing information from many studies to help arrive at a conclusion. So, expect to find considerable variation in the results of studies on most topics.

## Tip 7: Be Cautious of Research Reports in the Media

A recent survey indicated that medical stories on television and in newspapers often contained erroneous information. The benefits of new drugs are typically exaggerated and the risks minimized (Pugh & Borenstein, 2006). When realizing that news commentators and writers are not specifically trained in research, it isn't surprising. The authors have noted over the years a good many statements about exercise that seem exaggerated or are poorly explained.

## Tip 8: Be Wary of Studies Where Conflict of Interest May Exist

Increasingly researchers in the disciplines of HPER are involved in research with food supplements, exercise equipment, and medications. Typically, a company requests a researcher with expertise on a given topic to conduct a study testing the efficacy of the particular supplement, exercise device, or whatever. The researcher may agree and be paid a consultant fee for conducting the research and writing a research report for the company. The inherent problem, however, is conflict of interest. By being paid, the researcher may become biased in conducting the study and /or writing the research report as well as research paper submitted for publication. Consequently, the scientific integrity of the research may be compromised.

The issue is longstanding in medical research, but as more HPER faculty become involved in such research as well as research with other commercial enterprises, the problem grows. Some journals require authors to indicate in the publication if any relationship exists with the company. This at least warns the reader of possible conflict of interest. However, the reader should at least be aware of possible conflict of interest when no statement is made in a publication. Journals in our disciplines might well require such a statement. Some professional organizations and institutions advocate banning paid consultancies. Another breach of research integrity occurs in cases where the company prohibits publication or presentation of any research on the product without their approval. This caveat obviously prevents disseminating results that do not favor the interests of the company. Failure to publish such findings, however, is clearly incongruous with the purposes of research. Such contractual agreements should never be made between researchers and companies.

## Tip 9: Studies Reporting Statistically Significant Findings Are Published More Than those That Do Not

This means that some of the research literature is biased. The tendency to reject papers for publication that do not report significance probably stems from the feeling of editors and journal reviewers that limited internal validity is the likely cause of failing to achieve significance. Although this may be the case for some studies, it is likely not the reason in all cases. As expressed previously, the amount of change is expected to be small in some studies such as performance improvements in elite athletes. Thus, the small effects may prevent significance from occurring. Likewise, studies in which numerous extraneous variables exist, such as the worksite or school setting, may dampen the effect of an independent variable. The quality or internal validity of the studies may be sound, but the findings are simply the result of the conditions of the study. Acquisition of knowledge is hindered if researchers avoid investigating topics which by their very nature are difficult to yield significant findings. Obviously, studies should be judged by reviewers on quality and not on their results. Furthermore, concluding that an independent variable does not influence an outcome variable should be deemed as valuable as one that shows an effect. Hence, if a study has acceptable internal validity, its findings should be reported, regardless of whether or not statistical significance occurred. Lastly, the literature is biased in areas where researchers being paid as consultants were prohibited from publishing negative findings. We have no idea how many studies were never published because of this phenomenon, but in some areas of study where many researchers receive financial compensation the effect should be recognized.

## APPLICATION OF RESEARCH

The potential for applying the results of a study is called **external validity.** Most research in HPER is applied, so the potential for application is usually good. However, several precautions should be considered.

Technically, the only fully justified application of the results of a single study is to the subjects of that particular investigation. However, it is logical that people outside the study with similar traits as those of the original subjects may also be considered fair game for application. If this were not the case, applied research would be a misnomer and much research would have no purpose. For example, if a new medication to reduce blood pressure in hypertensive patients is found superior to current medications, the new medication might be used in hypertensive patients in general as long as they meet certain criteria for similarity, such as age, sex, and absence or presence of other medical characteristics.

*Technically, the only fully justified application of the results of a single study is to the subjects of that particular investigation.*

Good research includes a concern for appropriate application of results. The point is emphasized here because it is a common mistake to see results applied with little or no concern for matching the traits of research subjects with those of people outside the study. A group of weight lifters at a gym might read about a novel program used by the current Mr. America to build huge biceps. An article might go into great detail about the number of sets, repetitions, length of recovery, exercises, and so on. Is it scientifically defensible to assume that what worked for Mr. America will work for the readers of the magazine? (One of the authors knows it won't because he tried it; his arm circumference remained 12.5 firm inches!) Mr. America may possess some unique traits that allowed his biceps to grow massively with the program described. Unless others possess similar traits, such as previous years of training experience, a lifestyle in which weight training is the main task each day of the week, and a high responsiveness to training, they will most likely not experience the same results.

Advertisements are largely based on not understanding or failing to admit the principle of similarity of subjects. Advertisements depict remarkable changes as a result of using a certain drink, food, perfume, hair spray, or toothpaste. The assumption of such advertising is that we will purchase the product hoping that the same effect will happen to us.

A study shows that oatmeal lowers cholesterol 13%. Are you ready to buy some? First, the informed reader should know something about the subjects in the study. What if the subjects were men in their 50s and 60s with very high cholesterol levels at the start of the study? Are you still ready to head out the door to buy oatmeal? If you like oatmeal, fine. It is a wholesome food regardless of its impact on cholesterol levels. If you do not like oatmeal and you are in your 20s with a low cholesterol level, you certainly should not expect the same effect as that found in the study.

Most of us on occasion have violated common sense about applying the results of research (except for the authors!). However, when we make decisions on the job, more pressure may exist to make a sound decision. Unfortunately, no statistic or quantitative criterion is available to help determine when results of a study can be applied in a given situation. One must use good judgment in analyzing the similarity of subjects and those who may undergo the treatment. No statistic exists to indicate when application is sound.

Several factors make the results that occur in a study less likely to occur when applied to the clinical setting or work environment. The effects of being a volunteer, the history, pretest, and selection bias were discussed in Chapter 14. These factors do not preclude making applications from research. They merely indicate that the expected results may be a bit different (usually lower than subjects in a study).

Finally, realize that the results of a single study are only observations of a sample. Until the study is replicated one or more times and similar results are found, you cannot consider that you are dealing with facts. Replication is a basic part of research and science, and applying information from a single study is unscientific.

 **Summary**

The quality of a study should always be considered when reading and assessing research. Quality is largely determined by the internal validity and limitations. In addressing internal validity, the treatment, design, methods, data analysis, and sample size should be assessed. The results should be interpreted in terms of not only significance but also magnitude. The latter information is often omitted, but the insightful reader should at least estimate the effect size or variance explained because it is basic to interpreting the results of a study. Assessment should not be swayed by reputation and prestige.

Summarizing a vast number of studies is difficult but greatly enhanced by reading recent reviews of the literature. Meta-analysis is a means of quantifying the results of many separate studies and is likely to be used more frequently in the future to assess the state of knowledge in various topics. Making application from research to the real world requires judging the similarity of the subjects and conditions of a study to people and conditions outside the study. No statistical technique exists to aid the process of application, so common sense of the practitioner and researcher must prevail.

 **Learning Activities**

1. Have you accomplished the objectives stated at the beginning of the chapter? If not, reread the concepts you are uncertain about.
2. Using the checklist in Table 19-1, read and critique several published research studies in your discipline.

### TABLE 19-1. Checklist for Evaluating Research

| Yes or No | | Comments |
|---|---|---|
| _____ | 1. Purpose of research clearly stated | |
| _____ | 2. Need for study substantiated | |
| _____ | 3. Methods | |
| _____ |   a. Subjects described | |
| _____ |   b. Measurements described adequately for replication | |
| _____ |   c. Measures valid and reliable | |
| _____ |   d. Appropriate statistical procedures | |
| _____ | 4. Results | |
| _____ |   a. Clearly stated | |
| _____ |   b. Tables and figures aid comprehension | |
| _____ |   c. Significance levels given | |
| _____ | 5. Discussion and Conclusions | |
| _____ |   a. Results compared with other studies | |
| _____ |   b. Effect size or magnitude quantified | |
| _____ |   c. Limitations mentioned | |
| _____ |   d. Plausible speculations made | |
| _____ |   e. Conclusions based on data | |
| _____ |   f. Discussion of application sound | |
| _____ | 6. Internal Validity | |
| _____ |   a. Adequate treatment | |
| _____ |   b. Adequate sample size and power | |
| _____ |   c. If some comparisons not significant, is sample size mentioned? | |
| _____ |   d. Confounding variables | |
| _____ | 7. External Validity | |
| _____ |   a. To whom can the results of this study be applied? | |
| _____ |   b. Were subjects volunteers? | |

3. Scan a research journal in your discipline and determine whether the magnitude of the treatment effect or relationship using percent change or difference, omega squared, $r^2$, or effect size is expressed.
4. Read the Methods section of several articles and critique how well the authors justified the sample size.
5. Examine several articles in which no significant effect or relationship was reported. Do you feel that small sample size might have been a limitation? Do the authors comment on this possibility?

# Appendices

Appendix A: Statistics Tables

Appendix B: Answers to Statistics Exercises

Appendix C: Sample Consent Form and Sample Letters

# APPENDIX A

# Statistics Tables

## TABLE A-1. Critical Values of Chi Square

| df | .20 | .10 | .05 | .02 | .01 | .001 |
|----|------|------|------|------|------|------|
| 1 | 1.64 | 2.71 | 3.84 | 5.41 | 6.64 | 10.83 |
| 2 | 3.22 | 4.60 | 5.99 | 7.82 | 9.21 | 13.82 |
| 3 | 4.64 | 6.25 | 7.82 | 9.84 | 11.34 | 16.27 |
| 4 | 5.99 | 7.78 | 9.49 | 11.67 | 13.28 | 18.46 |
| 5 | 7.29 | 9.24 | 11.07 | 13.39 | 15.09 | 20.52 |
| 6 | 8.56 | 10.64 | 12.59 | 15.03 | 16.81 | 22.46 |
| 7 | 9.80 | 12.02 | 14.07 | 16.62 | 18.48 | 24.32 |
| 8 | 11.03 | 13.36 | 15.51 | 18.17 | 20.09 | 26.12 |
| 9 | 12.24 | 14.68 | 16.92 | 19.68 | 21.67 | 27.88 |
| 10 | 13.44 | 15.99 | 18.31 | 21.16 | 23.21 | 29.59 |
| 11 | 14.63 | 17.28 | 19.68 | 22.62 | 24.72 | 31.26 |
| 12 | 15.81 | 18.55 | 21.03 | 24.05 | 26.22 | 32.91 |
| 13 | 16.98 | 19.81 | 22.36 | 25.47 | 27.69 | 34.53 |
| 14 | 18.15 | 21.06 | 23.68 | 26.87 | 29.14 | 36.12 |
| 15 | 19.31 | 22.31 | 25.00 | 28.26 | 30.58 | 37.70 |
| 16 | 20.46 | 23.54 | 26.30 | 29.63 | 32.00 | 39.29 |
| 17 | 21.62 | 24.77 | 27.59 | 31.00 | 33.41 | 40.75 |
| 18 | 22.76 | 25.99 | 28.87 | 32.35 | 34.80 | 42.31 |
| 19 | 23.90 | 27.20 | 30.14 | 33.69 | 36.19 | 43.82 |
| 20 | 25.04 | 28.41 | 31.41 | 35.02 | 37.57 | 45.32 |
| 21 | 26.17 | 29.62 | 32.67 | 36.34 | 38.93 | 46.80 |
| 22 | 27.30 | 30.81 | 33.92 | 37.66 | 40.29 | 48.27 |
| 23 | 28.43 | 32.01 | 35.17 | 38.97 | 41.64 | 49.73 |
| 24 | 29.55 | 33.20 | 36.42 | 40.27 | 42.98 | 51.18 |
| 25 | 30.68 | 34.38 | 37.65 | 41.57 | 44.31 | 52.62 |
| 26 | 31.80 | 35.56 | 38.88 | 42.86 | 45.64 | 54.05 |
| 27 | 32.91 | 36.74 | 40.11 | 44.14 | 46.96 | 55.48 |
| 28 | 34.03 | 37.92 | 41.34 | 45.42 | 48.28 | 56.89 |
| 29 | 35.14 | 39.09 | 42.56 | 46.69 | 49.59 | 58.30 |
| 30 | 36.25 | 40.26 | 43.77 | 47.96 | 50.89 | 59.70 |

*Source*: Abridged from Table IV of R. A. Fisher and F. Yates: *Statistical tables for biological, agricultural, and medical research*, 6e, published by Pearson Education Ltd. UK, by permission of the authors and publishers.

### TABLE A-2. Critical Values of Spearman $r_s$ for the .05 and .01 Levels

| N | .05 | .01 | N | .05 | .01 |
|---|-----|-----|---|-----|-----|
| 6 | .886 | — | 19 | .462 | .608 |
| 7 | .786 | — | 20 | .450 | .591 |
| 8 | .738 | .881 | 21 | .438 | .576 |
| 9 | .683 | .833 | 22 | .428 | .562 |
| 10 | .648 | .818 | 23 | .418 | .549 |
| 11 | .623 | .794 | 24 | .409 | .537 |
| 12 | .591 | .780 | 25 | .400 | .526 |
| 13 | .566 | .745 | 26 | .392 | .515 |
| 14 | .545 | .716 | 27 | .385 | .505 |
| 15 | .525 | .689 | 28 | .377 | .496 |
| 16 | .507 | .666 | 29 | .370 | .487 |
| 17 | .490 | .645 | 30 | .364 | .478 |
| 18 | .476 | .625 | | | |

*Source*: Adapted from E. G. Olds, Distribution of sums of squares of rank differences for small numbers of individuals. *Annals of Mathematical Statistics 9,* 133–48 (1938), and E. G. Olds, The 5% significance levels for sums of squares of rank differences and a correction, *Annals of Mathematical Statistics 20:* 117–18 (1949). Copyright 1938 and Copyright 1949 by the Institute of Mathematical Statistics, Hayward, Calif. Permission to reprint was granted by the Institute of Mathematical Statistics.

## TABLE A-3. Critical Values of the Pearson Correlation Coefficient

| df | LEVEL OF SIGNIFICANCE FOR ONE-TAILED TEST | | | |
|---|---|---|---|---|
| | **.05** | **.025** | **.01** | **.005** |
| | LEVEL OF SIGNIFICANCE FOR TWO-TAILED TEST | | | |
| | **.10** | **.05** | **.02** | **.01** |
| 1 | .988 | .997 | .9995 | .9999 |
| 2 | .900 | .950 | .980 | .990 |
| 3 | .805 | .878 | .934 | .959 |
| 4 | .729 | .811 | .882 | .917 |
| 5 | .669 | .754 | .833 | .874 |
| 6 | .622 | .707 | .789 | .834 |
| 7 | .582 | .666 | .750 | .798 |
| 8 | .549 | .632 | .716 | .765 |
| 9 | .521 | .602 | .685 | .735 |
| 10 | .497 | .576 | .658 | .708 |
| 11 | .476 | .553 | .634 | .684 |
| 12 | .458 | .532 | .612 | .661 |
| 13 | .441 | .514 | .592 | .641 |
| 14 | .426 | .497 | .574 | .623 |
| 15 | .412 | .482 | .558 | .606 |
| 16 | .400 | .468 | .542 | .590 |
| 17 | .389 | .456 | .528 | .575 |
| 18 | .378 | .444 | .516 | .561 |
| 19 | .369 | .433 | .503 | .549 |
| 20 | .360 | .423 | .492 | .537 |
| 21 | .352 | .413 | .482 | .526 |
| 22 | .344 | .404 | .472 | .515 |
| 23 | .337 | .396 | .462 | .505 |
| 24 | .330 | .388 | .453 | .496 |
| 25 | .323 | .381 | .445 | .487 |
| 26 | .317 | .374 | .437 | .479 |
| 27 | .311 | .367 | .430 | .471 |
| 28 | .306 | .361 | .423 | .463 |
| 29 | .301 | .355 | .416 | .456 |
| 30 | .296 | .349 | .409 | .449 |
| 35 | .275 | .325 | .381 | .418 |
| 40 | .257 | .304 | .358 | .393 |
| 45 | .243 | .288 | .338 | .372 |
| 50 | .231 | .273 | .322 | .354 |
| 60 | .211 | .250 | .295 | .325 |
| 70 | .195 | .232 | .274 | .303 |
| 80 | .183 | .217 | .256 | .283 |
| 90 | .173 | .205 | .242 | .267 |
| 100 | .164 | .195 | .230 | .254 |

*Source:* Abridged from Table IV of R. A. Fisher and F. Yates: *Statistical tables for biological, agricultural, and medical research,* 6e, published by Pearson Education Ltd. UK, by permission of the authors and publishers.

## TABLE A-4. Critical Values of *t*

| df | LEVEL OF SIGNIFICANCE FOR ONE-TAILED TEST | | | | | |
|---|---|---|---|---|---|---|
| | .10 | .05 | .025 | .01 | .005 | .0005 |
| | LEVEL OF SIGNIFICANCE FOR TWO-TAILED TEST | | | | | |
| | .20 | .10 | .05 | .02 | .01 | .001 |
| 1 | 3.078 | 6.314 | 12.706 | 31.821 | 63.657 | 636.619 |
| 2 | 1.886 | 2.920 | 4.303 | 6.965 | 9.925 | 31.598 |
| 3 | 1.638 | 2.353 | 3.182 | 4.541 | 5.841 | 12.941 |
| 4 | 1.533 | 2.132 | 2.776 | 3.747 | 4.604 | 8.610 |
| 5 | 1.476 | 2.015 | 2.571 | 3.365 | 4.032 | 6.859 |
| 6 | 1.440 | 1.943 | 2.447 | 3.143 | 3.707 | 5.959 |
| 7 | 1.415 | 1.895 | 2.365 | 2.998 | 3.499 | 5.405 |
| 8 | 1.397 | 1.860 | 2.306 | 2.896 | 3.355 | 5.041 |
| 9 | 1.383 | 1.833 | 2.262 | 2.821 | 3.250 | 4.781 |
| 10 | 1.372 | 1.812 | 2.228 | 2.764 | 3.169 | 4.587 |
| 11 | 1.363 | 1.796 | 2.201 | 2.718 | 3.106 | 4.437 |
| 12 | 1.356 | 1.782 | 2.179 | 2.681 | 3.055 | 4.318 |
| 13 | 1.350 | 1.771 | 2.160 | 2.650 | 3.012 | 4.221 |
| 14 | 1.345 | 1.761 | 2.145 | 2.624 | 2.977 | 4.140 |
| 15 | 1.341 | 1.753 | 2.131 | 2.602 | 2.947 | 4.073 |
| 16 | 1.337 | 1.746 | 2.120 | 2.583 | 2.921 | 4.015 |
| 17 | 1.333 | 1.740 | 2.110 | 2.567 | 2.898 | 3.965 |
| 18 | 1.330 | 1.734 | 2.101 | 2.552 | 2.878 | 3.922 |
| 19 | 1.328 | 1.729 | 2.093 | 2.539 | 2.861 | 3.883 |
| 20 | 1.325 | 1.725 | 2.086 | 2.528 | 2.845 | 3.850 |
| 21 | 1.323 | 1.721 | 2.080 | 2.518 | 2.831 | 3.819 |
| 22 | 1.321 | 1.717 | 2.074 | 2.508 | 2.819 | 3.792 |
| 23 | 1.319 | 1.714 | 2.069 | 2.500 | 2.807 | 3.767 |
| 24 | 1.318 | 1.711 | 2.064 | 2.492 | 2.797 | 3.745 |
| 25 | 1.316 | 1.708 | 2.060 | 2.485 | 2.787 | 3.725 |
| 26 | 1.315 | 1.706 | 2.056 | 2.479 | 2.779 | 3.707 |
| 27 | 1.314 | 1.703 | 2.052 | 2.473 | 2.771 | 3.690 |
| 28 | 1.313 | 1.701 | 2.048 | 2.467 | 2.763 | 3.674 |
| 29 | 1.311 | 1.699 | 2.045 | 2.462 | 2.756 | 3.659 |
| 30 | 1.310 | 1.697 | 2.042 | 2.457 | 2.750 | 3.646 |
| 40 | 1.303 | 1.684 | 2.021 | 2.423 | 2.704 | 3.551 |
| 60 | 1.296 | 1.671 | 2.000 | 2.390 | 2.660 | 3.460 |
| 120 | 1.289 | 1.658 | 1.980 | 2.358 | 2.617 | 3.373 |
| ∞ | 1.282 | 1.645 | 1.960 | 2.326 | 2.576 | 3.291 |

*Source:* Abridged from Table IV of R. A. Fisher and F. Yates: *Statistical tables for biological, agricultural, and medical research,* 6e, published by Pearson Education Ltd. UK, by permission of the authors and publishers.

## TABLE A-5. Critical Values of F

5% (light face) and 1% (bold face) points for the distribution of F

DEGREES OF FREEDOM FOR GREATER MEAN SQUARE

| Degrees of freedom for lesser mean square | 1 | 2 | 3 | 4 | 5 | 6 | 7 | 8 | 9 | 10 | 11 | 12 | 14 | 16 | 20 | 24 | 30 | 40 | 50 | 75 | 100 | 200 | 500 | ∞ |
|---|---|---|---|---|---|---|---|---|---|---|---|---|---|---|---|---|---|---|---|---|---|---|---|---|
| 1 | 161 | 200 | 216 | 225 | 230 | 234 | 237 | 239 | 241 | 242 | 243 | 244 | 245 | 246 | 248 | 249 | 250 | 251 | 252 | 253 | 253 | 254 | 254 | 254 |
|  | **4052** | **4999** | **5403** | **5625** | **5764** | **5859** | **5928** | **5981** | **6022** | **6056** | **6082** | **6106** | **6142** | **6169** | **6208** | **6234** | **6258** | **6286** | **6302** | **6323** | **6334** | **6352** | **6361** | **6366** |
| 2 | 18.51 | 19.00 | 19.16 | 19.25 | 19.30 | 19.33 | 19.36 | 19.37 | 19.38 | 19.39 | 19.40 | 19.41 | 19.42 | 19.43 | 19.44 | 19.45 | 19.46 | 19.47 | 19.47 | 19.48 | 19.49 | 19.49 | 19.50 | 19.50 |
|  | **98.49** | **99.01** | **99.17** | **99.25** | **99.30** | **99.33** | **99.34** | **99.36** | **99.38** | **99.40** | **99.41** | **99.42** | **99.43** | **99.44** | **99.45** | **99.46** | **99.47** | **99.48** | **99.48** | **99.49** | **99.49** | **99.49** | **99.50** | **99.50** |
| 3 | 10.13 | 9.55 | 9.28 | 9.12 | 9.01 | 8.94 | 8.88 | 8.84 | 8.81 | 8.78 | 8.76 | 8.74 | 8.71 | 8.69 | 8.66 | 8.64 | 8.62 | 8.60 | 8.58 | 8.57 | 8.56 | 8.54 | 8.54 | 8.53 |
|  | **34.12** | **30.81** | **29.46** | **28.71** | **28.24** | **27.91** | **27.67** | **27.49** | **27.34** | **27.23** | **27.13** | **27.05** | **26.92** | **26.83** | **26.69** | **26.60** | **26.50** | **26.41** | **26.35** | **26.27** | **26.23** | **26.18** | **26.14** | **26.12** |
| 4 | 7.71 | 6.94 | 6.59 | 6.39 | 6.26 | 6.16 | 6.09 | 6.04 | 6.00 | 5.96 | 5.93 | 5.91 | 5.87 | 5.84 | 5.80 | 5.77 | 5.74 | 5.71 | 5.70 | 5.68 | 5.66 | 5.65 | 5.64 | 5.63 |
|  | **21.20** | **18.00** | **16.69** | **15.98** | **15.52** | **15.21** | **14.98** | **14.80** | **14.66** | **14.54** | **14.45** | **14.37** | **14.24** | **14.15** | **14.02** | **13.93** | **13.83** | **13.74** | **13.69** | **13.61** | **13.57** | **13.52** | **13.48** | **13.46** |
| 5 | 6.61 | 5.79 | 5.41 | 5.19 | 5.05 | 4.95 | 4.88 | 4.82 | 4.78 | 4.74 | 4.70 | 4.68 | 4.64 | 4.60 | 4.56 | 4.53 | 4.50 | 4.46 | 4.44 | 4.42 | 4.40 | 4.38 | 4.37 | 4.36 |
|  | **16.26** | **13.27** | **12.06** | **11.39** | **10.97** | **10.67** | **10.45** | **10.27** | **10.15** | **10.05** | **9.96** | **9.89** | **9.77** | **9.68** | **9.55** | **9.47** | **9.38** | **9.29** | **9.24** | **9.17** | **9.13** | **9.07** | **9.04** | **9.02** |
| 6 | 5.99 | 5.14 | 4.76 | 4.53 | 4.39 | 4.28 | 4.21 | 4.15 | 4.10 | 4.06 | 4.03 | 4.00 | 3.96 | 3.92 | 3.87 | 3.84 | 3.81 | 3.77 | 3.75 | 3.72 | 3.71 | 3.69 | 3.68 | 3.67 |
|  | **13.74** | **10.92** | **9.78** | **9.15** | **8.75** | **8.47** | **8.26** | **8.10** | **7.98** | **7.87** | **7.79** | **7.72** | **7.60** | **7.52** | **7.39** | **7.31** | **7.23** | **7.14** | **7.09** | **7.02** | **6.99** | **6.94** | **6.90** | **6.88** |
| 7 | 5.59 | 4.74 | 4.35 | 4.12 | 3.97 | 3.87 | 3.79 | 3.73 | 3.68 | 3.63 | 3.60 | 3.57 | 3.52 | 3.49 | 3.44 | 3.41 | 3.38 | 3.34 | 3.32 | 3.29 | 3.28 | 3.25 | 3.24 | 3.23 |
|  | **12.25** | **9.55** | **8.45** | **7.85** | **7.46** | **7.19** | **7.00** | **6.84** | **6.71** | **6.62** | **6.54** | **6.47** | **6.35** | **6.27** | **6.15** | **6.07** | **5.98** | **5.90** | **5.85** | **5.78** | **5.75** | **5.70** | **5.67** | **5.65** |
| 8 | 5.32 | 4.46 | 4.07 | 3.84 | 3.69 | 3.58 | 3.50 | 3.44 | 3.39 | 3.34 | 3.31 | 3.28 | 3.23 | 3.20 | 3.15 | 3.12 | 3.08 | 3.05 | 3.03 | 3.00 | 2.98 | 2.96 | 2.94 | 2.93 |
|  | **11.26** | **8.65** | **7.59** | **7.01** | **6.63** | **6.37** | **6.19** | **6.03** | **5.91** | **5.82** | **5.74** | **5.67** | **5.56** | **5.48** | **5.36** | **5.28** | **5.20** | **5.11** | **5.06** | **5.00** | **4.96** | **4.91** | **4.88** | **4.86** |
| 9 | 5.12 | 4.26 | 3.86 | 3.63 | 3.48 | 3.37 | 3.29 | 3.23 | 3.18 | 3.13 | 3.10 | 3.07 | 3.02 | 2.98 | 2.93 | 2.90 | 2.86 | 2.82 | 2.80 | 2.77 | 2.76 | 2.73 | 2.72 | 2.71 |
|  | **10.56** | **8.02** | **6.99** | **6.42** | **6.06** | **5.80** | **5.62** | **5.47** | **5.35** | **5.26** | **5.18** | **5.11** | **5.00** | **4.92** | **4.80** | **4.73** | **4.64** | **4.56** | **4.51** | **4.45** | **4.41** | **4.36** | **4.33** | **4.31** |
| 10 | 4.96 | 4.10 | 3.71 | 3.48 | 3.33 | 3.22 | 3.14 | 3.07 | 3.02 | 2.97 | 2.94 | 2.91 | 2.86 | 2.82 | 2.77 | 2.74 | 2.70 | 2.67 | 2.64 | 2.61 | 2.59 | 2.56 | 2.55 | 2.54 |
|  | **10.04** | **7.56** | **6.55** | **5.99** | **5.64** | **5.39** | **5.21** | **5.06** | **4.95** | **4.85** | **4.78** | **4.71** | **4.60** | **4.52** | **4.41** | **4.33** | **4.25** | **4.17** | **4.12** | **4.05** | **4.01** | **3.96** | **3.93** | **3.91** |
| 11 | 4.84 | 3.98 | 3.59 | 3.36 | 3.20 | 3.09 | 3.01 | 2.95 | 2.90 | 2.86 | 2.82 | 2.79 | 2.74 | 2.70 | 2.65 | 2.61 | 2.57 | 2.53 | 2.50 | 2.47 | 2.45 | 2.42 | 2.41 | 2.40 |
|  | **9.65** | **7.20** | **6.22** | **5.67** | **5.32** | **5.07** | **4.88** | **4.74** | **4.63** | **4.54** | **4.46** | **4.40** | **4.29** | **4.21** | **4.10** | **4.02** | **3.94** | **3.86** | **3.80** | **3.74** | **3.70** | **3.66** | **3.62** | **3.60** |
| 12 | 4.75 | 3.88 | 3.49 | 3.26 | 3.11 | 3.00 | 2.92 | 2.85 | 2.80 | 2.76 | 2.72 | 2.69 | 2.64 | 2.60 | 2.54 | 2.50 | 2.46 | 2.42 | 2.40 | 2.36 | 2.35 | 2.32 | 2.31 | 2.30 |
|  | **9.33** | **6.93** | **5.95** | **5.41** | **5.06** | **4.82** | **4.65** | **4.50** | **4.39** | **4.30** | **4.22** | **4.16** | **4.05** | **3.98** | **3.86** | **3.78** | **3.70** | **3.61** | **3.56** | **3.49** | **3.46** | **3.41** | **3.38** | **3.36** |
| 13 | 4.67 | 3.80 | 3.41 | 3.18 | 3.02 | 2.92 | 2.84 | 2.77 | 2.72 | 2.67 | 2.63 | 2.60 | 2.55 | 2.51 | 2.46 | 2.42 | 2.38 | 2.34 | 2.32 | 2.28 | 2.26 | 2.24 | 2.22 | 2.21 |
|  | **9.07** | **6.70** | **5.74** | **5.20** | **4.86** | **4.62** | **4.44** | **4.30** | **4.19** | **4.10** | **4.02** | **3.96** | **3.85** | **3.78** | **3.67** | **3.59** | **3.51** | **3.42** | **3.37** | **3.30** | **3.27** | **3.21** | **3.18** | **3.16** |
| 14 | 4.60 | 3.74 | 3.34 | 3.11 | 2.96 | 2.85 | 2.77 | 2.70 | 2.65 | 2.60 | 2.56 | 2.53 | 2.48 | 2.44 | 2.39 | 2.35 | 2.31 | 2.27 | 2.24 | 2.21 | 2.19 | 2.16 | 2.14 | 2.13 |
|  | **8.86** | **6.51** | **5.56** | **5.03** | **4.69** | **4.46** | **4.28** | **4.14** | **4.03** | **3.94** | **3.86** | **3.80** | **3.70** | **3.62** | **3.51** | **3.43** | **3.34** | **3.26** | **3.21** | **3.14** | **3.11** | **3.06** | **3.02** | **3.00** |
| 15 | 4.54 | 3.68 | 3.29 | 3.06 | 2.90 | 2.79 | 2.70 | 2.64 | 2.59 | 2.55 | 2.51 | 2.48 | 2.43 | 2.39 | 2.33 | 2.29 | 2.25 | 2.21 | 2.18 | 2.15 | 2.12 | 2.10 | 2.08 | 2.07 |
|  | **8.68** | **6.36** | **5.42** | **4.89** | **4.56** | **4.32** | **4.14** | **4.00** | **3.89** | **3.80** | **3.73** | **3.67** | **3.56** | **3.48** | **3.36** | **3.29** | **3.20** | **3.12** | **3.07** | **3.00** | **2.97** | **2.92** | **2.89** | **2.87** |
| 16 | 4.49 | 3.63 | 3.24 | 3.01 | 2.85 | 2.74 | 2.66 | 2.59 | 2.54 | 2.49 | 2.45 | 2.42 | 2.37 | 2.33 | 2.28 | 2.24 | 2.20 | 2.16 | 2.13 | 2.09 | 2.07 | 2.04 | 2.02 | 2.01 |
|  | **8.53** | **6.23** | **5.29** | **4.77** | **4.44** | **4.20** | **4.03** | **3.89** | **3.78** | **3.69** | **3.61** | **3.55** | **3.45** | **3.37** | **3.25** | **3.18** | **3.10** | **3.01** | **2.96** | **2.89** | **2.86** | **2.80** | **2.77** | **2.75** |
| 17 | 4.45 | 3.59 | 3.20 | 2.96 | 2.81 | 2.70 | 2.62 | 2.55 | 2.50 | 2.45 | 2.41 | 2.38 | 2.33 | 2.29 | 2.23 | 2.19 | 2.15 | 2.11 | 2.08 | 2.04 | 2.02 | 1.99 | 1.97 | 1.96 |
|  | **8.40** | **6.11** | **5.18** | **4.67** | **4.34** | **4.10** | **3.93** | **3.79** | **3.68** | **3.59** | **3.52** | **3.45** | **3.35** | **3.27** | **3.16** | **3.08** | **3.00** | **2.92** | **2.86** | **2.79** | **2.76** | **2.70** | **2.67** | **2.65** |

(continued)

## TABLE A-5. (continued)

**5% (light face) and 1% (bold face) points for the distribution of F**

**DEGREES OF FREEDOM FOR GREATER MEAN SQUARE**

| Degrees of freedom for lesser mean square | 1 | 2 | 3 | 4 | 5 | 6 | 7 | 8 | 9 | 10 | 11 | 12 | 14 | 16 | 20 | 24 | 30 | 40 | 50 | 75 | 100 | 200 | 500 | ∞ |
|---|---|---|---|---|---|---|---|---|---|---|---|---|---|---|---|---|---|---|---|---|---|---|---|---|
| 18 | 4.41 | 3.55 | 3.16 | 2.93 | 2.77 | 2.66 | 2.58 | 2.51 | 2.46 | 2.41 | 2.37 | 2.34 | 2.29 | 2.25 | 2.19 | 2.15 | 2.11 | 2.07 | 2.04 | 2.00 | 1.98 | 1.95 | 1.93 | 1.92 |
|  | **8.28** | **6.01** | **5.09** | **4.58** | **4.25** | **4.01** | **3.85** | **3.71** | **3.60** | **3.51** | **3.44** | **3.37** | **3.27** | **3.19** | **3.07** | **3.00** | **2.91** | **2.83** | **2.78** | **2.71** | **2.68** | **2.62** | **2.59** | **2.57** |
| 19 | 4.38 | 3.52 | 3.13 | 2.90 | 2.74 | 2.63 | 2.55 | 2.48 | 2.43 | 2.38 | 2.34 | 2.31 | 2.26 | 2.21 | 2.15 | 2.11 | 2.07 | 2.02 | 2.00 | 1.96 | 1.94 | 1.91 | 1.90 | 1.88 |
|  | **8.18** | **5.93** | **5.01** | **4.50** | **4.17** | **3.94** | **3.77** | **3.63** | **3.52** | **3.43** | **3.36** | **3.30** | **3.19** | **3.12** | **3.00** | **2.92** | **2.84** | **2.76** | **2.70** | **2.63** | **2.60** | **2.54** | **2.51** | **2.49** |
| 20 | 4.35 | 3.49 | 3.10 | 2.87 | 2.71 | 2.60 | 2.52 | 2.45 | 2.40 | 2.35 | 2.31 | 2.28 | 2.23 | 2.18 | 2.12 | 2.08 | 2.04 | 1.99 | 1.96 | 1.92 | 1.90 | 1.87 | 1.85 | 1.84 |
|  | **8.10** | **5.85** | **4.94** | **4.43** | **4.10** | **3.87** | **3.71** | **3.56** | **3.45** | **3.37** | **3.30** | **3.23** | **3.13** | **3.05** | **2.94** | **2.86** | **2.77** | **2.69** | **2.63** | **2.56** | **2.53** | **2.47** | **2.44** | **2.42** |
| 21 | 4.32 | 3.47 | 3.07 | 2.84 | 2.68 | 2.57 | 2.49 | 2.42 | 2.37 | 2.32 | 2.28 | 2.25 | 2.20 | 2.15 | 2.09 | 2.05 | 2.00 | 1.96 | 1.93 | 1.89 | 1.87 | 1.84 | 1.82 | 1.81 |
|  | **8.02** | **5.78** | **4.87** | **4.37** | **4.04** | **3.81** | **3.65** | **3.51** | **3.40** | **3.31** | **3.24** | **3.17** | **3.07** | **2.99** | **2.88** | **2.80** | **2.72** | **2.63** | **2.58** | **2.51** | **2.47** | **2.42** | **2.38** | **2.36** |
| 22 | 4.30 | 3.44 | 3.05 | 2.82 | 2.66 | 2.55 | 2.47 | 2.40 | 2.35 | 2.30 | 2.26 | 2.23 | 2.18 | 2.13 | 2.07 | 2.03 | 1.98 | 1.93 | 1.91 | 1.87 | 1.84 | 1.81 | 1.80 | 1.78 |
|  | **7.94** | **5.72** | **4.82** | **4.31** | **3.99** | **3.76** | **3.59** | **3.45** | **3.35** | **3.26** | **3.18** | **3.12** | **3.02** | **2.94** | **2.83** | **2.75** | **2.67** | **2.58** | **2.53** | **2.46** | **2.42** | **2.37** | **2.33** | **2.31** |
| 23 | 4.28 | 3.42 | 3.03 | 2.80 | 2.64 | 2.53 | 2.45 | 2.38 | 2.32 | 2.28 | 2.24 | 2.20 | 2.14 | 2.10 | 2.04 | 2.00 | 1.96 | 1.91 | 1.88 | 1.84 | 1.82 | 1.79 | 1.77 | 1.76 |
|  | **7.88** | **5.66** | **4.76** | **4.26** | **3.94** | **3.71** | **3.54** | **3.41** | **3.30** | **3.21** | **3.14** | **3.07** | **2.97** | **2.89** | **2.78** | **2.70** | **2.62** | **2.53** | **2.48** | **2.41** | **2.37** | **2.32** | **2.28** | **2.26** |
| 24 | 4.26 | 3.40 | 3.01 | 2.78 | 2.62 | 2.51 | 2.43 | 2.36 | 2.30 | 2.26 | 2.22 | 2.18 | 2.13 | 2.09 | 2.02 | 1.98 | 1.94 | 1.89 | 1.86 | 1.82 | 1.80 | 1.76 | 1.74 | 1.73 |
|  | **7.82** | **5.61** | **4.72** | **4.22** | **3.90** | **3.67** | **3.50** | **3.36** | **3.25** | **3.17** | **3.09** | **3.03** | **2.93** | **2.85** | **2.74** | **2.66** | **2.58** | **2.49** | **2.44** | **2.36** | **2.33** | **2.27** | **2.23** | **2.21** |
| 25 | 4.24 | 3.38 | 2.99 | 2.76 | 2.60 | 2.49 | 2.41 | 2.34 | 2.28 | 2.24 | 2.20 | 2.16 | 2.11 | 2.06 | 2.00 | 1.96 | 1.92 | 1.87 | 1.84 | 1.80 | 1.77 | 1.74 | 1.72 | 1.71 |
|  | **7.77** | **5.57** | **4.68** | **4.18** | **3.86** | **3.63** | **3.46** | **3.32** | **3.21** | **3.13** | **3.05** | **2.99** | **2.89** | **2.81** | **2.70** | **2.62** | **2.54** | **2.45** | **2.40** | **2.32** | **2.29** | **2.23** | **2.19** | **2.17** |
| 26 | 4.22 | 3.37 | 2.98 | 2.74 | 2.59 | 2.47 | 2.39 | 2.32 | 2.27 | 2.22 | 2.18 | 2.15 | 2.10 | 2.05 | 1.99 | 1.95 | 1.90 | 1.85 | 1.82 | 1.78 | 1.76 | 1.72 | 1.70 | 1.69 |
|  | **7.72** | **5.53** | **4.64** | **4.14** | **3.82** | **3.59** | **3.42** | **3.29** | **3.17** | **3.09** | **3.02** | **2.96** | **2.86** | **2.77** | **2.66** | **2.58** | **2.50** | **2.41** | **2.36** | **2.28** | **2.25** | **2.19** | **2.15** | **2.13** |
| 27 | 4.21 | 3.35 | 2.96 | 2.73 | 2.57 | 2.46 | 2.37 | 2.30 | 2.25 | 2.20 | 2.16 | 2.13 | 2.08 | 2.03 | 1.97 | 1.93 | 1.88 | 1.84 | 1.80 | 1.76 | 1.74 | 1.71 | 1.68 | 1.67 |
|  | **7.68** | **5.49** | **4.60** | **4.11** | **3.79** | **3.56** | **3.39** | **3.26** | **3.14** | **3.06** | **2.98** | **2.93** | **2.83** | **2.74** | **2.63** | **2.55** | **2.47** | **2.38** | **2.33** | **2.25** | **2.21** | **2.16** | **2.12** | **2.10** |
| 28 | 4.20 | 3.34 | 2.95 | 2.71 | 2.56 | 2.44 | 2.36 | 2.29 | 2.24 | 2.19 | 2.15 | 2.12 | 2.06 | 2.02 | 1.96 | 1.91 | 1.87 | 1.81 | 1.78 | 1.75 | 1.72 | 1.69 | 1.67 | 1.65 |
|  | **7.64** | **5.45** | **4.57** | **4.07** | **3.76** | **3.53** | **3.36** | **3.23** | **3.11** | **3.03** | **2.95** | **2.90** | **2.80** | **2.71** | **2.60** | **2.52** | **2.44** | **2.35** | **2.30** | **2.22** | **2.18** | **2.13** | **2.09** | **2.06** |
| 29 | 4.18 | 3.33 | 2.93 | 2.70 | 2.54 | 2.43 | 2.35 | 2.28 | 2.22 | 2.18 | 2.14 | 2.10 | 2.05 | 2.00 | 1.94 | 1.90 | 1.85 | 1.80 | 1.77 | 1.73 | 1.71 | 1.68 | 1.65 | 1.64 |
|  | **7.60** | **5.42** | **4.54** | **4.04** | **3.73** | **3.50** | **3.33** | **3.20** | **3.08** | **3.00** | **2.92** | **2.87** | **2.77** | **2.68** | **2.57** | **2.49** | **2.41** | **2.32** | **2.27** | **2.19** | **2.15** | **2.10** | **2.06** | **2.03** |
| 30 | 4.17 | 3.32 | 2.92 | 2.69 | 2.53 | 2.42 | 2.34 | 2.27 | 2.21 | 2.16 | 2.12 | 2.09 | 2.04 | 1.99 | 1.93 | 1.89 | 1.84 | 1.79 | 1.76 | 1.72 | 1.69 | 1.66 | 1.64 | 1.62 |
|  | **7.56** | **5.39** | **4.51** | **4.02** | **3.70** | **3.47** | **3.30** | **3.17** | **3.06** | **2.98** | **2.90** | **2.84** | **2.74** | **2.66** | **2.55** | **2.47** | **2.38** | **2.29** | **2.24** | **2.16** | **2.13** | **2.07** | **2.03** | **2.01** |
| 32 | 4.15 | 3.30 | 2.90 | 2.67 | 2.51 | 2.40 | 2.32 | 2.25 | 2.19 | 2.14 | 2.10 | 2.07 | 2.02 | 1.97 | 1.91 | 1.86 | 1.82 | 1.76 | 1.74 | 1.69 | 1.67 | 1.64 | 1.61 | 1.59 |
|  | **7.50** | **5.34** | **4.46** | **3.97** | **3.66** | **3.42** | **3.25** | **3.12** | **3.01** | **2.94** | **2.86** | **2.80** | **2.70** | **2.62** | **2.51** | **2.42** | **2.34** | **2.25** | **2.20** | **2.12** | **2.08** | **2.02** | **1.98** | **1.96** |
| 34 | 4.13 | 3.28 | 2.88 | 2.65 | 2.49 | 2.38 | 2.30 | 2.23 | 2.17 | 2.12 | 2.08 | 2.05 | 2.00 | 1.95 | 1.89 | 1.84 | 1.80 | 1.74 | 1.71 | 1.67 | 1.64 | 1.61 | 1.59 | 1.57 |
|  | **7.44** | **5.29** | **4.42** | **3.93** | **3.61** | **3.38** | **3.21** | **3.08** | **2.97** | **2.89** | **2.82** | **2.76** | **2.66** | **2.58** | **2.47** | **2.38** | **2.30** | **2.21** | **2.15** | **2.08** | **2.04** | **1.98** | **1.94** | **1.91** |
| 36 | 4.11 | 3.26 | 2.86 | 2.63 | 2.48 | 2.36 | 2.28 | 2.21 | 2.15 | 2.10 | 2.06 | 2.03 | 1.98 | 1.93 | 1.87 | 1.82 | 1.78 | 1.72 | 1.69 | 1.65 | 1.62 | 1.59 | 1.56 | 1.55 |
|  | **7.39** | **5.25** | **4.38** | **3.89** | **3.58** | **3.35** | **3.18** | **3.04** | **2.94** | **2.86** | **2.78** | **2.72** | **2.62** | **2.54** | **2.43** | **2.35** | **2.26** | **2.17** | **2.12** | **2.04** | **2.00** | **1.94** | **1.90** | **1.87** |
| 38 | 4.10 | 3.25 | 2.85 | 2.62 | 2.46 | 2.35 | 2.26 | 2.19 | 2.14 | 2.09 | 2.05 | 2.02 | 1.96 | 1.92 | 1.85 | 1.80 | 1.76 | 1.71 | 1.67 | 1.63 | 1.60 | 1.57 | 1.54 | 1.53 |
|  | **7.35** | **5.21** | **4.34** | **3.86** | **3.54** | **3.32** | **3.15** | **3.02** | **2.91** | **2.82** | **2.75** | **2.69** | **2.59** | **2.51** | **2.40** | **2.32** | **2.22** | **2.14** | **2.08** | **2.00** | **1.97** | **1.90** | **1.86** | **1.84** |

| df | | | | | | | | | | | | | | | | | | | | | | | | |
|---|---|---|---|---|---|---|---|---|---|---|---|---|---|---|---|---|---|---|---|---|---|---|---|---|
| 40 | 4.08 | 3.23 | 2.84 | 2.61 | 2.45 | 2.34 | 2.25 | 2.18 | 2.12 | 2.07 | 2.04 | 2.00 | 1.95 | 1.90 | 1.84 | 1.79 | 1.74 | 1.69 | 1.66 | 1.61 | 1.59 | 1.55 | 1.53 | 1.51 |
|  | **7.31** | **5.18** | **4.31** | **3.83** | **3.51** | **3.29** | **3.12** | **2.99** | **2.88** | **2.80** | **2.73** | **2.66** | **2.56** | **2.49** | **2.37** | **2.29** | **2.20** | **2.11** | **2.05** | **1.97** | **1.94** | **1.88** | **1.84** | **1.81** |
| 42 | 4.07 | 3.22 | 2.83 | 2.59 | 2.44 | 2.32 | 2.24 | 2.17 | 2.11 | 2.06 | 2.02 | 1.99 | 1.94 | 1.89 | 1.82 | 1.78 | 1.73 | 1.68 | 1.64 | 1.60 | 1.57 | 1.54 | 1.51 | 1.49 |
|  | **7.27** | **5.15** | **4.29** | **3.80** | **3.49** | **3.26** | **3.10** | **2.96** | **2.86** | **2.77** | **2.70** | **2.64** | **2.54** | **2.46** | **2.35** | **2.26** | **2.17** | **2.08** | **2.02** | **1.94** | **1.91** | **1.85** | **1.80** | **1.78** |
| 44 | 4.06 | 3.21 | 2.82 | 2.58 | 2.43 | 2.31 | 2.23 | 2.16 | 2.10 | 2.05 | 2.01 | 1.98 | 1.92 | 1.88 | 1.81 | 1.76 | 1.72 | 1.66 | 1.63 | 1.58 | 1.56 | 1.52 | 1.50 | 1.48 |
|  | **7.24** | **5.12** | **4.26** | **3.78** | **3.46** | **3.24** | **3.07** | **2.94** | **2.84** | **2.75** | **2.68** | **2.62** | **2.52** | **2.44** | **2.32** | **2.24** | **2.15** | **2.06** | **2.00** | **1.92** | **1.88** | **1.82** | **1.78** | **1.75** |
| 46 | 4.05 | 3.20 | 2.81 | 2.57 | 2.42 | 2.30 | 2.22 | 2.14 | 2.09 | 2.04 | 2.00 | 1.97 | 1.91 | 1.87 | 1.80 | 1.75 | 1.71 | 1.65 | 1.62 | 1.57 | 1.54 | 1.51 | 1.48 | 1.46 |
|  | **7.21** | **5.10** | **4.24** | **3.76** | **3.44** | **3.22** | **3.05** | **2.92** | **2.82** | **2.73** | **2.66** | **2.60** | **2.50** | **2.42** | **2.30** | **2.22** | **2.13** | **2.04** | **1.98** | **1.90** | **1.86** | **1.80** | **1.76** | **1.72** |
| 48 | 4.04 | 3.19 | 2.80 | 2.56 | 2.41 | 2.30 | 2.21 | 2.14 | 2.08 | 2.03 | 1.99 | 1.96 | 1.90 | 1.86 | 1.79 | 1.74 | 1.70 | 1.64 | 1.61 | 1.56 | 1.53 | 1.50 | 1.47 | 1.45 |
|  | **7.19** | **5.08** | **4.22** | **3.74** | **3.42** | **3.20** | **3.04** | **2.90** | **2.80** | **2.71** | **2.64** | **2.58** | **2.48** | **2.40** | **2.28** | **2.20** | **2.11** | **2.02** | **1.96** | **1.88** | **1.84** | **1.78** | **1.73** | **1.70** |
| 50 | 4.03 | 3.18 | 2.79 | 2.56 | 2.40 | 2.29 | 2.20 | 2.13 | 2.07 | 2.02 | 1.98 | 1.95 | 1.90 | 1.85 | 1.78 | 1.74 | 1.69 | 1.63 | 1.60 | 1.55 | 1.52 | 1.48 | 1.46 | 1.44 |
|  | **7.17** | **5.06** | **4.20** | **3.72** | **3.41** | **3.18** | **3.02** | **2.88** | **2.78** | **2.70** | **2.62** | **2.56** | **2.46** | **2.39** | **2.26** | **2.18** | **2.10** | **2.00** | **1.94** | **1.86** | **1.82** | **1.76** | **1.71** | **1.68** |
| 55 | 4.02 | 3.17 | 2.78 | 2.54 | 2.38 | 2.27 | 2.18 | 2.11 | 2.05 | 2.00 | 1.97 | 1.93 | 1.88 | 1.83 | 1.76 | 1.72 | 1.67 | 1.61 | 1.58 | 1.52 | 1.50 | 1.46 | 1.43 | 1.41 |
|  | **7.12** | **5.01** | **4.16** | **3.68** | **3.37** | **3.15** | **2.98** | **2.85** | **2.75** | **2.66** | **2.59** | **2.53** | **2.43** | **2.35** | **2.23** | **2.15** | **2.06** | **1.96** | **1.90** | **1.82** | **1.78** | **1.71** | **1.66** | **1.64** |
| 60 | 4.00 | 3.15 | 2.76 | 2.52 | 2.37 | 2.25 | 2.17 | 2.10 | 2.04 | 1.99 | 1.95 | 1.92 | 1.86 | 1.81 | 1.75 | 1.70 | 1.65 | 1.59 | 1.56 | 1.50 | 1.48 | 1.44 | 1.41 | 1.39 |
|  | **7.08** | **4.98** | **4.13** | **3.65** | **3.34** | **3.12** | **2.95** | **2.82** | **2.72** | **2.63** | **2.56** | **2.50** | **2.40** | **2.32** | **2.20** | **2.12** | **2.03** | **1.93** | **1.87** | **1.79** | **1.74** | **1.68** | **1.63** | **1.60** |
| 65 | 3.99 | 3.14 | 2.75 | 2.51 | 2.36 | 2.24 | 2.15 | 2.08 | 2.02 | 1.98 | 1.94 | 1.90 | 1.85 | 1.80 | 1.73 | 1.68 | 1.63 | 1.57 | 1.54 | 1.49 | 1.46 | 1.42 | 1.39 | 1.37 |
|  | **7.04** | **4.95** | **4.10** | **3.62** | **3.31** | **3.09** | **2.93** | **2.79** | **2.70** | **2.61** | **2.54** | **2.47** | **2.37** | **2.30** | **2.18** | **2.09** | **2.00** | **1.90** | **1.84** | **1.76** | **1.71** | **1.64** | **1.60** | **1.56** |
| 70 | 3.98 | 3.13 | 2.74 | 2.50 | 2.35 | 2.23 | 2.14 | 2.07 | 2.01 | 1.97 | 1.93 | 1.89 | 1.84 | 1.79 | 1.72 | 1.67 | 1.62 | 1.56 | 1.53 | 1.47 | 1.45 | 1.40 | 1.37 | 1.35 |
|  | **7.01** | **4.92** | **4.08** | **3.60** | **3.29** | **3.07** | **2.91** | **2.77** | **2.67** | **2.59** | **2.51** | **2.45** | **2.35** | **2.28** | **2.15** | **2.07** | **1.98** | **1.88** | **1.82** | **1.74** | **1.69** | **1.62** | **1.56** | **1.53** |
| 80 | 3.96 | 3.11 | 2.72 | 2.48 | 2.33 | 2.21 | 2.12 | 2.05 | 1.99 | 1.95 | 1.91 | 1.88 | 1.82 | 1.77 | 1.70 | 1.65 | 1.60 | 1.54 | 1.51 | 1.45 | 1.42 | 1.38 | 1.35 | 1.32 |
|  | **6.96** | **4.88** | **4.04** | **3.56** | **3.25** | **3.04** | **2.87** | **2.74** | **2.64** | **2.55** | **2.48** | **2.41** | **2.32** | **2.24** | **2.11** | **2.03** | **1.94** | **1.84** | **1.78** | **1.70** | **1.65** | **1.57** | **1.52** | **1.49** |
| 100 | 3.94 | 3.09 | 2.70 | 2.46 | 2.30 | 2.19 | 2.10 | 2.03 | 1.97 | 1.92 | 1.88 | 1.85 | 1.79 | 1.75 | 1.68 | 1.63 | 1.57 | 1.51 | 1.48 | 1.42 | 1.39 | 1.34 | 1.30 | 1.28 |
|  | **6.90** | **4.82** | **3.98** | **3.51** | **3.20** | **2.99** | **2.82** | **2.69** | **2.59** | **2.51** | **2.43** | **2.36** | **2.26** | **2.19** | **2.06** | **1.98** | **1.89** | **1.79** | **1.73** | **1.64** | **1.59** | **1.51** | **1.46** | **1.43** |
| 125 | 3.92 | 3.07 | 2.68 | 2.44 | 2.29 | 2.17 | 2.08 | 2.01 | 1.95 | 1.90 | 1.86 | 1.83 | 1.77 | 1.72 | 1.65 | 1.60 | 1.55 | 1.49 | 1.45 | 1.39 | 1.36 | 1.31 | 1.27 | 1.25 |
|  | **6.84** | **4.78** | **3.94** | **3.47** | **3.17** | **2.95** | **2.79** | **2.65** | **2.56** | **2.47** | **2.40** | **2.33** | **2.23** | **2.15** | **2.03** | **1.94** | **1.85** | **1.75** | **1.68** | **1.59** | **1.54** | **1.46** | **1.40** | **1.37** |
| 150 | 3.91 | 3.06 | 2.67 | 2.43 | 2.27 | 2.16 | 2.07 | 2.00 | 1.94 | 1.89 | 1.85 | 1.82 | 1.76 | 1.71 | 1.64 | 1.59 | 1.54 | 1.47 | 1.44 | 1.37 | 1.34 | 1.29 | 1.25 | 1.22 |
|  | **6.81** | **4.75** | **3.91** | **3.44** | **3.14** | **2.92** | **2.76** | **2.62** | **2.53** | **2.44** | **2.37** | **2.30** | **2.20** | **2.12** | **2.00** | **1.91** | **1.83** | **1.72** | **1.66** | **1.56** | **1.51** | **1.43** | **1.37** | **1.33** |
| 200 | 3.89 | 3.04 | 2.65 | 2.41 | 2.26 | 2.14 | 2.05 | 1.98 | 1.92 | 1.87 | 1.83 | 1.80 | 1.74 | 1.69 | 1.62 | 1.57 | 1.52 | 1.45 | 1.42 | 1.35 | 1.32 | 1.26 | 1.22 | 1.19 |
|  | **6.76** | **4.71** | **3.88** | **3.41** | **3.11** | **2.90** | **2.73** | **2.60** | **2.50** | **2.41** | **2.34** | **2.28** | **2.17** | **2.09** | **1.97** | **1.88** | **1.79** | **1.69** | **1.62** | **1.53** | **1.48** | **1.39** | **1.33** | **1.28** |
| 400 | 3.86 | 3.02 | 2.62 | 2.39 | 2.23 | 2.12 | 2.03 | 1.96 | 1.90 | 1.85 | 1.81 | 1.78 | 1.72 | 1.67 | 1.60 | 1.54 | 1.49 | 1.42 | 1.38 | 1.32 | 1.28 | 1.22 | 1.16 | 1.13 |
|  | **6.70** | **4.66** | **3.83** | **3.36** | **3.06** | **2.85** | **2.69** | **2.55** | **2.46** | **2.37** | **2.29** | **2.23** | **2.12** | **2.04** | **1.92** | **1.84** | **1.74** | **1.64** | **1.57** | **1.47** | **1.42** | **1.32** | **1.24** | **1.19** |
| 1000 | 3.85 | 3.00 | 2.61 | 2.38 | 2.22 | 2.10 | 2.02 | 1.95 | 1.89 | 1.84 | 1.80 | 1.76 | 1.70 | 1.65 | 1.58 | 1.53 | 1.47 | 1.41 | 1.36 | 1.30 | 1.26 | 1.19 | 1.13 | 1.08 |
|  | **6.66** | **4.62** | **3.80** | **3.34** | **3.04** | **2.82** | **2.66** | **2.53** | **2.43** | **2.34** | **2.26** | **2.20** | **2.09** | **2.01** | **1.89** | **1.81** | **1.71** | **1.61** | **1.54** | **1.44** | **1.38** | **1.28** | **1.19** | **1.11** |
| ∞ | 3.84 | 2.99 | 2.60 | 2.37 | 2.21 | 2.09 | 2.01 | 1.94 | 1.88 | 1.83 | 1.79 | 1.75 | 1.69 | 1.64 | 1.57 | 1.52 | 1.46 | 1.40 | 1.35 | 1.28 | 1.24 | 1.17 | 1.11 | 1.00 |
|  | **6.64** | **4.60** | **3.78** | **3.32** | **3.02** | **2.80** | **2.64** | **2.51** | **2.41** | **2.32** | **2.24** | **2.18** | **2.07** | **1.99** | **1.87** | **1.79** | **1.69** | **1.59** | **1.52** | **1.41** | **1.36** | **1.25** | **1.15** | **1.00** |

Reprinted, by permission, from G. W. Snedecor, *Statistical methods*, 5th ed. pp. 246–249, Blackwell Publishing (formerly Iowa State College Press), Ames, Iowa, 1956.

### TABLE A-6. Area of the Normal Curve Between the M and z

| z | Area from Mean to z | z | Area from Mean to z | z | Area from Mean to z |
|---|---|---|---|---|---|
| 0.00 | .0000 | 0.42 | .1628 | 0.84 | .2995 |
| 0.01 | .0040 | 0.43 | .1664 | 0.85 | .3023 |
| 0.02 | .0080 | 0.44 | .1700 | 0.86 | .3051 |
| 0.03 | .0120 | 0.45 | .1736 | 0.87 | .3078 |
| 0.04 | .0160 | 0.46 | .1772 | 0.88 | .3106 |
| 0.05 | .0199 | 0.47 | .1808 | 0.89 | .3133 |
| 0.06 | .0239 | 0.48 | .1844 | 0.90 | .3159 |
| 0.07 | .0279 | 0.49 | .1879 | 0.91 | .3186 |
| 0.08 | .0319 | 0.50 | .1915 | 0.92 | .3212 |
| 0.09 | .0359 | 0.51 | .1950 | 0.93 | .3238 |
| 0.10 | .0398 | 0.52 | .1985 | 0.94 | .3264 |
| 0.11 | .0438 | 0.53 | .2019 | 0.95 | .3289 |
| 0.12 | .0478 | 0.54 | .2054 | 0.96 | .3315 |
| 0.13 | .0517 | 0.55 | .2088 | 0.97 | .3340 |
| 0.14 | .0557 | 0.56 | .2123 | 0.98 | .3365 |
| 0.15 | .0596 | 0.57 | .2157 | 0.99 | .3389 |
| 0.16 | .0636 | 0.58 | .2190 | 1.00 | .3413 |
| 0.17 | .0675 | 0.59 | .2224 | 1.01 | .3438 |
| 0.18 | .0714 | 0.60 | .2257 | 1.02 | .3461 |
| 0.19 | .0753 | 0.61 | .2291 | 1.03 | .3485 |
| 0.20 | .0793 | 0.62 | .2324 | 1.04 | .3508 |
| 0.21 | .0832 | 0.63 | .2357 | 1.05 | .3531 |
| 0.22 | .0871 | 0.64 | .2389 | 1.06 | .3554 |
| 0.23 | .0910 | 0.65 | .2422 | 1.07 | .3577 |
| 0.24 | .0948 | 0.66 | .2454 | 1.08 | .3599 |
| 0.25 | .0987 | 0.67 | .2486 | 1.09 | .3621 |
| 0.26 | .1026 | 0.68 | .2517 | 1.10 | .3643 |
| 0.27 | .1064 | 0.69 | .2549 | 1.11 | .3665 |
| 0.28 | .1103 | 0.70 | .2580 | 1.12 | .3686 |
| 0.29 | .1141 | 0.71 | .2611 | 1.13 | .3708 |
| 0.30 | .1179 | 0.72 | .2642 | 1.14 | .3729 |
| 0.31 | .1217 | 0.73 | .2673 | 1.15 | .3749 |
| 0.32 | .1255 | 0.74 | .2704 | 1.16 | .3770 |
| 0.33 | .1293 | 0.75 | .2734 | 1.17 | .3790 |
| 0.34 | .1331 | 0.76 | .2764 | 1.18 | .3810 |
| 0.35 | .1368 | 0.77 | .2794 | 1.19 | .3830 |
| 0.36 | .1406 | 0.78 | .2823 | 1.20 | .3849 |
| 0.37 | .1443 | 0.79 | .2852 | 1.21 | .3869 |
| 0.38 | .1480 | 0.80 | .2881 | 1.22 | .3888 |
| 0.39 | .1517 | 0.81 | .2910 | 1.23 | .3907 |
| 0.40 | .1554 | 0.82 | .2939 | 1.24 | .3925 |
| 0.41 | .1591 | 0.83 | .2967 | 1.25 | .3944 |

(continued)

### TABLE A-6. (*continued*)

| z | Area from Mean to z | z | Area from Mean to z | z | Area from Mean to z |
|---|---|---|---|---|---|
| 1.26 | .3962 | 1.68 | .4535 | 2.10 | .4821 |
| 1.27 | .3980 | 1.69 | .4545 | 2.11 | .4826 |
| 1.28 | .3997 | 1.70 | .4554 | 2.12 | .4830 |
| 1.29 | .4015 | 1.71 | .4564 | 2.13 | .4834 |
| 1.30 | .4032 | 1.72 | .4573 | 2.14 | .4838 |
| 1.31 | .4049 | 1.73 | .4582 | 2.15 | .4842 |
| 1.32 | .4066 | 1.74 | .4591 | 2.16 | .4846 |
| 1.33 | .4082 | 1.75 | .4599 | 2.17 | .4850 |
| 1.34 | .4099 | 1.76 | .4608 | 2.18 | .4854 |
| 1.35 | .4115 | 1.77 | .4616 | 2.19 | .4857 |
| 1.36 | .4131 | 1.78 | .4625 | 2.20 | .4861 |
| 1.37 | .4147 | 1.79 | .4633 | 2.21 | .4864 |
| 1.38 | .4162 | 1.80 | .4641 | 2.22 | .4868 |
| 1.39 | .4177 | 1.81 | .4649 | 2.23 | .4871 |
| 1.40 | .4192 | 1.82 | .4656 | 2.24 | .4875 |
| 1.41 | .4207 | 1.83 | .4664 | 2.25 | .4878 |
| 1.42 | .4222 | 1.84 | .4671 | 2.25 | .4878 |
| 1.43 | .4236 | 1.85 | .4678 | 2.26 | .4881 |
| 1.44 | .4251 | 1.86 | .4686 | 2.27 | .4884 |
| 1.45 | .4265 | 1.87 | .4693 | 2.28 | .4887 |
| 1.46 | .4279 | 1.88 | .4699 | 2.29 | .4890 |
| 1.47 | .4292 | 1.89 | .4706 | 2.30 | .4893 |
| 1.48 | .4306 | 1.90 | .4713 | 2.31 | .4896 |
| 1.49 | .4319 | 1.91 | .4719 | 2.32 | .4898 |
| 1.50 | .4332 | 1.92 | .4726 | 2.33 | .4901 |
| 1.51 | .4345 | 1.93 | .4732 | 2.34 | .4904 |
| 1.52 | .4357 | 1.94 | .4738 | 2.35 | .4906 |
| 1.53 | .4370 | 1.95 | .4744 | 2.36 | .4909 |
| 1.54 | .4382 | 1.96 | .4750 | 2.37 | .4911 |
| 1.55 | .4394 | 1.97 | .4756 | 2.38 | .4913 |
| 1.56 | .4406 | 1.98 | .4761 | 2.39 | .4916 |
| 1.57 | .4418 | 1.99 | .4767 | 2.40 | .4918 |
| 1.58 | .4429 | 2.00 | .4772 | 2.41 | .4920 |
| 1.59 | .4441 | 2.01 | .4778 | 2.42 | .4922 |
| 1.60 | .4452 | 2.02 | .4783 | 2.43 | .4925 |
| 1.61 | .4463 | 2.03 | .4788 | 2.44 | .4927 |
| 1.62 | .4474 | 2.04 | .4793 | 2.45 | .4929 |
| 1.63 | .4484 | 2.05 | .4798 | 2.46 | .4931 |
| 1.64 | .4495 | 2.06 | .4803 | 2.47 | .4932 |
| 1.65 | .4505 | 2.07 | .4808 | 2.48 | .4934 |
| 1.66 | .4515 | 2.08 | .4812 | 2.49 | .4936 |
| 1.67 | .4525 | 2.09 | .4817 | 2.50 | .4938 |

(*continued*)

## TABLE A-6. (*continued*)

| z | Area from Mean to z | z | Area from Mean to z | z | Area from Mean to z |
|---|---|---|---|---|---|
| 2.51 | .4940 | 2.79 | .4974 | 3.07 | .4989 |
| 2.52 | .4941 | 2.80 | .4974 | 3.08 | .4990 |
| 2.53 | .4943 | 2.81 | .4975 | 3.09 | .4990 |
| 2.54 | .4945 | 2.82 | .4976 | 3.10 | .4990 |
| 2.55 | .4946 | 2.83 | .4977 | 3.11 | .4991 |
| 2.56 | .4948 | 2.84 | .4977 | 3.12 | .4991 |
| 2.57 | .4949 | 2.85 | .4978 | 3.13 | .4991 |
| 2.58 | .4951 | 2.86 | .4979 | 3.14 | .4992 |
| 2.59 | .4952 | 2.87 | .4979 | 3.15 | .4992 |
| 2.60 | .4953 | 2.88 | .4980 | 3.16 | .4992 |
| 2.61 | .4955 | 2.89 | .4981 | 3.17 | .4992 |
| 2.62 | .4956 | 2.90 | .4981 | 3.18 | .4993 |
| 2.63 | .4957 | 2.91 | .4982 | 3.19 | .4993 |
| 2.64 | .4959 | 2.92 | .4982 | 3.20 | .4993 |
| 2.65 | .4960 | 2.93 | .4983 | 3.21 | .4993 |
| 2.66 | .4961 | 2.94 | .4984 | 3.22 | .4994 |
| 2.67 | .4962 | 2.95 | .4984 | 3.23 | .4994 |
| 2.68 | .4963 | 2.96 | .4985 | 3.24 | .4994 |
| 2.69 | .4964 | 2.97 | .4985 | 3.25 | .4994 |
| 2.70 | .4965 | 2.98 | .4986 | 3.26 | .4994 |
| 2.71 | .4966 | 2.99 | .4986 | 3.27 | .4995 |
| 2.72 | .4967 | 3.00 | .4987 | 3.28 | .4995 |
| 2.73 | .4968 | 3.01 | .4987 | 3.29 | .4995 |
| 2.74 | .4969 | 3.02 | .4987 | 3.30 | .4995 |
| 2.75 | .4970 | 3.03 | .4988 | 3.40 | .4997 |
| 2.76 | .4971 | 3.04 | .4988 | 3.50 | .4998 |
| 2.77 | .4972 | 3.05 | .4989 | 3.60 | .4998 |
| 2.78 | .4973 | 3.06 | .4989 | 3.70 | .4999 |

# APPENDIX B

# Answers to Statistics Exercises

## Chapter 7

1. **a.** Nominal
   **b.** Ratio
   **c.** Ordinal
   **d.** Nominal
   **e.** Interval
   **f.** Nominal
   **g.** Ratio
   **h.** Interval
   **i.** Ratio
   **j.** Ordinal
   **k.** Absolute
   **l.** Absolute

2. **Group A**
   $\Sigma X^2 = 29$
   $\Sigma X = 175$
   $(\Sigma X)^2 = 841$

   **Group B**
   $\Sigma X = 27$
   $\Sigma X^2 = 155$
   $(\Sigma X)^2 = 729$

   **Group C**
   $\Sigma X = 21$
   $\Sigma X^2 = 99$
   $(\Sigma X)^2 = 441$

## Chapter 8

**Percent Body Fat**
$M = 8.4$
$MED = 8$
Range = 8 or 9

1. $SD = 2.61$
   $68\% = 5.8 - 11.0$
   $95\% = 3.3 - 13.5$
   $99\% = 1.7 - 15.1$

2. **a.** 6.68 %
   **b.** 30.15%
   **c.** 46.49%
   **d.** 8.57%
   **e.** 15.3%

**Percent Income**
$M = 12.5$
$MED = 11.5$
Range = 11 or 12
$SD = 3.35$
$68\% = 9.2 - 15.9$
$95\% = 5.9 - 19.1$
$99\% = 3.9 - 21.1$

**Stress Index for Recreation**
$M = 9.7$
$MED = 9$
Range = 10 or 11
$SD = 3.32$
$68\% = 6.4 - 13.0$
$95\% = 3.2 - 16.2$
$99\% = 1.1 - 18.3$

| 2. Health Test | Recreation Test | Better Score |
|---|---|---|
| **a.** $z = .42$ | $z = 1.25$ | Recreation |
| **b.** $z = 1.42$ | $z = 2.25$ | Recreation |
| **c.** $z = .71$ | $z = -.50$ | Health |
| **d.** $z = -1.42$ | $z = -1.25$ | Recreation |
| **e.** $z = -.43$ | $z = .50$ | Recreation |

## Chapter 9

1. There was a significant difference ($p \leq .05$) between the dieting group and the diet and exercise group. Dieting and exercising were better at lowering blood cholesterol.
2. There was a significant difference ($p \leq .05$) between Utahans and Nebraskans on the percent of their incomes spent on leisure activities. The Utahans spent more. (This is probably due to the excellent skiing in Utah!)
3. There was no significant difference ($p > .05$) between running 4 and 6 days per week on the improvement of $VO_{2max}$. Both training programs produce comparable results.
4. There was no significant difference ($p > .05$) between the two stress reduction techniques. Both techniques produce similar results.
5. There was a significant difference ($p \leq .01$) between body fat measures obtained by UWW and the skinfold method. The skinfold method is less accurate.

## Chapter 10

1. $r = .82$, which is significant at the .05 as well as .01 level. This means that a strong positive relationship exists between years of education and healthcare cost per family member; that is, as years of education increase, so does healthcare cost. The percent common variance is 67.2, and the percent specific variance is 32.8.
2. $r = .76$. The reliability of the test is moderately high; that is, the scores are consistent from trial to trial.
3. $r = -.85$, which is significant at the .05 as well as the .01 level. This indicates a strong negative relationship between the two variables: more years of attending the camp was associated with a lower GPA. The explained variance is 72.3%.
4. **a.** $Y' = .78X + 30.77$ is the equation to predict overall strength from grip strength.
   **b.** $SEE = 2.63$. About 68% of predicted scores will lie within 2.63 kg of the actual value.
   **c.** $Y' = 40.91$
5. **a.** $Y' = -1.13X + 58.6$ is the equation to predict $VO_{2max}$ from 1.5-mile run time. $SEE = 2.11$, which means that 68% of the predicted scores will be within 2.11 mL/kg/minute of the actual score.
   **b.** $Y' = 46.17$. The 68% confidence interval $= 46.17 \pm 1.0(2.11)$ or 44.06 to 48.28.
6. **a.** $Y' = 1.87X + 138.6$ is the equation to predict use of the lake area. $SEE = 57.12$, which means that 68% of the predicted scores will be within 57 persons of the actual value for use of the lake area.
   **b.** $Y' = 437.8$, or 438 in whole numbers. This is the predicted use of the lake area. The 95% confidence interval $= 437.8 \pm 1.96(57.12)$ or 326 to 550. About 95% of

predicted scores are expected to fall within this range. Note that the interval is rounded to the nearest **whole person.**

## Chapter 11

1. **a.** t = –2.37
   **b.** Yes; blood pressure was significantly reduced, and the probability of a type I decision error is less than or equal to 5%.
2. **a.** t = –1.18
   **b.** No; the differences are more than 5% likely to be due to chance.
3. **a.** t = –2.26, which is significant at the .05 level.
   **b.** Women in this study were more flexible than men. The probability of making a type I decision error is less than or equal to 5%.
   **c.** $\Omega^2$ = 18.6%, which means that 18.6% of the variance in flexibility between the groups is due to gender.
4. **a.** $\Omega^2$ = 3.8%.
   **b.** This means that 3.8% of the difference in salaries is due to the occupational group.
5. *t* = 4.75, which is significant at the .05 as well as .01 level. The chance of type I decision error is less than or equal to 5%.
6. **a.**

| Source | SS | df | MS | F |
|--------|------|-----|--------|-------|
| Between | 725 | 2 | 362.50 | 31.41 |
| Within | 150 | 13 | 11.54 | |
| Total | 875 | 15 | | |

   **b.** Yes
   **c.** It is 95% likely that a real difference in $VO_{2max}$ exists in the three groups of athletes.
   **d.** Perform a multiple comparison test to identify which groups are significantly different from each other.
   **e.** $\Omega^2$ = 79%, which indicates that 79% of the variance in scores is due to being a track athlete, basketball player, or volleyball player.
7. **a.** Yes
   **b.** The difference is 95% likely to be real and only 5% likely to be due to chance.
   **c.** Perform a multiple comparison test to identify which groups are significantly different from each other.
   **d.** $\Omega^2$ = 55%, which means that 55% of the variation among groups in bone mineral content can be attributed to estrogen replacement therapy, whereas 45% is due to other factors.

## Chapter 12

1. Chi square = 52.0, $p \leq .05$; therefore, there is a significant difference and relationship between type of athlete and exercise guidelines. Cramer's phi = .42, indicates a moderate relationship between type of athlete and compliance with exercise guidelines.

2. Chi square $= 27.2$, $p \leq .05$; therefore, there is a significant difference and relationship between gender type and approval of contact sports. Cramer's phi $= .48$, indicates a moderate relationship between gender and approval of contact sports.

3. Chi square $= 4.36$, $p \leq .05$; therefore, there is a significant difference and relationship between surface type and injury status. Cramer's phi $= .15$, indicates a weak relationship between surface type and injury status.

4. Spearman $r = .786$, $p \leq .05$; therefore, there is a strong positive relationship between team rank at the beginning and end of season. This suggests that teams with a high rank at the beginning tended to have a high rank at the end of season.

5. Spearman $r = -.901$, $p \leq .05$; therefore, there is a very strong negative relationship between $VO_{2max}$ rank and race time rank. This suggests that individuals with a high $VO_{2max}$ tended to have a lower (faster) race time.

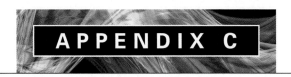

# APPENDIX C

# Sample Content Form and Sample Letters

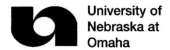

University of
Nebraska at
Omaha

School of Health, Physical
Education and Recreation
Omaha, Nebraska 68182-0216
(402) 554-2670

## SAMPLE INFORMED CONSENT FORM

XYZ Institution Review Board
Adult Informed Consent Form

## DETERMINANTS OF THE OXYGEN COST OF CYCLE ERGOMETRY

### Invitation to Participate

You are invited to participate in a research study that will determine the important factors that account for the oxygen cost of stationary cycling. Your participation in this study is completely voluntary.

### Basis for Subject Selection

You are being asked to participate in this study because you are a healthy male or female between the ages of 19 and 35. You may participate only if you are free from any cardiovascular, metabolic, and/or muscle or joint risk factors and you are a nonsmoker.

### Purpose of the Study

The purpose of this study is to determine the important factors that account for how much oxygen someone uses when pedalling a stationary cycle. It has been recently shown that men and women differ on how much oxygen they use when exercising at the same workload. This study will help to explain what accounts for this difference.

### Explanation of Procedures

You will be asked to come to the exercise physiology laboratory at Institution XYZ for two test sessions. Each will last about 1 hour. Before any testing you will be required to complete a medical questionnaire and read and sign a consent form.

During the first session, measurements of your height, weight, leg and thigh length, and inseam height will be made. An angle from your kneecap to your hip will be measured with a device that resembles a protractor. Inseam will be determined by measuring the height of a clipboard placed between your thighs at crotch level. This information will be used to establish an appropriate seat height. Next, you will be asked to perform an exercise test during which we will measure the amount of oxygen your body uses and your heart rate. Measurement of your oxygen consumption will be done through a mouthpiece attached to an electronic instrument known as a metabolic cart. You may find the mouthpiece slightly uncomfortable. Your heart rate will be measured by an electronic wristwatch from electrode belt attached to your chest.

The exercise test you will perform is submaximal and will be done on a stationary cycle. The exercise will begin with 5 to 10 minutes of rest on the cycle. If you are a male, you will perform three exercise stages lasting about 5 minutes each. One stage will be performed against no resistance, with the other two at light to moderate resistance levels. After the test you will pedal for about 5 minutes to cool down.

If you are a female, you will perform the same exercise tests as the males plus two additional stages at a light and moderate resistance.

To produce accurate test results, you will be asked to refrain from eating for at least 4 hours before testing and not to exercise or perform strenuous activity 12 hours before participating.

During the second visit to the laboratory, you will be asked to perform two strength tests on your dominant leg. In one test, performed at moderate speed, you will feel modest resistance. The other test will be done at a fast speed, and the resistance will feel very light. Both tests together require only about 5 minutes.

Finally, you will be weighed underwater to determine your percent of body fat. You will need to bring a swimsuit for this test. You will sit in a plastic chair that is suspended from a scale in a tank of warm water. You will be asked to submerge yourself while blowing out of your lungs all of the air that you can. After this is done, an underwater weight is taken. You will be asked to repeat this about 10 times. Afterward you will be asked to breathe into a device known as a spirometer to measure a lung volume. You will repeat this test twice. Underwater weighing and lung volume testing will take about 20 to 30 minutes.

### Potential Risks and Discomforts

The following are the risks and discomforts you may experience during this study:

**Cycle and Strength Tests** Possible risks include but are not limited to heart attack, abnormal heart rhythms, abnormal blood pressure, stroke, shortness of breath, dizziness, reduced coordination, and muscle soreness.

**Underwater Weighing and Lung Volume Test** Possible risks include but are not limited to swallowing water and apprehension of the water. The lung volume test may make you light-headed.

The risks of these occurring in healthy, younger subjects are very low. Most of the discomforts are relatively short-lived.

## Potential Benefits to Subjects

You will benefit by obtaining a predicted measure of your aerobic capacity, which is an important index of cardiovascular fitness, and a measure of your percent body fat.

## Potential Benefits to Society

Society would benefit by determining the important factors that account for the oxygen cost of cycle ergometry.

## Financial Obligations

The tests will be provided to you free of charge.

## In Case of Injury Compensation

In the unlikely event that you suffer an injury as a direct consequence of the research procedures described above, the emergency medical care required to treat the injury will be provided at the University of XYZ at no expense to you, provided that the cost of such medical care is not reimbursable through your health insurance. However, no additional compensation for physical care, hospitalization, loss of income, pain, suffering, or any other compensation will be provided. None of the above shall be construed as a waiver of any legal rights or redress you may have.

## Assurance of Confidentiality

Information obtained from you in this study will be treated confidentially. Your name will not be used in the publishing of the results of this study. Only grouped data will be reported.

## Rights of Research Subjects

Your rights as a research subject have been explained to you. If you have any additional questions concerning the rights of research subjects you may contact Institution XYZ Review Board at 555-555-5555.

## Voluntary Participation and Withdrawal

You are free to decide not to participate in this study or to withdraw at any time without adversely affecting your relationship with the investigators or the University of XYZ. Your decision will not result in loss of benefits to which you are otherwise entitled.

If any information develops or changes occur during the course of this study that may affect your willingness to continue participating, you will be informed immediately.

## Documentation of Informed Consent

YOU ARE VOLUNTARILY MAKING A DECISION WHETHER OR NOT TO PARTICIPATE IN THIS RESEARCH STUDY. YOUR SIGNATURE CERTIFIES THAT THE CONTENT AND MEANING OF THE INFORMATION ON THIS CONSENT FORM HAVE

BEEN FULLY EXPLAINED TO YOU AND THAT YOU HAVE DECIDED TO PARTICI-PATE HAVING READ AND UNDERSTOOD THE INFORMATION PRESENTED. YOUR SIGNATURE ALSO CERTIFIES THAT YOU HAVE HAD ALL YOUR QUESTIONS AN-SWERED TO YOUR SATISFACTION. IF YOU THINK OF ANY ADDITIONAL QUES-TIONS DURING THIS STUDY, PLEASE CONTACT THE INVESTIGATORS. YOU WILL BE GIVEN A COPY OF THIS CONSENT FORM TO KEEP.

_____          _____

Signature of Subject          Date

MY SIGNATURE AS WITNESS CERTIFIES THAT THE SUBJECT SIGNED THIS CONSENT FORM IN MY PRESENCE AS HIS OR HER VOLUNTARY ACT AND DEED.

_____          _____

Signature of Witness          Date


IN MY JUDGMENT, THE SUBJECT IS VOLUNTARILY AND KNOWINGLY GIVING IN-FORMED CONSENT AND POSSESSES THE LEGAL CAPACITY TO GIVE INFORMED CONSENT TO PARTICIPATE IN THIS RESEARCH STUDY.

_____          _____

Signature of Investigator          Date

(The investigators' names, titles, and phone numbers go here)

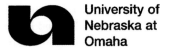 University of
Nebraska at
Omaha

School of Health, Physical
Education and Recreation
Omaha, Nebraska 68182-0216
(402) 554-2670

## SAMPLE SURVEY COVER LETTER

Dear (name of Athletic Trainer/Conditioning Coach):

We are surveying all NCAA Division I men's basketball teams to describe the size, strength speed, agility, and other characteristics of the modern player. Surprisingly little information has been published on this topic despite the great interest it undoubtedly has for coaches, athletic trainers, players, and fans. Therefore, we ask for your help to spend about 15 minutes in completing the attached form.

Because our pupose in doing this study is in concert with the efforts of the National Strength and Conditioning Association (NSCA) to promote effective conditioning of athletes, the NSCA Executive Director has written a letter endorsing the study (enclosed). We will send to every survey participant a summary report giving the average of all schools and the average scores for your own team. Thus, you can readily compare your players with those of the national average of each variable. We believe you will find this information interesting and useful.

Your assistance is greatly appreciated. Please return the survey in the enclosed self-addressed, stamped envelope by [specify the return date].

Sincerely,


(The investigators' names and titles)

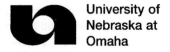 University of
Nebraska at
Omaha

School of Health, Physical
Education and Recreation
Omaha, Nebraska 68182-0216
(402) 554-2670

## SAMPLE THANK YOU LETTER

Dear Coach ——————— (Name of coach):

At last we are providing you with a copy of the results of the survey on NCAA Division I basketball players. Attached are two printouts of the data. One presents the mean, mode, median, standard deviation, and other findings for your team, while the second is the data for all teams combined. The columns are keyed as follows:

1. Height
2. Weight
3. Percent fat
4. Vertical jump
5. Power clean
6. Bench press
7. Squat
8. 1-mile run in minutes
9. 1.5-mile run in minutes
10. 40-yard dash in seconds
11. 30-yard dash in seconds
12. Agility run: T test in seconds
13. Power clean divided by weight
14. Bench press divided by weight
15. Squat divided by weight
16. Fat-free weight or lean weight
17. Power in vertical jump in kilograms per meter per second

Forty-five teams representing 437 players responded to the survey. We hope the information presented to you will be interesting and useful. You can compare how your team's players compare to those across the country. The 400-plus players' data represent a rather good cross-section of players in Division I.

We appreciate your assistance with this project and wish you and your team the best for the next season. Thanks again.

Sincerely,

(The investigators' names and titles)

# GLOSSARY

**absolute scale**   A level of measurement that allows distinguishing a difference and a direction of difference and that has a scale of discrete equal units.

**absolute zero**   A zero representing the absence of a trait or characteristic.

**abstract**   A source of reference information, including a summary; also, a summary appearing at the beginning of an article.

**alternative hypothesis**   A statistical hypothesis that is the logical alternative to the null hypothesis. It is written in such a way that if the null is not true, the alternative must be.

**American Psychological Association (APA) style**   A guideline for writing research papers and reports published by the APA. It includes information regarding organization, expression of ideas, editorial style, and typing instructions.

**analysis of variance (ANOVA)**   A statistic used to compare more than two mean scores.

**analysis of covariance (ANCOVA)**   A statistic used to compare more than two mean scores that adjusts mean scores on the basis of the effect of a third variable called a covariate.

**ANOVA**   See *analysis of variance*.

**ANCOVA**   See *analysis of covariance*.

**appendix**   Supplementary nonessential information to a research paper.

**applied research**   Research conducted with a specific application in mind.

**basic research**   Research with no specific application in mind; research for the sake of knowledge alone.

**bibliography**   A source of reference information from books, articles, and documents; also refers to sources not cited in a paper but related to the topic.

**blinded review**   Review of a research manuscript in which the reviewers do not know the identity of the author or institution and the author does not know the identity of the reviewers.

**cause-and-effect relationship**   A relationship in which one factor has been logically determined to have a predictable influence on another factor.

**central tendency**   Statistic used to express a score that is the most representative of all scores in a distribution.

**change score**   The difference between a pre-test and a post-test score.

**chi square**   A nonparametric statistic that compares frequency counts of what is theoretically expected to occur to what is empirically observed.

**coefficient of determination**   A statistic used to determine the strength of a relationship by accounting for the variance shared by two variables (common variance).

**coefficient of nondetermination**   A statistic used to determine the variance unaccounted for by a second variable (specific variance).

**Coefficient of variation**   A statistic used to show variability of a distribution. It may be used to compare the variability of two or more distributions when the means or the variables measured are not the same.

**computerized information retrieval**   Use of the computer to speed information retrieval.

**concurrent validity**   A type of statistical validity in which a proposed test is compared to a criterion standard within a short time to establish its accuracy.

**confidence interval**   A range of statistical values with stated probability that another statistic will be within the range. Typical interval probabilities are .68, .95, and .99.

**construct validity**   A type of statistical validity in which there is no definitive criterion. Typically, two groups that are distinctly different on the trait (construct) are compared with the use of the proposed test.

**content validity**   A type of logical validity that assumes an instrument accurately measures what it is supposed to measure.

**control group**   A group of subjects that is similar to the experimental group except that they do not receive the experimental treatment.

**correlated *t* test**   See dependent *t* test.

**correlation**   A statistic used to assess relationships between or among variables. There are several types, including Pearson and Spearman correlations.

**correlation matrix**   A table of correlation coefficients.

**correlational research**   A type of nonexperimental research in which the relationship between or among variables is studied.

**Cramer's phi**   A statistic used with a significant two-way chi square to determine the strength of a relationship.

**criterion-based validity**   A category of statistical validity in which a proposed test is compared to a criterion or gold standard.

**critical statistic or value**   A value in a statistics table (sampling distribution) to which a calculated statistic is compared to test the null hypothesis.

**deductive reasoning**   A logical method of reasoning moving from a generalization to specific conditions.

**degrees of freedom**   The number of variables that are free to vary in size. Degrees of freedom must be known to determine the critical statistic from a table.

**delimitations**   The scope of a study or a description of the subjects to be used, the location and duration of the study, and the variables studied.

**dependent *t* test**   A statistic used to compare two mean scores that are correlated with each other; also called a correlated *t* test.

**dependent variable**   A measure of some form of behavior; the effect of the independent variable.

**descriptive statistics**   Statistics that characterize only the subjects being observed.

**developmental research**   A type of nonexperimental research to study growth or maturation of subjects; may be cross-sectional (different subjects) or longitudinal (same subjects).

**discussion**   Section of a research paper that analyzes and interprets the results.

**Educational Research Information Center (ERIC)**   A data bank of indexed and abstracted reference information in the field of education.

**effect size**   A statistic used to assess the magnitude of the treatment effect or the effect of the independent variable on the dependent variable.

**empirical probability**   Probability that is based on the occurrence of past events.

**epidemiological research**   Research on the incidence and causes of diseases.

**equivalence reliability**   A type of reliability that is determined by repeated testing of the same subjects using alternative forms of a test that measures the same thing; also known as parallel forms reliability.

**error variance**   Variation in a dependent variable due to chance or sampling error.

**ex post facto research**   A type of nonexperimental research in which data collected in the past are used to address present problems.

**experimental group**   A group of subjects who receive the experimental treatment.

**experimental mortality**   A threat to internal validity due to subjects withdrawing from a study for nonrandom reasons.

**experimental research**   Research in which the researcher introduces an independent variable; the best way to establish a cause-and-effect relationship.

**external quality control**   Quality control measures for publishing or presenting research results.

**external validity**   The extent to which the results of a study may be applied to different conditions or subjects.

**face validity**   Logical validity that assumes an instrument accurately measures what it is supposed to measure.

**factor analysis**   A statistical procedure used to determine the commonality of a large number of measures or variables.

**field research**   Research conducted outside the laboratory or in the setting of the practitioner.

**Friedman's ANOVA**   A nonparametric statistical test used to determine whether a significant difference exists among more than two independent groups.

**general variance** The variation in scores explained by a second variable.

**generalizability** The ability to apply the results of a study to other conditions or situations.

**halo effect** An effect introduced when a researcher's expectation about the performance of a subject influences the subject's behavior.

**Hawthorne effect** The behavioral effect on a subject of participating in and being observed in a study.

**history** A threat to internal validity arising from events that happen to a subject outside the conditions of a study.

**hypothesis test** A statistical procedure used to objectively test the truth of the null hypothesis.

**independent *t* test** A statistic used to compare mean scores of two different or independent groups.

**independent variable** A variable that is manipulated by the researcher to determine the effect on behavior.

**index** A source of reference information limited to periodicals.

**inductive reasoning** A logical method of reasoning based on making generalizations from specific observations.

**inferential statistics** Statistics determined on a representative sample for the purpose of generalizing or inferring a trait to a population.

**informed consent** The process of clearly familiarizing a potential research subject about the purpose, risks, and benefits associated with a study, done so the subject can make an informed decision about participating in a study or not.

**institutional review board (IRB)** A committee of research experts that examines, approves, or disapproves research proposals at an institution. Its primary functions are to protect the rights of research subjects, the researcher, and the institution.

**interrater reliability** See *objectivity*.

**internal consistency reliability** A type of reliability that is determined by comparing half of the items on a single test to the other items; also known as split-half reliability.

**internal quality control** Research quality control measures up to the point of publishing or presenting research results.

**internal validity** A type of experimental validity: the extent to which an independent variable affects a dependent variable.

**interval scale** A level of measurement that allows distinguishing a difference and a direction of difference and that has a scale of equal units.

**introduction** Chapter or section of a research report that provides a background and justification of a study; may also include statement of the problem, hypothesis, delimitations, limitations, definition of terms, and significance.

**Kruskal-Wallis ANOVA** A nonparametric statistical test used to determine whether a significant difference exists among more than two independent groups.

**laboratory research** Research in which the treatment and data collection are conducted in a laboratory or highly controlled environment.

**limitations** Events that may interfere with the results of a study.

**logical validity** Validity that is qualitatively determined. Types include face and content.

**Mann-Whitney *U*** A nonparametric statistical test used to determine whether a significant difference exists between two independent groups.

**maturation** A threat to internal validity due to the natural growth of subjects during a study.

**mean** A measure of central tendency that is the arithmetic average of all scores in a distribution.

**measurement error** An error made in measurement of a variable; the difference between a score that is free from error and one that is actually measured. Measurement error always exists to some extent.

**median** A measure of central tendency that is the midpoint in distribution of scores.

**meta-analysis** A procedure using statistics to interpret the results of many studies by treating the results of each investigation as a discrete bit of information.

**methods** Section of a research paper that describes the subjects, procedures to collect data, research design, and data analysis.

**mode** A measure of central tendency that is the most frequently occurring score in a distribution.

**multiple regression** A statistical procedure used to predict one variable from knowledge about two or more variables.

**multiple treatment interference** A threat to external validity that occurs when treatments interact with one another, making any effect dependent on that order of testing.

**negatively skewed distribution** A nonnormal distribution with the majority of scores being high, with few low scores.

**nominal scale** A level of measurement that only allows comparisons distinguishing a difference.

**nonexperimental research** Research typified by observations or descriptions of the status of a given condition or situation. No independent variable is introduced or manipulated. Also known as descriptive research.

**nonparametric statistics** A variety of statistics based on nominal or ordinal data, with observed populations thought to be nonnormally distributed.

**normal curve** A model for statistical decision making. The unit normal curve has a mean equaling 0, a standard deviation equaling 1, and an area equaling 1.0 square unit; also referred to as the $z$ distribution.

**null hypothesis** A statistical hypothesis that states no difference or no relationship. It is always assumed to be true unless demonstrated otherwise.

**objectivity** A type of reliability that is determined by comparing the results between or among more than one evaluator; also known as interrater reliability.

**observational research** Nonexperimental research in which the researcher observes and records certain behaviors of subjects.

**omega squared** A statistic used to determine the strength of a treatment or independent variable; indicates the percent variance explained by the independent variable on the dependent variable.

**one-tailed hypothesis test** A statistical test in which the probability region for rejecting the null hypothesis is on one end of a sampling distribution; used when the researcher can predict the direction of outcome.

**operational definition** A definition that specifies the exact usage in a study. It should reflect common usage in the discipline.

**order effect** A change in behavior due to the sequence of testing.

**ordinal scale** A level of measurement that allows distinguishing a difference and a direction of difference.

**parallel forms reliability** See *equivalence reliability*.

**parameter** A trait of a population.

**parametric statistics** Statistics based on interval or ratio data, with observed populations thought to be normally distributed.

**partial correlation** A statistical procedure used to assess the relationship between two variables with the effects of a third variable removed.

**pedantic** Using uncommon terms to express oneself in hopes of being perceived as intellectual.

**placebo effect** An effect on a subject who participates in a study and who is in the group that receives no treatment.

**plagiarism** Use of the ideas, language, or thoughts of someone else and presenting them as your own.

**population** An all-inclusive group defined by the researcher.

**positively skewed distribution** A nonnormal distribution with the majority of scores being low, with few high scores.

**post hoc error** Attribution of any beneficial change in behavior to the influence of the independent variable when it is not known.

**post hoc tests** Statistics used to identify group differences after ANOVA indicates a main effect is significant; also known as follow-up, multiple comparison, or a posteriori tests. Examples are the Tukey and Scheffe tests.

**pre-experimental research designs** A type of experimental research design that is typified by using subjects in intact groups and introducing an independent variable. Control groups are typically not used.

**predictive validity**   A type of statistical validity in which a proposed test is used to accurately predict the occurrence of a future event.

**primary reference**   Direct mention of an original work.

**quasi-experimental research design**   Research design that is typified by using subjects in intact groups and introducing an independent variable. Control groups are used in some cases.

**random sampling**   An unbiased method of forming a representative sample from a population so that every element in the population has an equal probability of being selected. Methods include random numbers, systematic counting, and stratified samples.

**randomization**   The chance placement of subjects into groups.

**range**   A measure of variability that is the difference between the highest and lowest scores in a distribution.

**ratio scale**   A level of measurement that allows distinguishing a difference and a direction of difference; it has a scale of equal units and an absolute zero.

**reactive effects of pre-testing**   A threat to external validity that occurs when an independent variable is effective only if preceded by a particular pretest.

**regression line**   A line in a scattergram that allows prediction of a variable; commonly called the line of best fit.

**reliability**   The extent to which test scores are repeatable.

**research**   A logical, methodical procedure for solving problems.

**research hypothesis**   What the researcher thinks will occur in a study.

**research review**   Analysis of the literature on a specific topic.

**results**   Section of a research paper that reports the outcome.

**review of literature**   Section of a research paper that analyzes and interprets the literature.

**sample**   A representative subset of a population.

**sampling error**   Error that occurs when chance or random effects cause an event to occur in a manner different from the expected.

**sampling distribution**   A probability table that provides values for the chance occurrence of a particular statistic; may also be a data set obtained from a sampling procedure.

**scattergram**   A graph that depicts the relationship between two variables.

**scientific method**   A logical plan for solving problems and drawing conclusions. Components include the problem, hypothesis, determination of methods, gathering and analysis of data, and conclusion.

**secondary reference**   A reference to an original work in another source.

**selection bias**   A threat to internal validity that occurs when subjects may select being in an experimental group or control group.

**selection maturation**   A threat to internal validity that occurs when a subject has a unique condition that will improve naturally over the time of a study.

**simple linear regression**   A statistical procedure to predict one variable from knowledge about a second variable.

**Spearman *r***   A nonparametric statistic that determines the relationship between two distributions of ranked data.

**Spearman-Brown equation**   An equation that corrects a correlation calculated on halves of a test.

**specific variance**   The variation in scores not explained by a second variable.

**speculation**   A plausible explanation not directly supported by data.

**split-half reliability**   See *internal consistency reliability*.

**stability reliability**   A type of reliability that is determined by repeated testing of the same subjects using the same test; also known as test–retest reliability.

**standard deviation**   A measure of variability that is the approximate deviation of each score in a distribution from the mean.

**standard error of estimate (*SEE*)**   The error in a prediction equation or the standard deviation of scores around a regression line.

**statistical hypotheses**    The null and the alternative hypotheses. Statistical procedures are used to determine which one is true.

**statistical power**    The ability of a statistic to produce significance.

**statistical regression**    A threat to internal validity that occurs when an individual has an extreme pre-test score. The tendency is to regress toward a more typical performance on a subsequent test.

**statistical significance**    The statistical reference point that is selected for the purpose of testing the null hypothesis, also called the alpha level. Traditional probability levels are .05 and .01.

**statistical validity**    A type of validity that is quantitatively determined. Types include concurrent, predictive, and construct.

**subject–treatment interaction**    A threat to external validity that occurs when a treatment is effective only for a particular type of subject.

**survey research**    A type of nonexperimental research that is typified by broad-based data collection.

**test–retest reliability**    See *stability reliability*.

**testing**    A threat to internal validity; the effect of a pretest that may improve subsequent testing performance.

**theoretical probability**    Probability expressed as the ratio of the number of ways an event can occur divided by the number of possible events. Probability statements are commonly symbolized with small *p* and are expressed in proportions of 1.0.

**theory**    Integration of facts into a framework for explaining a phenomenon.

**thesaurus**    A list of synonyms.

**treatment**    The stimulus to which subjects in a study are exposed.

**treatment variance**    Variation in a dependent variable due to the treatment or independent variable.

**true experimental design**    Experimental research design that is typified by randomization of subjects into groups, use of control groups, and application of an independent variable.

**two-tailed hypothesis test**    A statistical test in which the probability regions for rejecting the null hypothesis are on both ends of a sampling distribution; used when the researcher cannot predict the direction of outcome.

**type I error**    Rejection of a null hypothesis when it is true. The probability of making a type I error is called the alpha level.

**type II error**    Acceptance of the null hypothesis when it is false. The probability of making a type II error is called the beta level.

**unblinded review**    Review of a research manuscript in which the reviewer knows the identity of the author or institution.

**validity**    The extent to which an instrument accurately measures what it is supposed to measure.

**variability**    Statistics that are used to express the dispersion of scores in a distribution.

**variance**    A measure of variability that is a squared standard deviation; the basis for calculating numerous inferential statistics.

**verbose**    Using excessive words to convey a thought.

**Wilcoxon matched pairs test**    A nonparametric statistical test used to determine whether there is a significant difference between two related groups.

*z score*    A standard score of the normal distribution expressed in standard deviation units. Most *z* scores range from −3.0 to 3.0.

# REFERENCES AND SELECTED READINGS

American Psychological Association (2001). *Publication manual of the American psychological association* (5th ed.). Washington: APA.

American Psychological Association (1973). *Ethical principles and the conduct of research with human participants*. Washington: APA Ad Hoc Committee on Ethical Standards.

Anderson, J. W., Konz, E. C., Frederich, R. C., & Wood, C. L. (2001). Long-term weight-loss maintenance: A meta-analysis of U. S. studies. *American Journal of Clinical Nutrition, 74*, 579–584.

Bartz, A. E. (1999). Basic statistical concepts. Upper Saddle River, NJ: Prentice-Hall.

Baumgartner, T. A., & Jackson, A. S. (1999). *Measurement and evaluation in physical education and exercise science*. Boston: WCB McGraw-Hill.

Best, J. W. (1981). *Research in education*. Englewood Cliffs, NJ: Prentice Hall.

Borg, W. R., & Gall, M. D. (1979). *Educational research: An introduction* (3rd ed.). New York: Longman, p. 200.

Borg, W. R., & Gall, M. D. (2006). *Educational research: An introduction* (8th ed.). New York: Longman.

Bradley, J. V. (1971). *Distribution-free statistical tests*. Englewood Cliffs, NJ: Prentice Hall.

Campbell, D. T., & Stanley, J. C. (1963). *Experimental and quasi-experimental designs for research*. Chicago: Rand McNally.

Ceci, S. J., & Peters, D. P. (1984). How blind is blind review? *American Psychologist, 39*, 1491–1494.

Christensen, J. E., & Christensen, C. E. (1977). Statistical power analysis of health, physical education, and recreation research. *Research Quarterly, 48*, 204–208.

Code of Federal Regulations 45 CFR 46. (1983). *Protection of human subjects*. Office of Protection from Research Risks (OPRR) Reports.

Code of Nuremberg. (1949). Reprinted in: *Trials of war criminals before the Nuremberg military tribunals under control council law No. 10*. Washington: U. S. Government Printing Office, 12, 81-82.

Cohen, J. (1969). *Statistical power analysis for the behavioral sciences*. New York: Academic Press.

Cohen, J. (1988). *Statistical power analysis for the behavioral sciences* (3rd ed.). New York: Academic Press.

Cook, D. (1962). The Hawthorne effect in educational research. *Phi Delta Kappan, 44*, 116–122.

*Council of Biology Editors Style Manual: A Guide for Authors, Editors, and Publishers in the Biological Sciences* (1978). (4th ed.) Arlington, VA: Published for the Conference of Biological Editors Inc.

Cronk, B. C. (1999). *How to use SPSS*. Los Angeles: Pyrczak.

Daniel, W. (1978). *Applied non-parametric statistics*. Boston: Houghton Mifflin.

Day, R. A. (1983). *How to write and publish a scientific paper*. Philadelphia: Institute for Scientific Information.

Eichorn, P., & Yankauer, A. (1987). Do authors check their references? A survey of accuracy of references in three public health journals. *American Journal of Public Health, 77*, 1011–1012.

Feinstein, A. R. (1983). Science, sanity, and "statistical significance." *Infectious Diseases, 13*, 5–8.

Fleishman, E. A. (1969). *The structure and measurement of physical fitness*. Englewood Cliffs, NJ: Prentice-Hall.

Fox, D. J. (1969). *The research process in education*. New York: Holt, Rinehart, and Winston.

Franks, B. D., & Huck, S. W. (1986). Why does everyone use the .05 level of significance? *Research Quarterly for Exercise and Sport, 57*, 245–249.

Glass, G. V., McGaw, B., & Smith, M. (1981). *Meta-analysis in social research*. Beverly Hills, CA: Sage.

Goodrich, J. E., & Roland, C. G. (1977). Accuracy of published medical reference citations. *Journal of Technical Writing and Communication, 7*, 15–19.

Green, L. W., & Lewis, F. M. (1986). *Measurement and evaluation in health education and health promotion*. Mountain View, CA: Mayfield.

Hanson, D. L. (1967). Influence of the Hawthorne effect upon physical education research. *Research Quarterly, 38*, 732.

Hays, W. L. (1981). *Statistics*. New York: CBS College.

Jackson, A., Pollock, M., & Ward, A.(1980). Generalized equations for predicting body density of women. *Medicine and Science for Sports and Exercise, 12*, 175–182.

Kachigan, S. K. (1986). *Statistical analysis*. New York: Radius Press.

Kelley, G. A., Kelley, K. S., & Vu Tran, Z. (2000). Exercise and bone mineral density in men: A meta-analysis. *Journal of Applied Physiology, 88*, 1730–1736.

Kerlinger, F. N. (1964). *Foundations of behavioral research*. New York: Holt, Rinehart, and Winston, pp. 258–259.

Kerlinger, F., & Pedhazar, E. (1973). *Multiple regression in behavioral research*. New York: Holt, Rinehart, and Winston, 446–447.

Kirk, R. E. (1968). *Experimental design: Procedures for the behavioral sciences*. Belmont, CA: Brooks/Cole.

Lemura, L. M., von Duvillard, S. P., & Mookerjee, S. (2000). The effects of physical training of functional capacity in adults ages 46 to 90: A meta-analysis. *Journal of Sports Medicine and Physical Fitness, 40,* 1–10.

McArdle, W., Katch, F., & Katch, V. (2001). *Exercise physiology.* Baltimore: Lippincott, Williams & Wilkins.

*Meet Minitab,* Release 13. (2000). State College, PA: Minitab.

*Merriam-Webster's Collegiate Dictionary* (1993). (10th ed.) Springfield, MA: Merriam-Webster.

Morrow, J. R., Bray, M. S., Fulton, J. E., & Thomas, J. R. (1992). Interrater reliability of 1987–1991. *Research Quarterly for Exercise and Sport, 63,* 200–204.

National Commission for the Protection of Human Subjects of Biomedical and Behavioral Research (1978). *The Belmont Report: Ethical principles for the protection of human subjects of research.* Washington: U. S. Government Printing Office.

Neutens, J. J., & Rubinson, L. (2002). *Research techniques for the health sciences.* San Francisco: Benjamin Cummings.

Norman, G. R., & Streiner, D. L. (1994). *Biostatistics: The bare essentials.* St. Louis: Mosby–Year Book.

Patten, M. L. (1998). *Questionnaire research: A practical guide.* Los Angeles: Pyrczak.

Pearson, D., & Shaw, S. (1982). *Life extension: A practical scientific approach.* New York: Warner.

Pelegrino, D. A. (1979). *Research methods for recreation and leisure.* Dubuque, IA: William C. Brown.

Peters, D. P., & Ceci, S. J. (1982). Peer review practices of psychological journals: The fate of articles submitted again. *Behavioral and Brain Sciences, 5,* 187–255.

Pugh, T. & Borenstein, S. (2004). American consumers suffering as more new drugs debut in U.S., analysis shows. Knight-Ridder, Available online at www.healthy skepticism.org/library/ref.php?id=268

Safrit, M. J., & Wood, T. M. (1995). *Introduction to measurement in physical education and exercise science.* St. Louis: Mosby–Year Book.

Sage, G. E. (1989). A commentary on qualitative research in sport and physical education. *Research Quarterly for Exercise and Sport, 60,* 204–207.

Schmidt, M. J. (1975). *Understanding and using statistics.* Lexington, MA: D. C. Heath.

Sparling, P. B. (1980). A meta-analysis of studies comparing maximal oxygen uptake in men and women. *Research Quarterly for Exercise and Sport, 51,* 542–552.

Strunk, W., & White, E. B. (1979). *The elements of style* (3rd ed.). New York: Macmillan.

Stull, G., Christina, R., & Quinn, S. (1991). Accuracy of references. *Research Quarterly for Exercise and Sport, 62,* 245–248.

Thomas, J. R., & French, K. E. (1986). The use of meta-analysis in exercise and sport: A tutorial. *Research Quarterly for Exercise and Sport, 57,* 196–204.

Thomas, J. R., & Nelson, J. K. (2001). *Research methods in physical activity.* Champaign, IL: Human Kinetics.

Thomas, J. R., Salazar, W., & Landers, D. M. (1991). What is missing in p <.05? Effect size. *Research Quarterly for Exercise and Sport, 62,* 344–348.

Tolson, H. (1980). An adjustment to statistical significance: V2. *Research Quarterly for Exercise and Sport, 51,* 580–584.

Tran, Z. V., Weltman, A., Glass, G. V., & Mood, D. P. (1983). The effects of exercise on blood lipids and lipoproteins: A meta-analysis. *Medicine and Science in Sports and Exercise, 15,* 393–402.

University of Nebraska Institutional Review Board for the Protection of Human Research Subjects. *IRB guidelines for the protection of human subjects in research studies.* Omaha: University of Nebraska.

Winer, B. J. (1962). *Statistical principles in experimental design.* New York: McGraw-Hill, p. 88.

World Medical Association. (1974). *Declaration of Helsinki.* World Medical Journal.

Yankauer, A. (1991). The accuracy of medical journal references: A follow-up study. *CBE Views, 14,* 23–24.

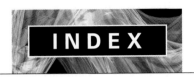

# INDEX

Note: Page numbers followed by f indicate figures; page numbers followed by t indicate tables.

## A

Abbreviation(s), in research
    writing, 67
Absolute scale, 75–76
    defined, 311
Absolute zero, defined, 311
Abstract(s), 28–29, 29t
    defined, 311
    of thesis, 37t, 38
Accuracy
    instrument, as threat to
        internal validity, 202t,
        204, 212t
    of references, 55
Age, as factor in strength
    in adults, 122, 123f
    in children, 122, 122f
Alpha level error, 109–110,
    110t
Alternate forms method, 193
Alternative hypothesis, 107
    defined, 311
American Alliance of Health,
    Physical Education,
    Recreation, and Dance, 30
American Cancer Society, 30
American College of Sports
    Medicine, 30, 276
American Heart Association,
    30
American Psychological
    Association (APA), 68
    guidelines for construction
        of tables, 49, 49t
    Publication Manual of, 68
American Psychological
    Association (APA) style,
    defined, 311
Analysis(es)
    chi-square, computer
        printout of, 172, 173f,
        174, 174t
    content, 251

in qualitative research,
    251–254, 252t
data, hypothetical
    computer output of,
    119f
data of, of thesis, 46
distribution-free, 77
factor, 140, 141t
    defined, 312
statistical, of thesis, 46
Analysis of covariance
    (ANCOVA), 165–166, 165t
    defined, 311
Analysis of variance (ANOVA),
    146, 152–165
    defined, 311
    factorial, 159–164, 160f,
        161t, 162f, 163f
    Friedman's, 182, 182t, 312
    interpretation of, 158–159,
        159t
    Kruskal-Wallis one-way,
        181, 182t, 313
    one-way, 152–153, 153t
    post hoc tests for, 155–158,
        156t, 157t
    randomized blocks,
        158–159
    with repeated measures,
        164–165, 164t
    statistical assumptions for,
        146
    two (2 x 2), 161
    two-way, 159–164, 160f,
        161t, 162f, 163f
        defined, 161
        sample computer
            printout of, 162, 162f
    two-way factorial, 222
ANCOVA. See Analysis of
    covariance (ANCOVA)
Anonymity, of research
    subjects, 21, 23t

ANOVA. See Analysis of
    variance (ANOVA)
APA. See American
    Psychological Association
    (APA)
Appendix(ces)
    defined, 311
    of thesis, 37t, 55–56
Applied research, 11– 12
    defined, 311
Arbitrary zero, 76
Article(s), research,
    publication of, 263–264
Artificial nature of
    experimental condition, as
    threat to external validity,
    202t, 209–210
Assumption(s), statistical,
    146
Audit trail, 253
Axial coding, 253

## B

Basic research, 11–12
    defined, 311
Belmont Report, 18
Beta level error, 110
Between-group variance,
    153
Bias(es), selection
    defined, 315
    as threat to interval validity,
        202t, 204–205, 212t
Biased sample, 79
Biased sampling, in research
    interpretation, 280– 281
Bibliography, 28, 29t
    defined, 311
Bimodal, 87
Blinded review, 264
    defined, 311
Blocking procedure, 158
Book(s), references for, 54

# C

Calculated statistic, in
  hypothesis testing, 111
Case studies
  defined, 247
  nonexperimental
    research–related,
    240–241, 244t
  qualitative
    research–related,
    247–248
Categorical response, 234
Causal relationship, 230–231
Cause-and-effect
  relationships, 128–130
  defined, 217, 311
  experimentation and,
    216–217
  nonexperimental research
    and, 230–231
Central tendency
  defined, 311
  mean, 86
  measures of, 86–87. *See also*
    *Median; Mode; specific*
    *mode, e.g.,* Mean
  median, 86–87
  mode, 87
Chain samples, 252
Change score, 221
  defined, 311
Chi square, 171–179,
    172t-176t, 173f, 176f, 178t,
    179f, 182t
  critical values of, 291
  defined, 311
  goodness of fit application
    of, 174–175, 174t
  interpretation of, 172–174,
    173f, 173t, 174t
  one-way, 171–172, 172t
  restrictions and
    assumptions for,
    178–179
  two-way, 175–176, 175t,
    176t
    applications of, 177–178,
      178t, 179f
    interpretation of,
      176–177, 176f
Children, strength in, age and,
    122, 122f

Chi-square analysis,
  computer printout of, 172,
    173f, 174, 174t
Citation location, in
  references, 55
Classical probability, 103
Cliche(s), in research writing,
    64, 64t
Closed-ended questions, 234
Code of Nuremberg, 18
Coding
  axial, 253
  open, 253
Coefficient of determination,
    128
  defined, 311
Coefficient of
  nondetermination, 128,
    129f
  defined, 311
Coefficient of variation, 90
  defined, 311
Coherence, 254
Comma(s), misused, in
  research writing, 65
Common variance, 128, 129f
Computerized information
  retrieval, 30–34, 32t, 33t
  defined, 311
Concurrent validity, 190
  defined, 311
Confidence interval, 93,
    134–135
  defined, 311
Confidentiality, of research
  subjects, 21, 23t
Confirmability, 254
Conflict of interest, in
  research interpretation,
    283
Consent, informed, 18–21.
  *See also* Informed consent
Consistency, internal, 193–194
Construct validity, 191
  defined, 311
Content analysis, 251
  in qualitative research,
    251–254, 252t
Content form, sample,
    305–308
Content validity, 189, 189t, 237
  defined, 312

Contingency table, 175, 175t
Control
  experimental, 201–215,
    217–218
  quality, 257–287. *See also*
    Quality control
Control group
  defined, 312
  internal validity and, 211,
    212t
Convenience sample, 80, 252
Correlated *t* tests, 146–149,
    147t, 148t, 149f
  calculation of, 147t
  defined, 312
  hypothesis testing for, 148t
  interpretation of, 148–149
  purpose of, 146
  results of, computer
    printout of, 148, 149f
Correlation(s)
  computer printout showing,
    127f
  concepts in, 122–124,
    122f-124f
  defined, 121, 312
  inverse, 122
  multiple, 137
  negative, 122
  partial, 139–140
    defined, 314
  Pearson, 124–131, 125t,
    126t, 127f, 129f, 130t.
    *See also* Pearson
    correlation
  positive, 122
  statistics and, in research
    interpretation, 282
Correlation matrix, 130, 130t
  defined, 312
Correlational research, 240,
    244t
  defined, 312
*Council of Biology Editors*
  *Style Manual*, 67
Counting, systematic, 79
Covariance, analysis of,
    165–166, 165t
Cover letter, in survey
  research, 235–236, 237t,
    239t
  sample, 309

Cramer's phi, defined, 312
Cramer's phi coefficient, 177
Credibility, 253
Criterion(a), inclusion, 45
Criterion-based validity,
    189–190
    defined, 312
Critical statistic
    defined, 312
    in hypothesis testing, 111
Critical value, 111
    defined, 312
Cross-sectional approach, 241
Curiosity, intellectual, of
    researcher, 14
Curve(s)
    nonnormal, 98–100, 98f, 99f
    normal, 90–96, 91f–96f. *See
    also* Normal curve

**D**

Data analysis
    hypothetical computer
        output of, 119f
    of thesis, 46
Data collection
    concepts of, 187–200
    in qualitative research,
        251–254, 252t
    of thesis, 46
Declaration of Helsinki, 18
Deductive reasoning, 9
    defined, 312
Defense(s), student, in
    internal quality control,
    260–261
Definition, operational,
    defined, 314
Degrees of freedom, 111
    defined, 312
Delimitation(s)
    defined, 312
    of thesis, 41–42
Department of Health and
    Human Services, 18
Dependability, 254
Dependent *t* tests, 146–149,
    147t, 148t, 149f. *See also*
    Correlated *t* tests
    defined, 312
Dependent variable, 13
    defined, 312

Descriptive research,
    229–239, 243, 244t
Descriptive statistics, 77–78
    defined, 312
Design(s)
    experimental, 216–228
        of thesis, 45–46
    true, 220–222
    defined, 316
    measurement, 185–255
    one-shot, 227
    post-nonrandom, 222–223
    post-test, 221–222
    post-test only, 220–221
    pre-experimental, 219,
        225–228, 228t
    pre-nonrandom, 222–223
    pre-random, 222–223
    pre-test, 221–222
    qualitative, in qualitative
        research, 152t, 251–254
    quasi, 219
    quasi-experimental,
        222–225
    repeated-measures,
        223–224
    research, 185–255
        experimental, 218–220
        pre-experimental,
            defined, 314
        quasi-experimental,
            defined, 315
    static group comparison,
        226
    time series, 224–225
    true, 219
Determination, coefficient of,
    128
    defined, 311
Developmental research, 241,
    244t
    defined, 312
Deviation(s), standard,
    defined, 315
Deviation score, 88
Dictionary, in research
    writing, 61
Discussion, defined, 312
Discussion chapter of thesis,
    37t, 49–52
Dishonesty, research,
    266–267, 267t

Distribution(s)
    nonnormal, 98–100, 98f, 99f
    sampling
        defined, 315
        in hypothesis testing, 111
    skewed
        negatively, defined, 314
        positively, defined, 314
Distribution-free analyses, 77
Dropout of subjects, 205
Duncan Multiple Range test,
    155

**E**

Educational Research
    Information Center
    (ERIC), defined, 312
Effect(s)
    main, 160–161, 160f
    order, 164
        defined, 314
    placebo, defined, 314
    reactive, of pre-testing,
        defined, 315
    treatment, assessment of
        research and, 273–275
Effect size, 274, 278
    defined, 312
Electronic resources, 32t
Empirical probabilities, 171
Empirical probability,
    defined, 312
Epidemiological research,
    241–242, 244t
    defined, 312
Equation(s), statistical, 81–82,
    82t
Equivalence reliability, 193
    defined, 312
ERIC. *See* Educational
    Research Information
    Center (ERIC)
Error(s)
    alpha level, 109–110, 110t
    beta level, 110
    measurement, 197–200. *See
    also* Measurement error
    post hoc, 275–276
        defined, 314
    sampling
        defined, 315
        in hypothesis testing, 107

Error(s) (*Contd.*)
   type I, 109–110, 110t
      defined, 316
   type II, 110–111, 110t
      defined, 316
Error variance, 153, 219–220
   defined, 312
Estimate, accuracy of,
   133–136
Ethics, in human subject
      research, 17–23
   anonymity, 21, 23t
   codes and guidelines,
      17–18
   confidentiality, 21, 23t
   informed consent, 18–21
   invasion of privacy, 21, 23t
   IRB's role in, 18
   knowledge of results, 22,
      23t
   researcher's role, 22
   safe and competent
      treatment, 22, 23t
Ex post facto research, 243,
   244t
   defined, 312
*Exercise and Sport Science
   Reviews*, 276–277
Experimental control,
   201–215, 217–218
Experimental control
   revisited, 217–218
Experimental designs,
   216–228
   of thesis, 45–46
   true, 220–222
      defined, 316
Experimental group, defined,
   312
Experimental mortality
   defined, 312
   as threat to internal validity,
      202t, 205–206, 212t
Experimental research,
   216–228
   defined, 312
Experimental research
   designs, 218–220
Experimental validity,
   201–215
Experimental variance,
   219–220

Experimentation
   cause-and-effect
      relationships and,
      216–217
   use of, 216–217
External quality control,
   defined, 312
External validity, 13, 284
   defined, 52, 208, 312
   internal validity vs.,
      213–214
   threats to, 202t, 208–210
      artificial nature of
         experimental
         condition, 202t,
         209–210
      controlling for, 212–213,
         213t
      multiple treatment
         interference, 202t, 210
      reactive effects of
         pre-testing, 202t, 209
      subject and retreatment
         interaction, 202t, 209
Extraneous variables, 218
Extrapolation, 254

**F**

*F* ratio, 154
Face validity, 188
   defined, 312
Fact(s), defined, 9–10
Factor(s), defined, 140
Factor analysis, 140, 141t
   defined, 312
Field research, 12
   defined, 312
Figure(s), in research
      interpretation, 281–282,
      281f, 282f
Fisher's Least Significant
   Difference test, 155
Focus groups, 248–250, 249t
Food and Drug
   Administration, 18
Friedman's ANOVA, 182, 182t
   defined, 312–313

**G**

General variance, defined, 313
Generalizability, defined, 313
Gold standard, 189

Goodness of fit application, of
   one-way chi square,
   174–175, 174t
Group(s)
   experimental, defined, 312
   focus, 248–250, 249t
   nominal, 250–251

**H**

Halo effect
   defined, 313
   as threat to internal validity,
      202t, 208, 212t
Hawthorne effect
   defined, 313
   as threat to internal validity,
      202t, 207–208, 212t
Health
   journals related to, 31t
   physical education, and
      recreation (HPER)
      journals related to, 31t
   references in, examples
      of, 28, 29t
   Websites for, 33t
History
   defined, 313
   as threat to internal validity,
      202t, 203, 212t
Holistic perspective, 246
Honesty, of researcher, 15
HPER. *See* Health, physical
   education, and recreation
   (HPER)
HSD test. *See* Tukey's
   Honestly Significant
   Difference (HSD) test
Human subject research,
   ethics in, 17–23. *See also*
   Ethics, in human subject
   research
Hypothesis(es)
   alternative, 107
      defined, 311
   defined, 41
   null, 107
      defined, 314
   research, 41
      defined, 315
   statistical, 41, 106
      defined, 316
   of thesis, 41

Hypothesis test
  defined, 313
  one-tailed, defined, 314
  two-tailed, defined, 316
Hypothesis testing, 106–119,
    109f, 110t, 113t, 114t,
    116t, 119f
  calculated statistics in, 111
  for correlated *t* tests, 148t
  critical statistic in, 111
  errors in
    type I, 109–110, 110t
    type II, 110–111, 110t
  factors in, 111–112
  interpretations following,
    117–118
  level of significance in,
    108–109, 109f
  null and alternative
    hypotheses in, 106–107
  one-tailed, 115–117, 116t
  practical, 118–119, 119f
    vs. statistical significance,
    117–118
  sampling distributions in,
    111
  sampling error in, 107–108
  steps in, 112–114, 113t, 114t
  two-tailed, 115–117

**I**

Implication(s), in thesis
    discussion, 51
Inclusion criteria, 45
Independent *t* test, 149–152,
    150t, 151f, 151t
  computer printout of, 150,
    151f
  defined, 313
  omega squared, 151–152,
    151t
Independent variable, 13
  defined, 313
  experimental research and,
    275–276
Index(es), 29, 29t
  defined, 313
Inductive reasoning, 9
  defined, 313
Inferential statistics, 78
  defined, 313
Information retrieval, 27–34

abstracts, 28–29, 29t
bibliographies, 28, 29t
computerized, 30–34, 32t,
    33t
  defined, 311
indexes, 29, 29t
journals, 30, 31t
primary references, 27–28
research reviews, 29t, 30
secondary references, 27–28
sources of information,
    27–28
Informed consent, 18–21
  background and invitation
    to participate in, 19, 19t
  components of, 19–20, 19t
  defined, 313
  explanation of procedures,
    19t, 20
  potential benefits of, 19t, 20
  potential risks and
    discomforts, 19t, 20
  rights of inquiry and
    withdrawal, 19t, 20
  in survey research, 239
  valid, 21
Informed consent form,
    sample, 305–308
Institutional review boards
    (IRBs)
  defined, 313
  described, 18
  in internal quality control,
    261–263
Instrument accuracy, as
    threat to internal validity,
    202t, 204, 212t
Intellectual curiosity, of
    researcher, 14
Interaction, defined, 160
Interference, multiple
    treatment, defined, 314
Internal consistency
    reliability, 193–194
  defined, 313
Internal quality control,
    259–263. *See also* Quality
    control, internal
Internal validity, 12–13,
    201–208, 202t
  critiquing research and, 269
  defined, 201–202, 313

external validity vs.,
    213–214
threats to, 202–208, 202t
  controlling for, 210–212,
    212t
  groups in, 211, 212t
  methods in, 212t,
    212–212
  randomization in,
    210–211, 212t
  experimental mortality,
    202t, 205–206, 212t
  halo effect, 202t, 208,
    212t
  Hawthorne effect, 202t,
    207–208, 212t
  history, 202t, 203, 212t
  instrument accuracy,
    202t, 204, 212t
  maturation, 202–203,
    202t, 212t
  placebo effect, 202t, 206,
    212t
  selection bias, 202t,
    204–205, 212t
  selection maturation,
    202t, 206, 212t
  statistical regression,
    202t, 204, 212t
  testing, 202t, 203–204,
    212t
Internet, 30
Interrater reliability, 194
  defined, 313
Interval, confidence, 93,
    134–135
  defined, 311
Interval scale, 76
  defined, 313
Introduction
  defined, 313
  of thesis, 37t, 38–39
Introductory concepts,
    1–23
Invasion of privacy, 21, 23t
IRBs. *See* Institutional review
    boards (IRBs)

**J**

Jargon, in research writing,
    65–66
Journal(s), 30, 31t

*Journal of Strength and Conditioning Research*, 30

**K**

Knowledge of results, 22, 23t
Knowledge of specific subject, of researcher, 14
Kruskall-Wallis ANOVA, defined, 313
Kruskal-Wallis ANOVA, one-way, 181, 182t

**L**

Laboratory research, 12
defined, 313
Level of significance, in hypothesis testing, 108–190, 109f
*Life Extension: A Practical Scientific Approach*, 275
Likert scales, 234
Limitation(s)
defined, 313
of study, in thesis discussion, 51
of thesis, 42
Line of best fit, 122f, 123
Listserve, 238
Literature
current reviews of, 276–277
review of, defined, 315
Literature review, of thesis, 37t, 43–44
Logical validity, 188–189, 189t
defined, 313
Loss of subjects, 205

**M**

Mail, survey by, steps in conducting, 232–238, 235t, 237t
Main effect, 160–161, 160f
Mann-Whitney *U*, 181, 182t
defined, 313
Matrix(es)
correlation, 130, 130t
defined, 312
defined, 156, 157t
Maturation
defined, 313
selection
defined, 315

as threat to internal validity, 202t, 206, 212t
as threat to internal validity, 202–203, 202t, 212t
Mean
application of, 87
defined, 313
importance of, 98
as measure of central tendency, 86
Mean scores, comparison of, 145–169
Mean square (MS), 153
Measurement, concepts of, 187–200
Measurement and research design, 185–255
Measurement error, 197–200
defined, 313
quantifying, 199–200
sources of, 198–199
Measurement scales, statistical, 74–76. *See also* Statistic(s), measurement scales in
Measures of variability, 87–90, 89t. *See also* Variability, measures of
Media, research reports in, caution with use of, 283
Median
application of, 87
defined, 313
as measure of central tendency, 86–87
*Medicine and Science in Sports and Exercise*, 30
*Merriam Webster's Collegiate Dictionary*, 62
Meta-analysis, 278–279
defined, 243, 313
Meta-analysis research, 243, 244t
Method(s), defined, 313
Methods section of thesis, 37t, 44–46
Minimax principle, 219
Mode
defined, 314
as measure of central tendency, 87

Mortality, experimental
defined, 312
as threat to internal validity, 202t, 205–206, 212t
MS. *See* Mean square (MS)
Multiple correlation *(R)*, 137
Multiple regression, 136–139, 138t
defined, 136, 314
interpretation of, 137–139, 138t
specificity of prediction, 139
Multiple treatment interference
defined, 314
as threat to external validity, 202t, 210

**N**

National Commission for the Protection of Human Subjects of Biomedical and Behavioral Research, of U.S. Congress, 17–18
National Institutes for Health (NIH), 218
National Strength and Conditioning Association, 30
Negatively skewed distribution, defined, 314
Network samples, 252
Newman-Keuls test, 155
NIH. *See* National Institutes for Health (NIH)
Nominal groups, 250–251
Nominal scale, 75
defined, 314
Nondetermination, coefficient of, 128, 129f
defined, 311
Nonexperimental research, 239–243, 244t
case studies, 240–241, 244t
cause-and-effect relationships and, 230–231
correlation research, 240, 244t
defined, 314
descriptive research, 243, 244t

developmental research, 241, 244t
epidemiological research, 241–242, 244t
ex post facto research, 243, 244t
meta-analysis research, 243, 244t
observational research, 242–243, 244t
Nonnormal curves, 98–100, 98f, 99f
Nonnormal distributions, 98–100, 98f, 99f
Nonparametric statistics, 77, 170–184
  chi square, 171–179, 172t-176t, 173f, 176f, 178t, 179f, 182t. *See also* Chi square
  defined, 314
  Friedman's ANOVA, 182, 182t
  Kruskal-Wallis one-way ANOVA, 181, 182t
  Mann-Whitney *U*, 181, 182t
  Spearman *r*, 179–181, 180f, 180t
  Wilcoxon matched pairs test, 181, 182t
Normal curve, 90–96, 91f-96f
  application of, 93–96, 93f-96f
  confidence intervals of, 93
  defined, 314
  between M and z, area of, 298–300
  probability and, 104–106
  selected areas of, 92, 92f
  unit, 91–92, 91f
Null hypothesis, 107
  defined, 314
Number(s), in research writing, 68

**O**

Objectivity, 131, 194
  defined, 314
Observational research, 242–243, 244t
  defined, 314
Observed score, 197

Omega squared, 151–152, 151t
  defined, 314
One-group pre- and post-design, 225–226
One-shot design, 227
One-tailed hypothesis test, defined, 314
One-way ANOVA, 152–153, 153t
One-way chi square, 171–172, 172t
Open coding, 253
Open-ended questions, 234
Open-mindedness, of researcher, 13
Operational definition, defined, 314
Operational procedures of thesis, 45
Order effect, 164
  defined, 314
Ordinal scale, 75
  defined, 314

**P**

Parallel forms method, 193
Parallel forms reliability, defined, 314
Parallelism, in research writing, 65
Parameter(s), defined, 78, 314
Parametric statistics, 76–77
  defined, 314
Partial correlation, 139–140
  defined, 314
Pearson correlation, 124–131, 125t, 126t, 127f, 129f, 130t
  calculation of, 125, 125t
  cause-and-effect relationships, 128–130
  correlation matrix, 130, 130t
  critical values of, 293
  interpretation of, 125–128, 126t, 127f, 129f
    positive vs. negative relationship, 127
    significance, 125–127, 126t
    strength, 127–128
  objectivity, 131

reliability, 130
validity, 131
Pedantic, defined, 314
Pedantic writing, in research writing, 63–64, 63t
Peer review, in internal quality control, 260
Periodical(s), references for, 54–55
Perseverance, of researcher, 14
Perspective, holistic, 246
Physical education, journals related to, 31t
Placebo effect
  defined, 314
  as threat to internal validity, 202t, 206, 212t
Plagiarism
  avoidance of, 62–63
  defined, 62, 314
Population, defined, 314
Population specificity, 139
Positive correlation, 122
Positively skewed distribution, defined, 314
Post hoc error, 275–276
  defined, 314
Post hoc tests, 155–158, 156t, 157t
  defined, 314
  results of, reporting of, 156–157, 156t, 157t
  *t* test as, limitations of, 155–156
  treatment effect of, magnitude of, 157–158
Post-design, one-group, 225–226
Post-nonrandom design, 222–223
Post-test design, 221–222
Post-test only design, 220–221
Power(s)
  defined, 170
  statistical
    critiquing research and, 269, 271
    defined, 316
Pre-design, one-group, 225–226

Prediction(s), 121–144
multiple regression,
136–139, 138t
simple linear regression,
131–136, 132t, 133f, 134f
specificity of, in multiple
regression, 139
Predictive validity, 190–191
defined, 315
Pre-experimental designs,
219, 225–228, 228t
Pre-experimental research
designs, defined, 314
Preliminary procedures, of
thesis, 45
Pre-nonrandom design,
222–223
Pre-test design, 221–222
Pre-testing, reactive effects of
defined, 315
as threat to external
validity, 202t, 209
Primary references
defined, 315
in information retrieval,
27–28
Principle, defined, 10–11
Privacy, invasion of, 21, 23t
Probability, 102–106
classical, 103
empirical, 171
defined, 312
normal curve and, 104–106
theoretical, 103
defined, 316
Problem section, of thesis,
37t, 39–43. *See also*
Thesis(es), problem
section
Procedures section of thesis,
37t, 44–46
Publication(s), limitations
with, 264–265
*Publication Manual*, of APA,
68
Publication of research
article, 263–264
Publish-or-perish, research
quality and, 265–266
Purpose of study of thesis,
40–41
Purposeful sampling, 252

**Q**
Qualitative design, in
qualitative research,
251–254, 252t
Qualitative research, 245–255
case studies, 247–248
content analysis in,
251–254, 252t
data collection in, 251–254,
252t
focus groups in, 248–250,
249t
interpretation of, 251–254,
252t
nominal groups in, 250–251
overview of, 245
qualitative design in,
251–254, 252t
quantitative research vs.,
246–247, 247t
sampling procedures in,
251–254, 252t
USDA guidelines for,
246
Quality, research
assessment of, 269–276
publish-or-perish and,
265–266
research quantity vs.,
266
Quality control, 257–287
external, 263–265
defined, 312
internal, 259–263
defined, 313
IRBs in, 261–263
peer review in, 260
student colloquia and
defenses in, 260–261
in research, 259–267
Quantitative research,
qualitative research vs.,
246–247, 247t
Quantity, research, research
quality vs., 266
Quasi designs, 219
Quasi-experimental research
design, defined, 315
Quasi-experimental research
designs, 222–225
pre- and post-nonrandom
design, 222–223

repeated-measures design,
223–224
time series design, 224–225
Question(s)
closed-ended, 234
open-ended, 234

**R**
*R See* Multiple correlation *(R)*
Random samples, in sampling
procedures, 79–81
Random sampling
defined, 315
stratified, 79, 80t
Randomization
defined, 315
internal validity and,
210–211, 212t
Randomized-blocks ANOVA,
158–159
Range(s), 88
defined, 315
restricted, 135
Ratio(s), *F*, 154
Ratio scale, 76
defined, 315
Reactive effects of pre-testing
defined, 315
as threat to internal validity,
202t, 209
Reasoning
deductive, 9
defined, 312
inductive, 9
defined, 313
Recreation, journals related
to, 31t
Reductionism, 246
Redundancy, in research
writing, 65
Reference(s)
for books, 54
components in, 54–55
for periodicals, 54–55
primary
defined, 315
in information retrieval,
27–28
secondary
defined, 315
in information retrieval,
27–28

styles for, 53
of thesis, 37t, 53–55
user-friendly, in research
  writing, 68
Reference material, collation
  of, 59–60
Regression
  multiple, 136–139, 138t. *See
    also* Multiple regression
  simple linear, 131–136,
    132t, 133f, 134f. *See also*
    Simple linear regression
  statistical
    defined, 316
    as threat to internal
      validity, 202t, 204,
      212t
Regression line, 122f, 123
  defined, 315
Relationship(s), 121–144
  causal, 230–231
  cause-and-effect. *See*
    Cause-and-effect
    relationships
Reliability, 130, 191–194
  coefficients for,
    interpretation of,
    195–197, 196t
  defined, 191, 315
  equivalence, 193
    defined, 312
  internal consistency,
    193–194
    defined, 313
  interrater, 194
    defined, 313
  parallel forms, defined, 314
  split-half, defined, 315
  stability, 192–193
  statistics for, 195–197, 196t
  test–retest, defined, 316
  validity and, relationship
    between, 194–195
Repeated-measures designs,
  223–224
Research. *See also specific
  components, e.g.,*
  Information retrieval
  application of, 257–287
  applied, 11–12
    defined, 311
    assessment of, 268–284

checklist for, 286t
internal validity in, 269
measurements in,
  critique of, 272
power in, 269
sample size in, 269–272
significance levels used
  and reported in,
  critique of, 272–273
statistical significance in,
  269
treatment effect in,
  determination of,
  273–275
variance of subjects in,
  examination of,
  critique of, 272
basic, 11–12
  defined, 311
consumers of, 7
correlational, 240, 244t
  defined, 312
daily uses of, 6–7
deductive reasoning in, 9
  defined, 315
descriptive, 229–239, 243,
  244t. *See also*
  Descriptive research
developmental, 241, 244t
  defined, 312
epidemiological, 241–242,
  244t
  defined, 312
ethics in, 17–23. *See also*
  Ethics, in human
  subject research
ex post facto, 243, 244t
  defined, 312
experimental, 216–228
  defined, 312
external validity in, 13
fact in, 9–10
field, 12
  defined, 312
human subject, ethics in,
  17–23. *See also* Ethics, in
  human subject research
independent variables in, 13
inductive reasoning in, 9
information retrieval in,
  27–34
internal validity in, 12–13

interpretation of
  abuse of statistics in,
    279–280
  biased sampling in,
    280–281
  conflict of interest and,
    283
  correlation and statistics
    in, 282
  figures in, 281–282, 281f,
    282f
  mixed findings in,
    282–283
  research reports in media
    and, 283
  sample size in, 280
  statistically significant
    findings and, 284
  tips for, 279–284, 281f,
    282f
introduction to, 3–16
laboratory, 12
  defined, 313
location of, 12
media reports about,
  caution with use of,
  283
meta-analysis, 243, 244t
misconception about, 4–5
nonexperimental, 239–243,
  244t. *See also*
  Nonexperimental
  research
observational, 242–243,
  244t
  defined, 314
principle in, 10–11
professionalism
  concerning, 6
purposes of, 4
qualitative, 245–255. *See
  also* Qualitative research
quality control in, 259–267
quality of, assessment of,
  269–276
quantitative, qualitative
  research vs., 246–247,
  247t
research paper and
  proposal, 35–47
results of
  interpretation of, 276–279

Research (*Contd.*)
  summarization of,
    276–279
  scientific method of, 7–8
  sound, 275
  staying current with, 6
  survey, 232–238, 235t, 237t,
    239t. *See also* Survey
    research
  theory in, 10
  writing of paper, 57–69. *See
    also* Research writing
Research article, publication
  of, 263–264
Research designs
  experimental, 218–220
  pre-experimental, defined,
    314
  quasi-experimental,
    defined, 315
Research dishonesty,
  266–267, 267t
Research findings, variation
  among, in research
  interpretation, 282–283
Research hypothesis, 41
  defined, 315
Research paper, 35–47. *See
  also* Thesis(es)
  components of, 36–56, 37t.
    *See also* Thesis(es)
  thesis vs., 35–36
Research quality
  assessment of, 269–276
  publish-or-perish and,
    265–266
  research quantity vs., 266
Research quantity, research
  quality vs., 266
*Research Quarterly for
  Exercise and Sport
  (RQES)*, 30, 264, 274
Research reviews, 29t, 30
  defined, 315
Research writing, 25–69
  collating reference
    material, 59–60
  common faults in, 63–68,
    63t, 64t
  abbreviations, 67
  active vs. passive voice,
    67–68

cliches, 64, 64t
jargon, 65–66
misuse of commas, 65
misuse of words, 66
numbers, 68
parallelism, 65
pedantic style, 63–64, 63t
redundancy, 65
subject-verb agreement,
  64
symbols, 66
tense, 67
unemotional tone, 68
user-friendly references,
  68
verbosity, 63, 63t
vogue words, 65
dictionary use, 61
discuss plans, 59
get something down on
  paper, 59
organize references, 60
outlines in, 60–61, 61t
plagiarism and, 62–63
review paper several times,
  61–62
study feasibility, 58
study simplification, 59
thesaurus use, 61
tips for, 60–63, 61t
topic selection, 57–58
Researcher(s)
  characteristics of, 13–15
  role in ethical treatment, 22
Residual, defined, 133–134
Resource(s), electronic, 32t
Response(s)
  categorical, 234
  scaled, 234
Restricted range, 135
Result(s), defined, 315
Results of study, application
  of, in thesis discussion, 52
Results section of thesis, 37t,
  48–49, 49t
Review(s)
  blinded, 264
  defined, 311
  research, defined, 315
  unblinded, defined, 316
Review of literature, defined,
  315

Review process, limitations
  with, 264–265
RQES. *See Research Quarterly
  for Exercise and Sport
  (RQES)*

**S**
Safe and competent
  treatment, 22, 23t
Sample(s)
  biased, 79
  chain, 252
  convenience, 80, 252
  defined, 78, 315
  network, 252
  random, 79–81
    stratified, 79, 80t
  in sampling procedures, 78
  snowball, 252
Sample informed consent
  form, 305–308
Sample size
  critiquing research and,
    269–272
  in research interpretation,
    280
Sample survey cover letter,
  309
Sample thank you letter, 310
Sampling
  biased, in research
    interpretation, 280–281
  purposeful, 252
  random
    defined, 315
    stratified, 79, 80t
Sampling distribution
  defined, 315
  in hypothesis testing, 111
Sampling error
  defined, 315
  in hypothesis testing, 107
Sampling procedures, 78–81,
  80t
  populations in, 78
  in qualitative research,
    251–254, 252t
  randomization into groups,
    81
  samples in, 78
    convenience, 80
    random, 79

Scale(s)
  absolute, 75–76
    defined, 311
  interval, 76
    defined, 313
  Likert, 234
  measurement, 74–76. *See also* Statistic(s), measurement scales in
  nominal, 75
    defined, 314
  ordinal, 75
    defined, 314
  ratio, 76
    defined, 315
Scaled responses, 234
Scattergram(s), 122–124
  defined, 315
  for line of best fit interpretation, in simple linear regression, 132–133, 134f
Scheffe test, 155
Scientific method(s), 7–8
  defined, 315
  facts in, 9–10
  less, 11
Score(s)
  change, 221
    defined, 311
  deviation, 88
  mean, comparison of, 145–169
  observed, 197
  standard, 97
  true, 197
  z, 97–98
    defined, 316
Secondary references
  defined, 315
  in information retrieval, 27–28
SEE. *See* Standard error of estimate (SEE)
Selection bias
  defined, 315
  as threat to internal validity, 202t, 204–205, 212t
Selection maturation
  defined, 315
  as threat to internal validity, 202t, 206, 212t

SEM. *See* Standard error of measurement (SEM)
Sensitivity, 191
Significance, statistical
  critiquing research and, 269
  defined, 316
Significance level, of Pearson correlation, 125–127, 126t
Significance of study, of thesis, 43
Simple linear regression, 131–136, 132t, 133f, 134f
  accuracy of estimate, 133–136
  defined, 315
  equation for, 131–132, 132t
  line of best fit, 132–133, 134f
Skewed distributions, 98–100, 98f, 99f
  negatively, 98–100, 98f, 99f
    defined, 314
  positively, 98–100, 98f, 99f
    defined, 314
Snowball samples, 252
Spearman *r*, 179–181, 180f, 180t
  critical values of, 292
  defined, 315
  interpretation of, 180–181, 180f
Spearman-Brown equation, defined, 315
Specific variance, 128, 129f
  defined, 315
Specificity, population, 139
Specificity of prediction, in multiple regression, 139
Speculation
  defined, 315
  in thesis discussion, 51
Split-half method, 193
Split-half reliability, defined, 315
SS. *See* Sum of squares (SS)
Stability reliability, 192–193
Standard deviation, 88–89, 89t
  defined, 315
  importance of, 98
  interpretation of, 89, 89t

Standard error of estimate (SEE), 133–136
  defined, 315
Standard error of measurement (SEM), 199
Standard score, 97
Static group comparison design, 226
Statistic(s), 71–184
  abuse of, 279–280
  assumptions in using, 124
  basic concepts in, 73–84
  calculated, in hypothesis testing, 111
  computational notations and tips, 81–82, 82t
  correlation-based, 141t
    in research interpretation, 282
  critical
    defined, 312
    in hypothesis testing, 111
  defined, 73, 78
  descriptive, 77–78
    defined, 312
  inferential, 78
    defined, 313
  measurement scales in, 74–76
    absolute scale, 75–76, 311
    characteristics of, 77, 77t
    interval scale, 76, 313
    nominal scale, 75, 314
    ordinal scale, 75, 314
    ratio scale, 76, 315
  nonparametric, 77, 170–184. *See also* Nonparametric statistics
  overview of, 73–74
  parametric, 76–77
    defined, 314
  in research interpretation, 279–280
  sampling procedures, 78–81, 80t. *See also* Sampling procedures
  tables of, 291–300
  for validity and reliability, 195–197, 196t
Statistical analysis of thesis, 46
Statistical assumptions, 146

Statistical equations, 81–82, 82t
Statistical hypotheses, 41, 106
  defined, 316
Statistical power
  critiquing research and, 269, 271
  defined, 316
Statistical regression
  defined, 316
  as threat to internal validity, 202t, 204, 212t
Statistical significance
  critiquing research and, 269
  defined, 316
Statistical validity, 189–191
  defined, 316
Statistically significant findings, published studies using, in research interpretation, 284
Stratified random sampling, 79, 80t
Strength
  in adults, age and, 122, 123f
  in children, age and, 122, 122f
Student colloquia, in internal quality control, 260–261
Student defenses, in internal quality control, 260–261
Study(ies)
  results of, significant and nonsignificant, tallying of, 278
  summary table of, construction of, 278
Subject(s)
  loss of, 205
  of thesis, 45
Subject–retreatment interaction, as threat to external validity, 202t, 209
Subject–treatment interaction, defined, 316
Subject–verb agreement, in research writing, 64
Sum of squares (SS), 153
Summary of thesis, 37t, 52–55
Survey cover letter, sample, 309
Survey research

  assessment in, 236–237, 239t
  cover letter for, 235–236, 237t, 239t
  defined, 316
  follow-up for, 237–238, 239t
  informed consent in, 239
  instrument development in, 233–235, 235t, 239t
  mailing of, 237, 239t
  methods in, 238–239
  planning for, 232, 239t
  sample selection in, 232–233, 239t
  steps in conducting, 232–238, 235t, 237t, 239t
  summarize results of, 238, 239t
  thank participants in, 238, 239t
  trial run in, 236–237, 239t
Symbol(s), in research writing, 66
Systematic counting, 79

**T**

$t$, critical values of, 294–297
$t$ tests, 145–146
  correlated, 146–149, 147t, 148t, 149f. *See also* Correlated $t$ tests
  dependent, 146–149, 147t, 148t, 149f. *See also* Correlated $t$ tests
  defined, 312
  independent. *See* Independent $t$ test
  as post hoc test, limitations of, 155–156
Table(s), of thesis, 49, 49t
Tendency, central, defined, 311
Tense, in research writing, 67
Terminology, thesis-related, 42–43
Test(s). *See also specific types*
  post hoc, defined, 314
  $t$ *See* $t$ tests
Testing
  defined, 316
  as threat to internal validity, 202t, 203–204, 212t

Test–retest method, 192
Test–retest reliability, defined, 316
Thank you letter, sample, 310
*The 120 Year Diet and Nutrition Plan*, 275
*The Elements of Style*, 68
Theoretical probability, 103
  defined, 316
Theory(ies), defined, 10, 316
Thesaurus
  defined, 316
  in research writing, 61
Thesis(es), 35–47
  abstract, 37t, 38
  appendix, 37t, 55–56
  components of, 36–56, 37t
  discussion section, 37t, 49–52
    application of results of study, 52
    comparison of results, 50
    implications, 51
    limitations of study, 51
    main findings, 50
    relating results, 50–51
    speculation, 51
  introduction, 37t, 38–39
  literature review, 37t, 43–44
  problem section, 37t, 39–43
    definition of terms, 42–43
    delimitations, 41–42
    hypotheses, 41
    limitations, 42
    purpose of study, 40–41
    significance of study, 43
  procedures section, 37t, 44–46
    data analysis, 46
    data collection, 46
    experimental design, 45–46
    subjects, 45
  references, 37t, 53–55
    accuracy, 55
    citation location, 55
    components in, 54–55
    styles for, 53
  research paper vs., 35–36
  results section, 37t, 48–49, 49t
    tables, 49, 49t

summary, 37t, 52–55
timetable for, 36t
title, 37–38, 37t
Time series design, 224–225
Title of thesis, 37–38, 37t
Tone, unemotional, in
  research writing, 68
Topic selection, 57–58
  feasibility of study, 58
  reading about, 58
Total variance, 153
Transferability, 254
Treatment, defined, 316
Treatment effect, assessment
  of research and, 273–275
Treatment variance, 219–220
  defined, 316
Trial run, in survey research,
  236–237, 239t
Triangulation, 253
Trimodal, 87
True designs, 219
True experimental designs,
  220–222
  defined, 316
True score, 197
Trustworthiness, 253
Tukey's Honestly Significant
  Difference (HSD) test, 155
Two-tailed hypothesis test,
  defined, 316
Two-way chi square, 175–176,
  175t, 176t
  applications of, 177–178,
    178t, 179f
  interpretation of, 176–177,
    176f
Two-way factorial ANOVA,
  222
Type I error
  defined, 316
  in hypothesis testing,
    109–110, 110t
Type II error
  defined, 316
  in hypothesis testing,
    110–111, 110t

**U**

Unblinded review, defined, 316
Underlining method, defined,
  156

Unemotional tone, in
  research writing, 68
Unit normal curve, 91–92, 91f
United States Department of
  Agriculture (USDA),
  guidelines for qualitative
  research, 246
U.S. Air Force, 18
U.S. Congress, National
  Commission for the
  Protection of Human
  Subjects of Biomedical
  and Behavioral Research
  of, 17–18
USDA. *See* United States
  Department of Agriculture
  (USDA)
User-friendly references, in
  research writing, 68

**V**

Validity, 131, 188–191, 189t
  coefficients for,
    interpretation of,
    195–197, 196t
  concurrent, 190
    defined, 311
  construct, 191
    defined, 311
  content, 189, 189t, 237
    defined, 312
  criterion-based, 189–190
    defined, 312
  defined, 188, 316
  described, 197
  experimental, 201–215
  external. *See* External
    validity
  face, 188
    defined, 312
  internal. *See* Internal
    validity
  logical, 188–189, 189t
    defined, 313
  pace, 188
  predictive, 190–191
    defined, 315
  reliability and, relationship
    between, 194–195
  statistical, 189–191
    defined, 316
  statistics for, 195–197, 196t

Value(s), critical, 111
  defined, 312
Variability
  defined, 316
  measures of, 87–90, 89t
    coefficient of variation,
      90
    range, 88
    standard deviation,
      88–89, 89t
    variance, 90
Variable(s)
  dependent, 13
    defined, 312
  extraneous, 218
  independent, 13
    defined, 313
  experimental research
    and, 275–276
Variance(s), 90
  analysis of, 146, 152–165.
    *See also* Analysis of
    variance (ANOVA)
  between-group, 153
  common, 128, 129f
    defined, 316
  error, 153, 219–220
    defined, 312
  experimental, 219–220
  general, defined, 313
  specific, 128, 129f
    defined, 315
  total, 153
  treatment, 219–220
    defined, 316
  within-group, 153
Variation, coefficient of, 90
  defined, 311
Venn diagram, 128, 129f
Verbose, defined, 316
Verbosity, in research writing,
  63, 63t
Vogue words, in research
  writing, 65
Voice, active vs. passive, in
  research writing, 67–68

**W**

Website(s), in HPER, 33t
Wilcoxon matched pairs test,
  181, 182t
  defined, 316

Within-group variance, 153
Word(s)
    misuse of, in research
        writing, 66
    vogue, in research writing,
        65

Wordiness, in research
    writing, examples of, 63,
    63t
World War II, 18
Writing, research, 25–69. *See
    also* Research writing

**Z**
*Z* score, 97–98
    defined, 316
Zero
    absolute, defined, 311
    arbitrary, 76